INSTITUTIONALIZING GENDER

Institutionalizing Gender

*Madness, the Family, and Psychiatric Power
in Nineteenth-Century France*

Jessie Hewitt

CORNELL UNIVERSITY PRESS

ITHACA AND LONDON

First published 2020 by Cornell University Press

Library of Congress Cataloging-in-Publication Data
Names: Hewitt, Jessie, 1981– author.
Title: Institutionalizing gender: madness, the family, and psychiatric power in nineteenth-century France / Jessie Hewitt.
Description: Ithaca [New York]: Cornell University Press, 2020. | Includes bibliographical references and index.
Identifiers: LCCN 2020009249 (print) | LCCN 2020009250 (ebook) | ISBN 9781501753312 (paperback) | ISBN 9781501753435 (pdf) | ISBN 9781501753329 (epub)
Subjects: LCSH: Gender expression—France—History—19th century. | Mental illness—Treatment—France—History—19th century. | Sex role—France—History—19th century. | Psychiatry—France—History—19th century. | Power (Philosophy)
Classification: LCC HQ1075.5.F8 H49 2020 (print) | LCC HQ1075.5.F8 (ebook) | DDC 305.30944/09034—dc23
LC record available at https://lccn.loc.gov/2020009249
LC ebook record available at https://lccn.loc.gov/2020009250

Cover image: Honoré Daumier, *Le médecin: Pourquoi, diable! mes malades s'en vont-ils donc tous?* (Courtesy of the U.S. National Library of Medicine, http://resource.nlm.nih.gov/101393661)

CONTENTS

Acknowledgments ix

INTRODUCTION 1

CHAPTER 1
Gender and the Founding "Fathers" of French Psychiatry 19

CHAPTER 2
Medical Controversy and Honor among (Mad)Men 43

CHAPTER 3
Domesticating Madness in the Family Asylum 67

CHAPTER 4
Scandalous Asylum Commitments and Patriarchal Power 92

CHAPTER 5
Rehabilitating a Profession under Siege 117

CHAPTER 6
Reforming the Asylum and Reimagining the Family 141

CONCLUSION
The "Mad" Woman in a Man's World 166

Notes 177

Bibliography 207

Index 225

ACKNOWLEDGMENTS

Writing a scholarly monograph is a labor of love, but it is also labor. I would have never completed this book without the privilege of full-time employment. It was only after several years as a contingent faculty member that I secured a tenure-track job and with it, the financial security and time to work on this book. I am grateful to have had the chance to complete it at all. Acknowledging the luck involved in my being able to do so seems both obvious and necessary.

I am thrilled to thank those who supported me over the years, beginning with Ted Margadant at the University of California, Davis. Ted is extremely knowledgeable and endlessly curious. Our many hours of conversation have shaped my thinking about French history in countless ways, and I will always be grateful for his willingness to supervise work so thematically distinct from his own. Catherine Kudlick likewise left her mark on this project, introducing me to disability history and serving as an inspiring example of how to mesh scholarly priorities with political ones. I have also been lucky to have Edward Ross Dickinson as a reader, sounding board, mentor, and friend. More recently Kathleen Feeley has proven a most generous departmental colleague at the University of Redlands, reading and commenting on my entire manuscript, not to mention welcoming me from the moment I arrived on campus.

Many individuals have helped clarify the arguments presented in this book. Some of my first readers include Liz Covart, Alison Steiner, and Shelley Brooks. I will always think fondly of my time spent talking about history with Robyn Douglas and Kim Hogeland. Andrew Denning sat with me though many a seminar and has offered extremely useful feedback on this project. I have also presented parts of this book at numerous conferences, including the Society for French Historical Studies and the Western Society for French History, where I've been fortunate to find colleagues who have become friends. I would like to single out Andrew Israel Ross, Sun-Young Park, Naomi Andrews, Jo Burr Margadant, Nina Kushner, Rachel Chrastil, Denise Davidson, Anne Verjus, Stephen Harp, Jonathyne Briggs, Aude Fauvel, and Jann Matlock for offering generous comments at just the right time.

My editor at Cornell, Emily Andrew, has been a dream to work with, as has acquisitions assistant Alexis Siemon. I thank them both for all they have done to bring this project to fruition, as well as the two anonymous readers whose comments have transformed this work so much for the better. I am also grateful to the Mellon Foundation. Their grant in support of the Sustainable History Monograph Pilot has made this work accessible to more readers than I ever imagined possible. A version of Chapter 3 originally appeared in "Women Working 'Amidst the Mad': Domesticity as Psychiatric Treatment in Nineteenth-Century Paris," *French Historical Studies* 38, no. 1 (2015): 105–137. Part of Chapter 4 was first published in "Married to the 'living dead': madness as a cause for divorce in late nineteenth-century France," *Contemporary French Civilisation* 40, no. 3 (2015): 311–330.

I have likewise been lucky to receive indispensable research support from the Department of History, the College of Arts and Sciences, and the Institute for Women and Research at the University of California, Davis; the Institute for German and European Studies at the University of California, Berkeley; the Society for French Historical Studies; the Western Society for French History; the University of San Francisco; the University of Redlands; and the Rotary Foundation. Equally vital has been the work of librarians and archivists in France, especially those of the Bibliothèque Nationale, the Archives de l'Assistance Publique – Hôpitaux de Paris, the Archives de Paris, and the municipal archives at Saint-Mandé.

Finally, I would like to thank my family. My dad, Frank, is the most generous person I know. His sense of empathy inspires my approach to history and life. My mom, Kim, is my dearest friend. She introduced me to my first bits of historical knowledge watching *Jeopardy!* with me as child, and she continues to handily beat me at trivia on a regular basis. The support, creativity, and intelligence of my little brother, Matt, blows me away, as does the adorableness of my sweet niece Vedette. My husband, Brian, is equal parts smart and kind. He has read every word and listened to every rant, entertaining me and loving me all the while. I adamantly do not thank our cats. If they had their way, I would spend all my time feeding them, snuggling them, and allowing them to trot upon my keyboard.

INSTITUTIONALIZING GENDER

Introduction

IN 1840, THE ASYLUM DOCTOR François Leuret published an account of what he considered the successful treatment of a particularly willful patient named Dupré. The middle-aged man, a former army officer who found himself committed to a series of French mental institutions throughout the 1820s and 1830s, supposedly held onto a number of delusional thoughts and had not responded to the usual methods of treatment. He alternated between claiming that he was the Emperor Napoleon and the head of a "tartar clan"—a leader much renowned for his sexual prowess and for "constantly tasting the pleasures of love."[1] Furthermore, Dupré claimed he was the only man in the Bicêtre asylum, having long insisted that the other patients, the employees, and even his doctors were actually women (some of whom, he conceded, wore masks and fake beards). The doctor, Leuret, took a special interest in this case, engaging his patient in strategically planned dialogues, punctuated with the threat of force, in order to convince the recalcitrant inmate to renounce his beliefs and reclaim his identity as the former soldier Dupré. Leuret defended his aggressive tactics against critics within the profession, implying that the ends justified the means. "I had reason to celebrate my conviction," he wrote, "because having begun the treatment of Monsieur Dupré on 15 June, 1838, he called me him and not her on the 20th. On the 21st, he began to obey; on the 22nd, he worked the land and occupied himself that evening with reading."[2]

At first glance, it would appear Leuret and his patient had very little in common. Dupré spent much of his life sequestered by French authorities for failing to live up to contemporary standards of rationality. Leuret, for his part, reached the height of his profession despite coming from a relatively humble background. One of these men was a postrevolutionary success story—a self-made *bourgeois*, the famous doctor son of a bread baker—while the other was a cautionary tale, a veteran officer of the Napoleonic Wars unable to thrive in the society he once called home. Yet their interactions, like so many that occurred inside the mental institutions of nineteenth-century France, reveal not only the creation of cruel new hierarchies but the constraints imposed on all Frenchmen, even those fortunate enough to find themselves on top. To be precise, the ability to adhere to

fluctuating and sometimes contradictory gender expectations determined the
fates of doctor and patient alike.

For Michel Foucault, the gender dimensions of Dupré's experience were not
worthy of note. When discussing this case at the Collège de France in 1973,
Foucault focused on the ways in which Dupré's treatment at Bicêtre produced
and supported an imbalance of power in the doctor-patient relationship. Leuret's
actions showed how asylum doctors aimed to aggrandize their personal authority—both through violence and less overtly repressive means—in order to break
down "the omnipotence of madness . . . by demonstrating a different, more vigorous will endowed with greater power."[3] Although there is much to be said
for this argument, it also overstates the all-encompassing nature of psychiatric
authority by taking Leuret too fully at his word. As we shall see, rereading the
history of madness with an eye toward the inconsistencies inherent in gender,
disability, and class ideologies often reveals the fragility of psychiatric power
as much as its omnipotence. It also exposes the shaky foundations upon which
dominant ideas about men, women, and irrationality rested over the course of
the long nineteenth century.

Psychiatric treatment at this time regularly reflected the gender values associated with the French bourgeoisie, an occupationally diverse elite joined together
through their adherence to particular cultural norms and a shared insistence
that they owed their elevated social positions to merit rather than noble birth.
Perhaps the most significant aspect of bourgeois class distinction was their promotion of the ideal of gendered separate spheres. Women were expected to focus
their energies on the home while men held responsibility in the "outside" world
owing to their supposedly superior sense of reason. This ideal rarely mapped
onto the realities of daily life, but it nonetheless helped to justify its proponents'
social status. The actions of alienists—as specialists in mental medicine were
called until the late 1800s—propped up separate spheres ideology by reifying
assumed connections between masculinity and rationality and femininity with
its opposite, most obviously by pathologizing gender nonconformity and framing the patient's acceptance of gender norms as proof of cure (a tendency I have
termed "institutionalizing gender").[4]

Challenges posed by mental patients to normative gender values were rarely as
direct as Dupré's fixation on his sexual prowess or his refusal to acknowledge the
manliness of his caretakers. The exaggerated nature of his claims, however, and
his doctor's preoccupation with countering them, highlights the centrality of
gender to all asylum interactions. Leuret depicted Dupré as irrational, yes, but he
also emphasized the impropriety of his patient's claim to have bedded numerous

women because this obsession with sexual virility contradicted Leuret's own class- and race-based notions of masculine self-control (recall that Dupré insisted he was not French, but a "tartar" leader instead). The patient's "cure," on the other hand, involved the expression of traits the doctor associated with a particularly nonthreatening form of masculine behavior (productively working during the day and calmly reading at night). With a circular logic, Leuret's actions suggest rationality required conforming to certain gender expectations whereas masculinity meant the ability to appear rational. Furthermore, Dupré's return to reason necessitated more than simply re-inscribing his own proper gender comportment. It also entailed affirming the gender identities of other rational men: Leuret's first priority was to persuade Dupré to admit that the doctor himself was not a woman, despite his patient's attachment to numerous other false beliefs.

Doctors in nineteenth-century France did not recognize a distinction between sex and gender. The idea that masculinity was a construct rather than a fact of nature would have struck them as absurd, as would the notion that Leuret's actions constituted an attempt to "defend" or affirm his own identity as a man. Of all the people in Bicêtre, the inmate Dupré came closest to acknowledging that sex and gender might be uncoupled, and this was taken as evidence of insanity by his doctor.[5] It is nonetheless possible for historians to productively make use of such theorizations to analyze gender's operation in the past. This is especially true for the nineteenth century, as evidence of the un-naturalness of bourgeois gender ideology increasingly rubbed up against "scientific" claims to the contrary in the decades preceding World War I, even inside institutional spaces that had long supported widespread assumptions about men and women's purportedly natural roles. This book examines the transition from a world in which gender and sex appeared straightforward and uncomplicated to one in which this was not so much the case. Yet it also highlights the ways that medical understandings of gender and madness were always less assured than they might have seemed to those espousing them.

Psychiatric attempts to institutionalize gender had horrific consequences for those, such as Dupré, who did not fit the mold. Nonetheless, such efforts also drew attention to the malleability of gendered behaviors that most people at the time claimed were natural and permanent. Leuret highlighted the constructed nature of both gender and psychiatric disability by staging a precisely choreographed treatment scenario to convince Dupré to accept him as a man. He sought to return the patient to what Leuret considered a readily apparent gender order, but the treatment relied so heavily and so purposefully on the performative aspects of psychiatric care that he implied normative behavior was first and foremost an act. All clinical encounters in the asylum exposed this fundamental contradiction: the attempt to return patients back to "normal" highlighted the fact that there was no such thing.[6]

This study therefore examines the workings of the asylum and its role in both the elaboration and deterioration of bourgeois gender values during France's long nineteenth century, a period defined by the contested but steady advance of political liberalism, the social dislocations of industrialization and urbanization, and the seemingly triumphal professionalization of medicine. Each of these long-term processes were inflected by and had consequences for the emergence of new gender ideals promoted and embodied by the French bourgeoisie, as well as new conceptions of madness and rationality. Examining the historical interplay of these developments from the vantage point of the asylum reorients our understanding of the nineteenth century in three key ways. First, it disrupts popular understandings of psychiatric authority during the profession's so-called golden age, showing how doctors were beholden to powerful gender expectations even as they benefited from them. At the same time, the ways asylum doctors used gender ideals such as masculine self-control and feminine domesticity in the process of patient treatment also indicate that medicine regularly undermined these very norms in spite of itself, especially with respect to the widespread belief in the inherent rationality of men. Finally, and relatedly, considering gender and madness side by side situates the nineteenth century as a transitional moment in the history of the family, in which gendered conceptions of reason supplanted biological sex as the primary justification for masculine authority within the home and beyond.

Gendering Madness and Institutionalizing Gender

The treatment of the ex-soldier Dupré occurred in the 1830s, the apogee of a psychiatric method known as the moral treatment, so called because it emphasized the "moral" (i.e., mental) aspects of insanity. Developed by the physician and asylum director Philippe Pinel in the late eighteenth century and spread throughout the burgeoning psychiatric profession during the first half of the nineteenth, the moral treatment entailed the enactment of personalized and highly calculated interactions between doctors and patients inside specialized institutions for the insane.[7] Few formal regulations existed in the first three decades of the nineteenth century regarding the operation of asylums or the procedures through which a person might find him- or herself interned. The influence of the moral treatment nonetheless grew during this period, and many of its tenets were eventually embedded in the national law on asylum commitment passed by French legislators in 1838. Although there were certainly disagreements among doctors as to how to best implement treatment inside asylum walls, particularly with respect to balancing the psychological and the somatic elements of care, most doctors before the 1850s believed the production of elaborate interactive scenes could help persuade patients to realign their behaviors and accept reality. The asylum's staff performed the moral treatment by engaging the patient in premeditated dialogues meant to elicit a specific psychological response. This often meant providing emotional support, but it also involved trickery and intimidation.

The numbers of specialized French psychiatric institutions and patients treated therein rose precipitously between the start and the end of the century. According to Pinel's student and colleague Jean-Étienne-Dominique Esquirol, there were eight asylums dedicated to the treatment of mental illness in France in 1818, with 5,153 patients in total.[8] That figure rose to over 64,000 by 1899.[9] This increase largely reflected the growth of the public asylum system, although there also existed numerous private institutions geared toward the needs of wealthy patients and their families (these were typically smaller, more intimate, and sometimes run by the same doctors who held positions in the public sector). The moral treatment remained influential throughout this time, in that both public and private asylum doctors proclaimed their allegiance to the teachings of Pinel and Esquirol.

The cutting edge of the profession, however, moved on by the second half of the nineteenth century, as it became clear that doctors had failed to cure the vast majority of the ever-growing numbers of asylum patients. It was not possible to truly perform the individualized regimen required by the moral treatment in large institutions in any case. The asylum system increasingly came to be viewed by critics as a solution in search of a problem, an excuse to aggrandize the power of doctors at the expense of those they labeled mad.[10] Neurologists such as Jean-Martin Charcot eventually replaced alienists as the most innovative medical professionals dedicated to the treatment of disorders such as hysteria, and most doctors who continued to work in asylums turned toward biological, hereditary explanations for madness by the fin-de-siècle,[11] spelling the death knell of Pinel's method once and for all.

Yet the rise and fall of the moral treatment is much more than a footnote in the history of psychiatry, a minor blip on the path toward our current focus on chemical solutions to psychological problems. Instead, its fate highlights the interdependency of gender and disability ideologies that characterized the birth of modernity in France.[12] The emergent class society of the nineteenth century simultaneously provided new opportunities and imposed new limitations based on the perceived rationality of political and economic actors. As those who defined the boundary between lucidity and madness, asylum doctors played an essential—though by no means exclusive—role in the solidification and spread of pernicious class and gender assumptions that limited the opportunities of women and workers while elevating the status of bourgeois men. Indeed, their professional fortunes depended on their willingness to define irrationality in ways that gave credence to class-based ideals of masculinity and femininity—to justify the status quo by turning cultural constructs into supposed facts about human nature. Yet, despite causing great harm to the women and men ensnared by their efforts, doctors were never able to fix the definitions of femininity and masculinity (or even rationality) any more than they could resolve the numerous medical controversies that popped up in the pages of their professional journals. Instead, they revealed the nineteenth-century gender system to be a house of cards, built with care but always at risk of crashing down around its occupants.

Mental patients claiming to be people they were not proliferated in postrevolutionary France. Laure Murat has written about other men who, like Dupré, thought they were Napoleon, using this time- and place-bound manifestation of mental illness to ask big questions about the relationship between madness, psychiatry, and its historical contexts. She wonders, "What does madness make of history?" and concludes that the content of delusions—along with evolving interpretations of them—both shaped and were shaped by politics in nineteenth-century France.[13] I ask, in turn: What does madness make of gender? Did shifting conceptions of madness and rationality inform the development of gender norms, and vice versa? How did understandings of masculinity and femininity affect the behaviors of doctors and their patients? And what does the relationship between gender and madness reveal about the expansion and the subversion of medical, masculine, and bourgeois power?[14]

Previous scholarship weighs heavily on the history of French psychiatry: Foucault, in particular, casts a long shadow. His early work on the "Great Confinement" of the seventeenth century, in which he argued the mad were institutionalized en masse alongside paupers and criminals, has been criticized by historians for inaccuracy and lack of specificity.[15] Yet Foucault's insights into the disciplining nature of the Enlightenment, and of modernity more generally, stand up to scrutiny. His discussions of the medical profession's role in the inculcation of self-discipline as a cultural ideal and a bodily habit constitute an essential starting point for my own interpretation of nineteenth-century psychiatry. That said, the Foucauldian vision of psychiatric power is oddly de-personalized, with individual doctors acting as stand-ins for the dispersed yet ever-present nature of modern "authority" rather than as historical agents in their own right. This tends to shield them from responsibility despite Foucault's critical stance toward the psychiatric profession and, perhaps more important, obscure doctors' own submission to the disciplining forces of which they were a part. Imagining alienists as classed and gendered subjects therefore reorients our understanding of medical power writ large.

So too does approaching the history of psychiatry in a fashion that consis-tently seeks to give voice to those labeled insane. This is a notoriously difficult task. Roy Porter called on historians of psychiatry to write histories from "the patient's view" over thirty years ago, yet, as a recent assessment of the field notes, "Porter's exhortation, for the most cynical, has acted as little more than a se-ductive proposal to lure audiences without bringing anything new to the un-derstanding of medical practices or the patient experience."[16] The discovery of patient writings from the nineteenth century makes constructing a "bottom up" psychiatric history of this era possible. As Alexandra Bacopoulos-Viau and Aude Fauvel point out, however, Porter himself failed to address precisely how historians of mental medicine might move beyond histories that consider patient writers as exceptions to the rule, "giving no real clue as to how one could go about studying more 'ordinary' patients."[17]

This book represents an attempt to allow mental patients to speak—not from the "bottom up," or from the "patient's perspective," but as active and necessary participants in an ongoing cultural conversation. This conversation took place in vast public asylums and more intimate *maisons de santé*, in the halls of the National Assembly and the meeting rooms of the *Société Médico-Psychologiques*, in family homes and on public streets. The meanings of masculinity, femininity, rationality, and madness were produced and reproduced through the course of innumerable personal interactions in a multitude of settings. Using patients' own words whenever possible highlights their engagement in this process. So too does using alienists' writings (which are far more plentiful) with an eye toward the limits of medical power, showing how doctors and patients were all beholden to cultural expectations outside the control of any one individual. Thus, in re-imagining Leuret as a man rather than simply a doctor, we likewise reposition Dupré: he too now enters the conversation as a man, not only a patient.[18]

Teasing out the relationship between masculinity, femininity, and madness during the nineteenth century requires us to step back and consider the French

Revolution, which set the stage for both the rise of the psychiatric profession and the spread of new class and gender expectations. The birth of psychiatry in France was intimately tied to the death of absolutism. Although those considered insane were confined in general hospitals and private *maisons de santé* throughout the eighteenth century, these institutions rarely specialized in the treatment of insanity and instead housed mad people alongside the indigent, the sick, and the physically disabled. More significantly, those who ran such institutions in the early modern period did not view institutional spaces as vectors of cure (although they did believe physical treatments such as bloodletting, baths, and purgatives could soothe troubled minds). This began to change in the mid-to-late-1700s as Enlightened optimism concerning innate human potential contributed to a growing faith in the curability of insanity.

France was hardly alone in its embrace of this idea—those who would come to be recognized as the forerunners of the psychiatric profession emerged nearly simultaneously in France, England, Scotland, Italy, and Central Europe—but the Revolution of 1789 provided unique opportunities to put previously haphazard medical innovations into practice on a wider scale. The young doctor Philippe Pinel became director of the Parisian asylum Bicêtre in 1793 in recognition of his medical skill and his political commitment to republicanism, inaugurating an era noteworthy for the medicalization of mental illness and the state's involvement in psychiatric treatment. Pinel supposedly released the mad from their shackles shortly after his appointment, identifying them as patients rather than prisoners for the first time.[19] This foundational moment of French psychiatry would be immortalized in art and through the testimonies of Pinel's followers in the century that followed. It hardly mattered that the event never occurred in the precise form recalled by posterity. The self-taught guardian and former inmate of Bicêtre, Pussin, unshackled the patients in 1797, two years after Pinel had moved to another post.[20]

The myth, however, was exceedingly useful, for it promoted an image of the profession that connected Pinel's treatment methods to the ideals of revolutionary France. In suggesting people perceived as mad deserved treatment rather than punishment, the story of the chains of Bicêtre situated the alienist as a liberator, a healer, and as someone capable of transforming the insane into citizens. Pinel did in fact free the patients of the women's hospital the Salpêtrière in 1800, acknowledging their humanity and their ability to eventually rejoin French society in the process. Furthermore, doctors inspired by the real and imagined Pinel emphasized their commitment to the humane treatment of mad people throughout the nineteenth century, even when the actual conditions that reigned in psychiatric institutions firmly contradicted the liberationist ideal. From the start, the asylum symbolized the possibilities and the limitations of political liberalism, as doctors envisioned a more inclusive society while recreating old hierarchies on new foundations, particularly with respect to gender, disability, and class.

Psychiatric pronouncements mattered during and after the Revolution because an individual's perceived rational capacity determined the allotment of political and social prerogatives. Mental patients effectively lost both the rights of citizenship and control over their finances for the duration of their asylum stays.[21] In this sense, male patients were legally feminized. Revolutionary and Napoleonic-era lawmakers insisted that women, as the less rational sex, were best suited for domestic roles, whereas men were natural breadwinners and active citizens because they could more effectively control their emotions.[22] This gender construct had deep roots. As Christopher Forth explains, a man's ability to master both his body and his feelings has represented a central element of ideal masculinity since the early modern period, when monarchs consolidated their authority and curbed the violent tendencies of the nobility. Self-restraint constituted an important social lubricant in developing court societies and a form of distinction among aristocratic men (despite their nostalgia for an imagined past free of such constraints).[23] The expectation of masculine self-control spread to the non-noble elite by at least the eighteenth century, when Enlightenment-era thinkers argued that differences between men and women determined their suitability for public life on this very basis.[24] The replacement of absolutism with a government based on the social contract served to amplify the gendering of reason by tying it to the practice of citizenship.[25]

Moreover, although France was somewhat slow to industrialize compared with other Western European societies, opportunities to succeed in business and the liberal professions nonetheless increased in the opening decades of the nineteenth century. This economic context further bolstered ideals of feminine domesticity and masculine self-control, as diverse segments of the middle classes readily subscribed to these gender expectations as a means of distinction. Unlike self-indulgent aristocrats or disorderly workers, bourgeois men supposedly exhibited the self-mastery required to lead in the realms of business, politics, and the family.[26] Bourgeois wives, for their part, exemplified feminine virtue by behaving in a fashion untenable for lower-class women, who could not afford to spend their time or their family's money on purely domestic pursuits.[27] Although the term "bourgeois" generally connoted upper-class non-noble status in nineteenth-century France, members of the middle strata of French society likewise subscribed to such norms when possible as a way to signal their differentiation from the popular classes.

The gendering of reason therefore accomplished a great deal of cultural work, simultaneously legitimating the authority of the bourgeoisie and excluding women from the political sphere. Yet despite its apparent taken-for-grantedness, separate spheres ideology was marked by internal contradictions, as well as persistent attempts to gloss over them by making gender differences appear natural. Explanations for mental illness in women often reflected this duality. The doctor Legrand du Saulle, for example, claimed women were biologically predisposed to hysteria and that particular moments in a woman's life cycle, including pregnancy, could aggravate her mental state.[28] Such beliefs served to reinforce associations between womanliness and mental instability, but they also implied that a woman's "natural" role as wife and mother was perhaps not so natural after all. Medical men themselves rarely acknowledged the relevance—or even the existence—of ideological contradictions, but those interned in asylums against their will often exploited such inconsistencies, both in day-to-day interactions with their doctors and when publicly defending themselves.

The institutionalization of middle-class and bourgeois men likewise undermined the profession's articulation of gender difference. New cultural understandings of meritocracy, in particular, strengthened associations between manliness and self-control that alienists would help sustain, while also creating expectations that not all men could meet. The elimination of noble privilege by the National Assembly in 1789 and the Chapelier Law's ban on guilds two years later were both intended to eradicate corporate prerogatives and create conditions more favorable to individual initiative. The *lycée* system and the *grandes écoles* similarly helped open bureaucratic careers to talent. Underlying each of these shifts was the belief that citizens should be free to apply their natural abilities without arbitrary limitations.[29] Ironically, the chance for men to freely make use of their reason multiplied potential sources of psychological distress, and postrevolutionary asylums housed many men whose failure to succeed professionally inspired or aggravated their conditions. Merit functioned not only as a potentially equalizing force but also as a new criterion for the allotment of privileges based on the possession of vaguely defined talent rather than noble birth or corporate membership.[30] This fact profoundly shaped the behaviors of men, as they sought to prove their worth in a society stripped of traditional markers of status by comporting themselves in a "reasonable" (i.e., self-possessed) manner. Consider Balzac's Rastignac, whose efforts to climb the social ladder in *Père Goriot* succeed in large part because he learns how to hide and control his emotions—a skill Goriot himself sorely lacks, which ultimately abets his downfall.

A man's ability to exhibit self-control in his efforts to move up in the world helped him navigate the disconnect between the meritocratic ideal and the competitive and often unforgiving reality in which he lived. The meritocratic thrust of the revolutionary era therefore lost none of its potency in a postrevolutionary world defined by class divisions and inequalities. If anything, the myth of meritocracy helped to maintain class distinctions by framing economic barriers to social mobility as personal defects.[31] Asylum doctors upheld the cultural potency of meritocracy by labeling men who failed to live up to its standards as insane and then working to reintegrate them back into society. In this sense, their actions represented an extreme form of the everyday policing of masculine behavior typical among the bourgeoisie that occurred in schools, businesses, barracks, and households throughout France. Yet, owing to their constant interaction with men who failed to conform to new class and gender expectations, doctors regularly drew attention to the instability of this entire edifice in spite of themselves.

Many such men were heads of household whose encounters with the psychiatric establishment revealed long-term alterations in the basis of paternal power. The patriarchal nature of family life was a constant that spanned the pre- and postrevolutionary eras, but its justification changed over time in that the power of fathers and husbands required little justification at all before French revolutionaries tied the possession of reason to the practice of citizenship. The legal and conceptual link between manliness and rational self-control legitimated the right of elite Frenchmen to rule long after the end of the Old Regime. Yet it also suggested that men's authority derived less from their physicality than from their ability to appear reasonable. Asylum doctors played a hand in the development of this cultural expectation through their theorizations of madness in men and their development of treatment regimens (even if they still maintained that reasonableness itself was an element of manliness, not masculinity per se). This new formulation threatened traditional hierarchies of gender and generation within families and, eventually, society at large.[32] In this way, the elevation of masculine rationality represents an underappreciated aspect of the transition from patriarchy—defined by Annette Timm and Joshua Sanborn as a social or political system "in which fathers or father figures exercise ultimate authority"—to a fraternity in which younger men shared authority among themselves.[33]

Part of this process involved the idealization of affective family ties, but the degree to which bourgeois and middle-class families actually lived these values is an open question. The writings of both doctors and patients, which vividly dramatize marital and intergenerational conflicts, serve as ideal entry points into the inner workings of the so-called sentimental family at its historic peak. Rachel Fuchs has examined the subtleties of familial authority in the nineteenth century, exploring the strategies undertaken by women and "natural children" to persuade the state to recognize paternity at a time when fathers had the legal right to abandon their illegitimate offspring. She concludes that courts were more inclined to support the rights of women and children than a straightforward reading of the legal codes would suggest, although officially men still maintained nearly complete control within and outside the home.[34] Asylum writings similarly reveal a disconnect between the law and shifting cultural values, while still underlining the very real power that men—especially fathers—continued to wield over women and children throughout the 1800s. Men were both more capable of institutionalizing others against their will and best prepared to defend themselves against unjust institutionalization. Nonetheless, the gendering of reason transformed masculine authority in ways that allowed wives and children to increase their own power vis-à-vis husbands and fathers on the basis of a man's perceived mental incapacity.

Finally, although this book pays more attention to the experiences of male patients and male doctors, it is also in conversation with pathbreaking studies in the history of psychiatry that emphasize the ways in which medical and gender ideologies worked, in tandem, to limit women's opportunities.[35] Not only did the psychiatric profession give credence to the persistent assumption that women were less capable than men but alienists played an essential role in the institutionalization of women who did not fit the feminine ideal in one way or another. Disability scholars, for their part, have argued that disability represents a "baseline" inequality which has been used historically to uphold hierarchies of gender, class, and race.[36] Like gender history, disability history analyzes how meanings attributed to bodily difference change over time—in this case physical, cognitive, or psychological impairments rather than biological sex—although the two categories often intersect. As Douglas Baynton has shown, prejudice against disability was so pervasive in the nineteenth century that disenfranchised groups regularly pressed for political rights on the basis that they were not physically weak or irrational.[37] One particularly egregious example of British suffragist propaganda actually made its case by highlighting "what a woman may be, and yet not have the vote" (such as a doctor, a teacher, a mayor, or a mother) and "what a man may have been, and yet not lose the vote"—including a "lunatic."[38]

The history of French asylum psychiatry likewise reveals the mutually constitutive nature of gender and disability ideologies, which has served to justify the unequal status of both women and people considered mad. The legal and cultural privileging of rationality legitimated the exclusion of women from politics while simultaneously propping up the authority of any elite man who remained untarnished by an accusation of insanity. Nonetheless, historians have shown that bourgeois gender ideals were far less rigid than once presumed. Studies of nineteenth-century French femininity call attention to the flexibility of separate spheres ideology, noting how women made use of dominant gender values to justify their own ambitions and authority despite legal and cultural constraints.[39] Coming from another vantage point, histories of bourgeois and middle-class manhood have increasingly focused on the insecurity of masculinity during this same period.[40] Historians of psychiatry have even debunked the popular notion that women were sent to asylums in significantly greater numbers than men.[41] All this suggests it is time to reassess the meaning of gender inside the nineteenth-century asylum, to ask whether the authority of doctors and of men—and doctors *as* men—was truly as hegemonic as is often imagined.

Two prominent interventions in the history of masculinity have shaped my approach to this endeavor. The first involves questioning the so-called crisis narrative. This directive has been put forth most recently by Mary Louise Roberts, who impels historians to abandon the idea that masculinity experiences periods of crisis when threatened in some way by current events (such as women's rights movements or war), and insists, as do I, that gender fixity can never be taken for granted even in less chaotic times.[42] Roberts avoids falling into a postmodernist rabbit hole where uncertainty is the only certainty, concluding "'stable' narratives *can* be built on the notion of normative instability itself."[43] The attempt to build a stable narrative on the notion of normative instability encapsulates one aim of this project. Yet, where Roberts suggests the notion of gender crisis might be productively replaced with that of gender damage, I trace long-term changes in the very nature of gender instability by heeding Toby Ditz's call to remember the ways that "masculinity articulates with femininity to confirm the 'privilege, power, and authority' that men have over women."[44] By foregrounding the mutual dependency between femininity and masculinity—and by taking a long view of psychiatry's engagement with gender over the course of the entire nineteenth century—I underscore the fundamental unnaturalness of gender-medical ideologies without forgetting their very real role in the creation and sustenance of multiple forms of inequality.

Women, in particular, were profoundly and uniquely victimized by the psychiatric system. Their legal and familial subordination already put them at a distinct disadvantage when trying to defend themselves against those who sought to commit them. Furthermore, doctors benefited personally when they perpetuated the already widespread cultural association between women and irrationality. For one, they justified the existence of the asylum system as a necessary bedrock against the dangers posed by insanity to domestic tranquility—the heart of bourgeois class distinction—which proved rather convenient with respect to their own professional aspirations. They strengthened the related association between men and reason in the process, which furthered the ambitions of French alienists while bolstering the authority of bourgeois men writ large. Nonetheless, as the case the ex-army officer Dupré suggests, upholding the lie of man's inherent rationality was not easy even when backed up by the combined forces of medicine and the state. This book tells the story of doctors' efforts to "institutionalize" this fiction, among others, and the consequences when they failed to do so.

THE FOLLOWING SIX CHAPTERS are arranged chronologically and thematically, each presenting one piece of the nineteenth-century history of the French asylum system: from its comparatively optimistic origins, to its midcentury consolidation, to its fin-de-siècle deterioration in the face of attacks from within the profession and without. The chapter topics do not constitute an exhaustive history of French psychiatry. Instead, they represent particular moments and clinical contexts in which psychiatry's relationship to bourgeois gender ideology either revealed itself or significantly changed. As a whole, these chapters point to the importance of asylum documents as windows into changing notions of masculinity, femininity, and family life. They also show how paying close attention to gender—as it pertained to male doctors, but also women practitioners and patients of both sexes—reframes the history of psychiatry.

The opening chapter examines the role of gender in the origins and treatment of insanity according to the discipline's founders, Philippe Pinel and Jean-Étienne-Dominique Esquirol, from the 1790s through the 1830s. Early alienists developed a theory of mental illness that was both universalizing—in that it assumed all people were susceptible to the derangement of the "passions"—and particular—in that the patient's class and gender background helped determine the precise contours of their alienation. This formulation led doctors to make use of gender in the development of treatment scenarios and in the construction of their own therapeutic personae. Psychiatric theories perpetuated the notion that men were inherently rational and that women's proper place was inside the home, but doctors consistently undermined these widespread assumptions.

Chapter 2 takes a case-study approach, homing in on the contradictory relationship between psychiatry and emergent notions of masculinity through the analysis of a contentious debate over the use of the "cold shower" in the treatment of delusions. This method became increasingly controversial in the decade surrounding the 1838 legislative decision to implement a state-run asylum system, as doctors eager to prove their professional legitimacy argued that the simulated drowning the process entailed constituted a form of punishment instead of a potential cure. The debate exposed intra-psychiatric conflicts over how to best embody professional and personal honor, the display of which represented a key element of class distinction for bourgeois men. Yet the cold shower controversy also showed that doctors believed their male patients' attachment to honor could both inspire and cure insanity, suggesting it held the potential to integrate men of diverse disability and class statuses into the postrevolutionary order.

Chapter 3 similarly zooms in on one particular gendered element of bourgeois class distinction, in this case feminine domesticity, by turning to the role of women in the direction of private mental institutions in the middle decades of the century. The focus here is on the Brierre de Boismont family, who lived alongside their patients and involved them in the household routine so as to encourage those deemed insane to return to rationality. Bourgeois domestic ideology sanctioned the participation of the Brierre de Boismont women in asylum operations despite cultural proscriptions against elite women's labor. As exemplars of ideal womanhood, they were central to the enactment of the treatment process, and their activities within the family's asylums often naturalized the gendered division of the public and private spheres. But they also gave lie to such beliefs by performing domesticity in an environment so unlike the typical bourgeois home.

The first chapters of this book highlight contradictions inherent in both the psychiatric system and the gender and class ideologies it served to uphold. At the same time, the profession undeniably rose in stature between the first French Revolution and the end of the July Monarchy, and the ways in which doctors made use of gender throughout this era tended to be consistent with the universalizing claims of the moral treatment. The psychiatric establishment faced mounting criticisms by the second half of the nineteenth century, however, as many French began to view the asylum as a threat to individual liberty. Attacks on the profession regularly evidenced the power of gender ideology to shape public opinion, as did expressions of self-defense from within the psychiatric community. Nonetheless, doctors de-emphasized the connection between gender and cure—and doubled down on more purely biological explanations for mental illness—at this very moment.

Chapter 4 therefore begins to delve into the decline of the moral treatment, using examples of unjust institutionalization to explore shifting notions of medical and patriarchal power. Doctors continued to prop up bourgeois gender ideology by incarcerating men and women who did not conform to its expectations, but patients seeking release wielded these same notions of proper behavior against relatives who sought to commit them and against the psychiatric profession itself. The cultural association between masculinity and rational self-control, in particular, proved dangerous to men accused of insanity while simultaneously providing a powerful form of resistance against those who aimed to institutionalize them. Scandalous asylum commitments also featured conflicts among family members, whose intricacies often indicated a gradual, multivalent move away from an "authoritarian" family ideal to something more benevolent or sentimental.

As criticisms of the psychiatric profession reached a boiling point, the nation found itself in a period of intense and prolonged crisis. France confronted both foreign invasion and civil war between 1870 and 1871. The linked national emergencies of the Franco-Prussian War and the Paris Commune constituted a blow to the moral treatment regime, as well as an opportunity for the psychiatric profession to partake in some much-needed self-promotion. As in the case of the Revolutionary era, national traumas inflected the theories and behaviors of psychiatric professionals during this time. Chapter 5 therefore examines how doctors used these disruptive events as opportunities to craft and promote new visions of psychiatric masculinity that connected the interests of the profession to those of the Third Republic. Crucially, the events of 1870–1871 also led doctors to rearticulate their theories of mental illness in ways that both challenged long-standing beliefs in its curability and pathologized the behaviors of women and workers to an unprecedented degree.

In the anxiety-ridden atmosphere of the fin-de-siècle, biological hereditary explanations for insanity served to pinpoint the supposed roots of national decline, and many French increasingly came to believe that asylum doctors had failed in their mission to rehabilitate those deemed insane. Not only did the public bemoan the hypocrisies of a system that incarcerated and rarely cured but specialists in the physical, rather than mental, origins of alienation solidified their professional ascendancy at this time. Eventually, asylum doctors expressed their own reservations towards the moral treatment, choosing to view most of their patients as "incurables" indifferent to the gender-based methods of the early- and mid-nineteenth century. The sixth and final chapter explores innovations in asylum psychiatry in this new context. The most ambitious responses to this onslaught against the profession involved placing patients with caregivers in the community. In most cases, this practice was not meant to teach patients how to live outside asylum walls so much as to clear institutions of patients who doctors deemed beyond rehabilitation. Such efforts therefore exhibited a new relationship between gender, class, and psychiatry—one that denied the healing power of bourgeois gender and family values and eroded the notion of cure itself.

This book's stable narrative built on the notion of normative instability therefore goes something like this: Doctors naturalized bourgeois gender values at the start of the century with the aim of greater inclusion of mad people into French society. Their efforts reflected the optimism of the psychiatric enterprise, but alienists were also extremely inflexible when it came to enforcing patients' compliance with expected gendered behaviors. Even so, psychiatric theories and practices regularly broke down distinctions of gender, class, and ability, a fact that constituted a persistent if unintended blow to traditional notions of patriarchal power. Doctors faced multiple challenges that threatened their professional standing as time wore on. Alienists continued to spread sexist and classist stereotypes about the inherent irrationality of women and the reasonableness of bourgeois men, but they also increasingly insisted that insanity was rooted in biology rather than circumstance. Asylum doctors thus abandoned the moral treatment's emphasis on gender as cure while instrumentalizing psychiatry in the name of class and gender distinction to a greater degree than ever before. The conclusion considers why this was the case, arguing that the abandonment of the moral treatment represented one response to the challenges posed by early mass culture, working-class politics, and women's rights to bourgeois male hegemony.

Nineteenth-century asylums featured sustained, well-documented interactions between men and women from a variety of class backgrounds and levels of psychiatric disability. Descriptions of these encounters provide a comprehensive view of the gender system in action, revealing how abstract conceptions of gender and reason affected real people—as individuals, as members of families, and as professionals and patients. It is no secret that the psychiatric profession has historically reflected common prejudices regarding gender and class, not to mention race.[45] Nonetheless, the gendering of rationality had the power to upset—rather than simply reinforce—prevailing dynamics between men and women, parents and children, and experts and amateurs. Not only did the asylum hold the unique capacity to reflect, in microcosm, processes occurring throughout French society more broadly but doctors quite purposefully took it upon themselves to solidify notions of gender difference by embedding them in their attempts to bring insane people back to the fold. That they failed to do so in the most "totalitarian" of modern institutions goes to show the impossibility of this task.

CHAPTER I

Gender and the Founding "Fathers" of French Psychiatry

THE FIRST FRENCH ASYLUM DOCTORS aimed to cure patients of
mental alienation and professionalize their medical subspecialty at a
time when change represented the only constant, working against a
backdrop of political turmoil, fluctuating class norms, and the rapid expansion
of the centralized nation-state. These alienists, like their patients, experienced
the early decades of the nineteenth century as if it were a new world—one
in which doctors themselves helped define French society's core values while
attempting to impose order amid chaos. In the process, they formulated theories
of the mind that intertwined with and gave force to emergent class-based standards regarding gender and family life.

Psychiatric assumptions about healthy families often served to reinforce bourgeois gender values by treating them as normative. Like postrevolutionary legislators, doctors believed the relationship between the individual and the state
was mediated through the family and that the home ideally served as a bedrock
against the frightening changes afflicting French society as a whole.[1] The famil-
ialist thrust of French law and medicine held strong throughout the nineteenth
century despite considerable differences between various governments (which
included three republics, two empires, and several monarchies). Indeed, the dramatic political shifts that occurred from 1789 to 1871 help explain why the source
of social stability would have to come from outside the realm of politics proper.
The (re)creation of seemingly happy families—economically productive, loving, and secure—had the power to stabilize the individual as well as the nation.
Asylum doctors considered the professionally successful married bourgeois the
rational man par excellence. His happily domesticated wife represented the ideal
woman, and bonds of genuine affection supposedly linked husband to wife and
parents to children.

It is tempting to interpret early alienists' efforts to enforce these values among
their patients as attempts to discipline the popular classes and reinforce restrictive norms among their own. Yet, psychiatric understandings of the home—and

the gender- and class-based social expectations it came to symbolize—were decidedly ambivalent. The most significant stresses during the nineteenth century, particularly for bourgeois and middle-class people such as asylum doctors, revolved around family life. Early alienists therefore suggested mental patients had the greatest chance of regaining sanity when they were far from their relatives. They likewise never tired of pointing out that the sources of mental alienation often resided in the "breast of the family."[2] Asylum doctors nevertheless argued a patient's resumption of his or her familial role constituted the end goal of all treatment measures and even proof of cure. In other words, doctors recognized that social pressures related to home life often contributed to mental collapse, but they also implied a rational person would not appear to struggle with these challenges at all. In the meantime they traversed this unsettled gender landscape and began to construct their own identities as professional men.

This chapter explores the early history of French psychiatry and serves as an introduction to themes that will be picked up in later chapters. Each section represents a stage of the patient experience, from the onset of mental illness, to the patient's arrival in the asylum, to the actual enactment of the moral treatment. The first decades of the nineteenth century established doctors' hopes for the asylum system and their own place within it, and early alienists clearly linked the incipient specialty to the perpetuation of family and gender norms associated with the middle classes. Nonetheless, their theories and actions presaged irresolvable contradictions between the practice of asylum psychiatry and the maintenance of bourgeois class distinction.

Inventing the Patient

The insane became human sometime in the late eighteenth century—that is, at least, according to their self-appointed caregivers within the nascent psychiatric profession. Whereas those considered mad had once been enchained like "ferocious beasts" and treated with "violence and blind brutality," Philippe Pinel and his disciples sought to approach asylum inmates with firmness and kindness.[3] This alteration in perspective represented a central element of the moral treatment, a method of care first theorized by Pinel during the revolutionary era that asylum doctors continued to refine throughout the first several decades of the 1800s.

Although those considered mad had long lived within institutions, their incarceration did not serve a medical function until the eighteenth century. Relatively few prerevolutionary practitioners believed in the curability of mental illness, and the absolutist state had little interest in reintegrating mad people into society. Pinel, like his predecessors, believed those who behaved irrationally should be separated from their communities, especially their families. Yet he also advocated the removal of physical restraints in all but the most dangerous situations and insisted that insanity could be overcome by regimenting and supervising patients' lives within asylums. In time, through a series of strategically planned interactions between doctor and patient, he expected the symptoms of madness to dissipate. The moral treatment was an individualized but routinized method of care intended to bring patients back into the community of citizens by redirecting their emotions in a normative fashion. Doctors left little to chance within their institutions, seeking instead to purposefully cultivate an atmosphere that would disorient their patients' senses and lead them toward the path of recovery.

The first alienists believed everyone possessed a sense of reason, even those experiencing symptoms of insanity. The flip side to this professed faith in human rationality was their assumption that all people—men and women of all social backgrounds—were liable to bouts of madness under the right circumstances. Pinel suggested as much in his writings on the Revolution. He pinpointed situations that triggered extreme emotional response when discussing the causes of mental alienation among the male patients of Bicêtre during that time, including various reactions to the Terror; the reversal of fortunes; and domestic distress.[4] These particular inspirations for the onset of mental illness were eminently relatable to Pinel's readers, who had themselves witnessed and experienced the same turmoil as had the asylum's patients. Far from labeling the insane as outside the bounds of the community, Pinel implied that those driven to the brink by the vicissitudes of political and social change were perhaps all too human, rather than the supposedly incomprehensible animals of the Old Regime.

Even during less dramatic historical interludes, psychiatry's founders emphasized the distortion and exaggeration of universal emotional states when discussing the onset of mental illness. Pinel and his influential student Jean-Étienne-Dominique Esquirol both cited unchecked emotions as especially relevant sources of insanity, Pinel going so far as to ask how any doctor could remain ignorant of the "the most lively human passions" when "they are the most frequent causes of alienation."[5] Esquirol wrote his doctoral thesis, "Des passions considérée comme causes, symptômes, et moyens curatifs de l'aliénation mentale," on the passions, using a combination of Pinel's case notes and his own as principal sources of evidence. He focused on how particular emotions—from tenderness and the desire for love to hate, fear, and anger—might wreak havoc on the minds of the mad. Both Pinel and Esquirol acknowledged that physical states such as lesions on the brain could cause psychological turmoil, but they consistently foregrounded the emotional dimensions of insanity in discussions of diagnosis and treatment. Madness represented a distortion of everyday "passions," an extreme and unhealthy manifestation of the feelings experienced by all people. As such, both doctors began their attempts at cure with the belief that everyone had access to the same emotional register, arguing that if the passions constituted symptoms of mental illness, then they could inspire cure when properly manipulated. Far from merely replacing passion with reason, the founders of French psychiatry considered emotion the key feature of the human condition, connecting those diagnosed as insane to the rest of society.

Although distorted passions represented a seemingly universal source of insanity, doctors argued that emotional life was itself historically and socially determined. For Esquirol, primal emotional responses concerning self-preservation and reproduction—notably love, anger, terror, and vengeance—could easily be taken to excess. But he additionally linked mental illness to the advance of civilization and the multiplication of wants that defined modern life, explaining that needs engender desires and that desires "represent the most fertile source of the moral and physical disorders that afflict man."[6] No less treacherous for their comparative lack of urgency, new needs "attached themselves to the first," thereby increasing the possibilities for the excitation of the passions. The feelings furthest removed from the instincts concerned those "born of our social ties," such as ambition, greed, glory, celebrity, and honor. Like baser passions related to reproduction or survival, these so-called secondary needs related to the individual's relationship to his or her family, whose reputation hinged on that of each individual member. Opportunities for the aggravation of such passions were especially numerous in a nominally meritocratic society such as that of postrevolutionary France, where class identities were in the process of replacing corporate ones and where one might move down the social hierarchy as readily as one might climb up. In elucidating this historically informed conception of the passions, Esquirol gave voice to a tendency already present in Pinel's writings: emotion was universal, but its expression and its potential for unhealthy distortion was intimately tied to an individual's social and familial role. This meant that a patient's class and gender background inevitably influenced their diagnosis and treatment.

Psychiatric conceptions of the passions nonetheless resided at the nexus of nature and culture, where physical inspirations for insanity worked in concert with situational ones. Asylum doctors most obviously perpetuated notions of gender difference in their discussions of the relationship between the body and the emotions. The relative weight attributed to physical versus emotional causes of mental illness depended on a number of factors, the most important being the patient's sex. Whereas the founders of French psychiatry found myriad chances for a woman's body to betray her mind, puberty was the only moment in a man's life when biology alone left him open to excessive or distorted passions. Doctors consistently identified male patients as more constrained by social norms than by physical states.

Esquirol's interpretation of the role of age in the onset of insanity is a case in point. Childhood constituted the only life stage in which individuals were truly shielded from the stirrings of mental illness, presumably because the passions had the fewest objects to attach themselves to at this time, while puberty in both boys and girls could lead to an excess of emotion owing to physical changes taking place in the body. Esquirol and his contemporaries viewed masturbation as especially pernicious proof that the emotions had been disturbed. Yet although age represented a series of physical states, it additionally implied a particular set of social and familial expectations that changed over the course of one's lifetime. In men, Esquirol thought mental illness more likely to originate in adulthood than in old age or even adolescence because those in the prime of life were especially focused on the outward trappings of success. In a similar vein, he often cited thwarted ambition as the source of madness in professional men, whereas "instinctual" emotions such as love and fear more often aggravated the minds of his working-class patients.

Felix Voisin, one of Esquirol's students, expanded on his mentor's discussion of madness in men, noting that particular lifestyles and their attendant cultural norms helped determine the form of mental alienation. Voisin insisted that physical causes were far more significant than mental ones, yet he still cited the passions—especially pride and vanity—as central "sources of our misery," and echoed Pinel by stating doctors should seek to "combat the passions with the passions."[7] More cynical than his notable contemporaries, Voisin argued that the lifestyles of rich and poor alike led vulnerable individuals almost inevitably toward mental breakdown. The dissolute upbringing of working-class children created a class of immoral men ruled by their passions: they became madmen or criminals. The emotional lives of so-called "superior" men, however, could also be carried astray. A man of great intelligence might go mad out of boredom; the indolent lifestyles of the financially secure proved especially fraught. Soldiers likewise found themselves vulnerable to aggravated passions. In their case, an excess of excitement—and numerous opportunities for pride and vanity to find outlets on the field of battle—created difficulties when attempting to acclimate to civilian life. Middle-class and bourgeois men were also at risk, as Esquirol had insisted, and insane merchants who could not help succumbing to the psychological pressures of their unstable occupations supposedly proliferated in the opening decades of the nineteenth century. Expectations for success had risen in the postrevolutionary decades, alongside new opportunities, and some men reacted to the uncertainty of professional life with emotional outbursts and mental collapse. The importance of the family to bourgeois class identity, as a means of both cultural distinction and wealth creation, must be understood in the context of these social and financial pressures.

Doctors were less likely to consider insanity in women as a psychological reaction to cultural expectations despite the notoriously rigid requirements of bourgeois domestic ideology. Alienists partook in the spread of particularly insidious attitudes regarding women and irrationality by presenting their theories concerning the female body's effect on the mind as scientific inevitabilities rather than acknowledging them as historically situated products of culture (as they were so willing to do in the case of men). All doctors in postrevolutionary France conceived of the typical body as a male one and the female body as an aberration from the norm, and the first alienists fixated on biological differences between the sexes when developing their approach to insanity in women. This was certainly the case for Voisin, who treated many women patients as the cofounder of a private *maison de santé* outside Paris; his first major work, dedicated to his mother of all people, examined the subject of erotic alienation in women.

Pinel and Esquirol similarly claimed the passions were more animated, and often more sexually tinged, for women than for men. The onset of menses supposedly provided the first chance for madness to appear, and a woman's period would continue to offer a key to her mental state during her entire life. Throughout the nineteenth century, asylum doctors cited an irregular cycle as one piece of evidence among many that a woman patient's constitution had been disturbed by insanity. They claimed the return to rationality generally coincided with the regulation of a woman's period and that pregnancy and childbirth represented moments of danger in a woman's life because these physical states aggravated the passions to a potentially pathological degree. Menopause brought similar concerns.[8]

Yet despite alienists' seemingly deterministic understanding of the relationship between biology and insanity in women, they also emphasized cultural attributes of the female life cycle when identifying the moments in which a woman's emotional state might cross the boundary from normal to pathological. For example, Esquirol explained that the education of young women dangerously excited the passions. This had supposedly not been the case in antiquity, an era in which he claimed women were actually less likely than men to go mad. Esquirol found bourgeois habits especially jarring to a girl's senses. Music, balls, and dancing all primed the female brain for emotion, and thus mental illness, at the precise moment when their adolescent bodies already encouraged passionate feelings. Moreover, reading novels could "inspire ideas of imaginary perfection" in young women, setting them up for disappointment when life failed to live up to their fantasies.[9] Biological facts thus combined with cultural habits to make women especially vulnerable to mental alienation.

Case notes and treatises describing women patients implicate psychiatric professionals in the promotion of attitudes that had been used since the Revolution to deny women the rights of citizenship. The writings of early alienists, however, also reflect the very real concerns of women at an historical moment when legal and cultural strictures focused their emotional lives on marriage and family. In contrast to their discussions of bourgeois men, Pinel and Esquirol never cited frustrated professional ambitions as a source of insanity in women (it never would have occurred to them that women might hold professional ambitions at all). Instead, they tied women's insanity most closely to aggravations within the home; a child's birth or death, disruptions of household routines, the dissipation of familial affections, and complications in the process of courtship could all inspire madness in women. Women whose reactions to their families appeared out of line with bourgeois understandings of femininity were often labeled insane, as were those who took such norms to apparently unhealthy extremes. Those who became "lovesick" and obsessed with the objects of their affection rather than simply attached, concerned, and devoted were judged to need their passions redirected and controlled.

For early asylum doctors this state of affairs was only natural, for marriage and family constituted the loci of women's emotional lives, and madness was above all a reflection of emotional distress. This tendency is seen most clearly in the writings of the celebrated young alienist Étienne-Jean Georget, another doctor who insisted that all people—regardless of class or gender—were susceptible to feelings that "wound our sense of self by contradicting our needs or wants."[10] Georget was one of Esquirol's most promising students before he died in 1828 at the age of thirty-three. His major work, titled simply *De la folie*, bore the imprint of Esquirol's teachings, yet he focused more sustained attention on the relationship between the body and the mind than had his mentor. Georget believed madness was an illness of the brain and even called the moral treatment "direct cerebral treatment" for this reason.[11] He also claimed bodily distress led to psychological disturbance and vice versa. Georget thus emphasized treating the emotional aspects of madness alongside the physical ones—such as insomnia or digestive difficulties—because new bodily symptoms would inevitably arise if the affliction's psychological cause was not discovered and overcome.

As was the case for Pinel and Esquirol, Georget's conception of the passions led him to create a class- and gender-based understanding of insanity and its treatment. Although feelings such as jealousy, love, hate, fear, sadness, and anger were comprehensible to all people and could serve as triggers for mental illness, the circumstances that aggravated such emotions in each individual patient differed. As a physician working at the Salpêtrière, Georget dealt with women patients of a variety of class backgrounds. Most women, he argued, experienced madness owing to frustrations in their family lives, but those of the popular classes dealt with more regular and more extreme forms of domestic distress. Poverty, of course, made it difficult to support a family and also compounded daily tensions between husbands and wives. Domestic violence ("brutality in marriage") received special mention by Georget as a source of mental alienation in working women.

Conversely, he emphasized emotional responses to scandalous love affairs, thwarted marriage plans, and secret jealousies (of their brothers, sisters, and prettier friends!) when assessing the origins of women's insanity more broadly. He believed madness struck women of the lower classes most often but that these patients were also more readily cured. In their case, he found it appropriate to use physical labor as a method of distraction, whereas he argued that the diversions associated with middle- and upper-class lifestyles actually contributed to the aggravation of the passions. Still, he considered the reincorporation of women patients into the family home—regardless of class—the end goal of psychiatric treatment. Sentiments supposedly held by all women would aid in this result: "The mother," wrote Georget, "will desire to care for her children, the wife to return to her household routine."[12] Georget's understanding of women and madness undoubtedly reinforced the ideal of domestic motherhood, although one wonders why a woman's supposedly natural condition would bring about so much psychological turmoil.

Psychiatry's founders also linked insanity in men to disordered behavior in family life, beyond the already mentioned pressure to assure the family's well-being through professional success. The perversion of what doctors considered normal affections constituted one of the clearest signs a man had gone mad, and Esquirol and Pinel both provided numerous examples of men whose love for their parents and wives seemed to transform into hate or indifference for no apparent reason. A male patient, for example, who had long been considered a "respectful son" began to "ignore the entreaties of his dear father."[13] The "tears of his lover" left him equally unmoved. As was the case for their women patients, the behavioral repertoires doctors associated with sanity in men conformed to the family ideals of the bourgeoisie, a class that promoted self-possessed yet sentimental relations between all members of the family. Men who did not adapt to nineteenth-century expectations of fatherly and husbandly behavior, in particular, risked being seen as insane. The disturbance of affective ties therefore represented a symptom of insanity in men and women both. What differed was the comparative emphasis doctors placed on male and female biology in the diagnostic process, in that they found cases of mental illness in women more likely—although not exclusively—to be connected to physical states unique to their sex.

In sum, doctors' attitudes toward the passions perpetuated bourgeois values concerning family life by identifying gender and class nonconformity as a sign of mental illness. They additionally reflected middle-class assumptions regarding the popular classes, whose expressions of insanity were supposedly less complex than those of their bourgeois counterparts. Yet, the ways that doctors utilized these class- and gender-based notions in the treatment process suggested they held integrative potential. Pinel believed all people—even those deep in the throes of madness—held inside of them a kernel of rationality.[14] Their sense of self remained, even if it was hidden. Accordingly, any patient could gradually attain self-mastery by redirecting the aggravated passions that acted as source and symptom.

Neither Pinel nor Esquirol sought to replace emotion with reason because they believed rationality existed under the surface all along, and because they considered emotion an essential part of the human personality. Controlling and redirecting emotion, not eliminating it, would allow individuals to prosper within the community, the polity, and the home. After all, as the title of Esquirol's dissertation made clear, the passions were not simply causes and reflections of mental alienation, but they were *moyens curatifs* as well. This belief in the healing properties of the emotions applied equally to men and women of all class backgrounds. For if the diagnosis of mental illness appears to have simply reproduced dominant assumptions related to men, women, and class, the treatment methods theorized and enacted by psychiatry's founding fathers made use of nineteenth-century gender values in order to heal *all* patients—in so doing, they undermined the very same class and gender distinctions they helped to create.

Isolating Madness

Psychiatry's founders spent the start of the nineteenth century trying, under less than ideal political conditions, to institutionalize legally their positions as the rightful guardians of the insane.[15] Those whose conceptions of individual liberty had been influenced by the French and North American revolutions began to view the humane treatment of mad people as essential. Yet without a specific government policy dictating the terms of the treatment process, there was no way to enforce new styles of patient care. The establishment of the conservative Restoration monarchy—ushered in by victorious European powers after the defeat of Napoleon in 1815—proved hostile to the creation of such a system. The regime of Charles X, which strongly linked its own authority to that of the rehabilitated Catholic Church, was particularly disinclined to support the liberal, anticlerical alienists in their efforts to standardize psychiatric treatment.[16] As Esquirol noted in 1819 after surveying numerous private and public institutions, many patients still lived in conditions much like those criticized by Pinel nearly three decades earlier.[17] Patient abuse remained a distinct possibility without passage of a law outlining the rights of patients and the exact legal mechanisms regulating the commitment process; unscrupulous family members, in particular, could still commit relatives with ease until legislators put safeguards in place. Furthermore, even well-meaning families could prove dangerous to those experiencing the symptoms of insanity.

Psychiatric attitudes toward the family—especially the belief that all patients should be "isolated" from their families in order to be cured—proved central to doctors' conceptualizations of asylum reform and to the performance of the moral treatment. The asylum served as a source of seclusion from all the cares of work and home, a space apart from public and private sphere alike, where doctors controlled all aspects of their patients' daily lives, including their interpersonal interactions. The promotion of familial isolation conveniently legitimated the alienist's professional services; for example, someone such as Esquirol served as director of the public facility Bicêtre and also operated a private institution dedicated to the treatment of wealthy patients. Professional self-interest cannot fully explain the emphasis doctors placed on isolating madness, however, for it was possible to imagine the deployment of psychiatric expertise in settings beyond the asylum (by sending patients to general hospitals and convalescent homes with an alienist on staff, by encouraging doctors to make house calls, or by having patients visit doctors on an appointment basis in private offices). Members of the psychiatric profession at the start of the nineteenth century nonetheless championed sequestration in specialized institutions as the only way to cure individuals of insanity.

Doctors' faith in the utility of isolation logically stemmed from their belief that the passions could be useful in the treatment of mental alienation. As shown, Pinel considered "domestic distress" one of several typical causes of mental illness; he further claimed that living in the family home represented an "eternal obstacle" to a patient's recovery.[18] Citing various British sources, including the "mad" King George's physician Willis, he insisted that a patient would be best served by the moral treatment if he or she were kept away from their relatives for its duration. Pinel thought the presence of loved ones could lead to the interruption of the treatment process, inspire feelings of irritation in the patient, disturb the calm atmosphere of the institution, and even cause a relapse.[19] In short, family life aggravated the passions, familiarity often bred contempt, and only a stranger would be able to effectively shift the orientation of a patient's emotional state. Early alienists aimed to restore what they considered normalcy to the household, but doing so depended on the cultivation of spatial and emotional distance between patients and their families. Thus, much like their gendered formulation of the passions, doctors' reliance on isolation simultaneously propped up bourgeois family values and indicated some ambivalence toward the family itself.

That said, doctors' actions tended to undermine authoritarian manifestations of familial power reminiscent of the Old Regime rather than the sentimental relations more firmly associated with the rising bourgeoisie. Bourgeois families celebrated affective relationships between relatives, especially within the nuclear family. Marriage strategies continued to revolve around economic security and the development of family alliances in the nineteenth century, but the ideal marriage was one that accomplished these goals while maintaining genuine friendship between spouses,[20] especially because the bourgeois home represented a site of tranquility in a chaotic world. As infant mortality rates declined, closeness between children and parents became increasingly central to family routines, and domestic architecture encouraged a sense of intimacy and privacy through the use of individual bedrooms, nurseries, and separate family wings where outside guests rarely if ever congregated.[21] Furthermore, although fathers still held ultimate authority within the home, there were many signs that members of the middle classes expected this authority to be wielded more justly and less violently than in previous centuries. As Loftur Guttormsson notes, "the mood was shifting away from beating as a routine punishment (except in schools) towards the application of moral and emotional pressures developing in children a capacity for self-government."[22] Novel approaches to child-rearing paralleled new attitudes toward the mentally ill, who were likewise now expected to learn how to control themselves rather than merely submit to physical compulsion.

The work that ultimately had the greatest long-term impact on the practice of asylum psychiatry in nineteenth-century France reflected the profession's alignment with bourgeois family values, although it did so in a way that often drew attention to the dangers posed by the family to a patient's mental health. Esquirol wrote *Memoire sur l'isolement d'aliénés* in 1832 in order to convince lawmakers of the recently established July Monarchy to create national regulations concerning the construction and administration of insane asylums, and the comparatively liberal atmosphere of the new regime proved conducive to the alienist's plans. In his memoir on isolation, Esquirol insisted that doctors, rather than families, knew what was best for the patient. He nevertheless built his case for professional intervention around the notion that family life represented the most essential element of a person's identity—an assumption bourgeois families would certainly have shared. Sequestration in a mental institution was a traumatic process, and Esquirol argued that the terms by which someone might find himself in such a place should be tightly regulated:

> The question of isolation attaches itself to the interests most dear to man, considered as a patient, as a member of the family and of society. Herein lies the gravity of an illness that puts [the] affected at risk of being deprived of the objects of his most dear affections, of being thwarted in his desires and in the exercise of his civil rights and his liberty.[23]

In other words, madness threw a patient's world into disarray by destroying his sense of self, disrupting his family relations, and splintering his social bonds. Isolation could restore not just a person's sanity, but their familial, communal, and civic identities as well.

In the most general sense, isolation could be used as a synonym for confinement or sequestration, and sometimes Esquirol did just that.[24] The term isolation is more historically useful than these alternatives, however, for it raises the question: isolation from what? Although "sequestration" emphasizes the space where a patient might be confined, isolation forces one to think of the space— and in this case, the people—he or she is being taken from. Esquirol defined isolation as "removing the mad person from all his habits, taking him far from the place he lives, separating him from his family, his friends, and his servants while surrounding him with strangers and changing completely his manner of life."[25] Treatment entailed a complete break from the home because its familiarity inhibited the patient's return to rationality. While Esquirol considered the asylum a curative space in which material surroundings and human interactions represented two complementary aspects of the same rehabilitative process, he suggested a similar sense of harmony between architecture, social relations, and individual recovery could not exist inside the family home owing to "the presence of individuals who awaken or irritate the . . . passions, [who] provoke the disturbance of reason and are insurmountable obstacles to its reestablishment."[26] Shocking, confounding, and redirecting a patient's senses required separation from everything and everyone he or she found familiar and familial.

Strangers therefore played a special part in the moral treatment. The presence of unfamiliar people in an unfamiliar environment encouraged a novel interplay among the patient's senses, which constituted the first step on the path toward recovery. Discombobulation and distraction presented doctors with an opportunity to start the healing process, to teach the patient how to resume their expected familial role. If patients expressed intense anger toward those closest to them, lashing out or becoming indifferent when in contact with the source of their rage, doctors claimed that a sense of pride encouraged them to act agreeably when meeting new people. Esquirol reported having witnessed patients interacting with their physicians in a very calm fashion while simultaneously cursing their family members under their breath. The company of other patients could also prove beneficial because the example of other madmen encouraged self-reflection.[27] Ordinary people and situations no longer made much of an impression on the insane person. The "extravagances of their peers," however, would prove shocking and distracting.[28] The strangeness of their new situation forced patients to momentarily forget themselves, to interact with others, and to live outside their minds. In the process, their former "mad desires" would eventually be replaced by ennui and hopes to go back home—the purpose of isolation in the first place.[29]

Esquirol presented numerous examples meant to prove the indispensability of isolation, most of which emphasized the negative influence of close family and friends on his patients' emotional states. Through his descriptions, the renowned alienist suggested the performance of behaviors one would reasonably expect within any middle-class home were precisely those that caused insane people the greatest disturbance. He noted that wives of depressed men sometimes could not hide the sadness they felt over the progression of their husbands' conditions. For many a head of household, "the tears of his wife (and) her sad countenance, are new motives that persuade the unfortunate that there is nothing better to do than to destroy himself."[30] Already depressed, such men viewed the suffering of their wives as further proof they had not lived up to societal expectations regarding their husbandly duties. Esquirol noted that one patient in particular, a twenty-seven-year-old man who had become depressed after losing his fortune, attempted suicide when faced with "the despair and the cares of his wife."[31] It was only when taken into Esquirol's asylum that the man ceased his self-destructive activities owing to enforced isolation from his family and friends, as well as his relocation to a ground-floor room where it would be impossible to jump to his death. An example of a young man who had recently displayed signs of depression is similarly revealing. According to his doctor, the man purportedly exclaimed, "Ah! My mother, how you torment me! I will never heal near you."[32] He had grown impatient with his mother's questions about the state of his health and her constant requests for him to follow the treatment regimen prescribed to him. Esquirol presented these cases and others as proof that patients should be kept away from their families—even, and perhaps especially, from those with good intentions.

Still, the reintegration of the patient into the seemingly natural workings of the household represented the primary goal of the moral treatment, and all commentators recognized that families held intense interest in the treatment of their loved ones regardless of the doctor's recently enhanced role. Although doctors went to great lengths to prove the damage that might be caused if an insane person lived in the family home instead of entering a specialized institution for treatment, they never blamed families for the psychological distress of their intimates even if they insisted that family life could aggravate the passions.[33] As seen in the above example of the meddlesome mother, Esquirol did not cite pathological family relations as the justification for isolation. It was not *her* behavior that he considered unhealthy. Instead, it was the son's response to seemingly innocuous and unremarkable mother-child interactions that needed to be identified, contained, and redirected. The son's perceived inability to react to his mother in a normative fashion labeled Esquirol's patient as irrational; removal from her company would be the first step in his recovery process. Isolation thus propped up sentimental family relations while nonetheless drawing attention to the fragility of the nineteenth-century construct of the bourgeois home as a place of refuge.

In a century that emphasized the tranquility of the bourgeois home and the familial relationships articulated therein as primary elements of class distinction, the suggestion that the family might be a source of mental illness would have been controversial. Esquirol thus framed his assertions carefully and rarely mentioned patients whose relatives' behaviors could be construed as cruel or even atypical. The only family members he depicted in a negative light were people who attempted to incarcerate sane relatives. Such individuals behaved in a fashion more akin to families of the Old Regime, a time when parents could institutionalize children without due process and husbands wielded greater legal power over wives, rather than those of a liberal era more reflective of psychiatric principles.[34] Doctors attempted a precarious balancing act by drawing attention to the dangers of family life. Implementing their theories of psychiatric treatment necessitated them doing so. Yet securing alienists' roles as the rightful caretakers of the insane also depended on their ability to preserve bourgeois class distinctions—the cult of domesticity ranking high among them.

The profession managed to walk this tightrope, at least at first, by pathologizing authoritarian household dynamics and celebrating benevolent ones.[35] Not only did doctors condemn families who attempted to institutionalize relatives without cause but they also implied that "unsentimental" behavior actually constituted evidence of insanity. Esquirol's discussions of heads of household afflicted with mental alienation were often indicative of this tendency. The above example of the suicidal husband involved a patient whose love for his family intensified his depression and who seemingly fared best when kept away from them. Esquirol also worried, however, that men were particularly needful of isolation because they were used to considering themselves "master(s) of the land."[36] These husbands had previously inspired the obedience of their families "through respect or through affection" and would become infuriated when their demands were not met in the same fashion following the onset of insanity.[37] Esquirol argued the man of the house should be forced to cede his authority if deemed insane, even though he had once reasonably expected his wife, children, and servants to bend to his will.

The doctor explained that a mad husband often failed to come to terms with his new role in the family:

> Like a despot, he is ready to punish with the greatest severity whomever will dare make the least remonstrance; whatever he demands is impossible; it doesn't matter . . . the affliction of his family, the sorrow of his friends, the eagerness of everyone, their deference to his will . . . all serve to support this madman in his ideas of power and domination.[38]

Men like this misunderstood the cultural basis of paternal power in the nineteenth century. Although his patients acted as if their authority naturally stemmed from their sex, Esquirol reasoned that the demands of male heads of household should be respected because men were the most rational members of the family. These capricious "despots" would therefore need to regain their sanity before their expectation of familial obedience was once again socially acceptable. The act of isolating an irrational husband—"outside his empire, far from his subjects"—would humble him and thereby help reorient the tone of his social interactions.[39]

Esquirol aimed to eventually return patients to their former lives. Accordingly, he did not envision asylums as permanent living spaces, but as necessary sites of repose and rehabilitation. While the household might serve as a source of respite from the outside world, mental patients needed respite from the home itself. The fact that they did not experience home life in the same way as their "normal" counterparts signaled their irrationality to a great degree. Isolation, in and of itself, did not produce a cure. It is better understood as a necessary precondition for the cultivation of new, healthy social relations between the mad person and other members of the community, most importantly their family. In order for a healthy family dynamic to reemerge, alienists insisted, an entirely new and equally significant relationship must be cultivated between the patient and the doctor himself.

Performing Treatment

Most descriptions of early French asylums come from the doctor's perspective and therefore tell us much more about the assumptions undergirding the behaviors of professional men than those of the people over whom they held power. The moral treatment was nonetheless a two-way—if always heavily imbalanced—process that occurred between doctor and patient. Doctors focused considerable care on formulating treatments they thought might appeal to their patients' hidden, rational selves and on developing personae they believed patients would respond to in a rehabilitative fashion. Psychiatric theories concerning the passions and familial isolation heavily influenced asylum doctors' step-by-step formulation of the treatment scenario, as well as their own behaviors, in ways that placed gender at the heart of every asylum interaction.

The first stage of the treatment process always involved shocking the patient's system in order to redirect their emotional state; as shown, the necessity of such surprise constituted the raison d'être of familial isolation, since familiar sensations supposedly kept patients from reconsidering their pathological behaviors. After having instilled what he considered the proper degree of shock (through isolation from family and interaction with new people, but also through more obviously repressive means), the doctor began to more fully immerse his patient in the mutual performance of the moral treatment by drawing on shared under-standings of proper feminine and masculine comportment. The development of gendered treatment scenarios stemmed from the importance doctors placed on the passions in the origins and the presentation of mental illness: although all people were capable of experiencing the same sentiments, and were susceptible to mental collapse if those feelings somehow went awry, the precise circumstances that aggravated the passions were highly individualized. Each case of madness depended on a person's temperament, their upbringing, and their class and gender background. Furthermore, doctors believed that certain codes of con-duct—such as those related to masculine honor or feminine virtue—remained comprehensible to all patients despite their symptoms.

Alienists staged elaborate scenes in which they used pertinent aspects of pa-tients' gender and class identities to convince them to return to rationality. For example, Esquirol thought a man's occupational background and past experi-ences could be used as an entry point for treatment, as his interpretation of a case of madness in a former soldier shows. Numerous fighting men found them-selves incarcerated in asylums during the 1790s and the decades that followed. After becoming depressed after losing his fortune during the Revolution, one such individual moved to Paris from the countryside at his wife's urging. Ap-parently growing bored with his new location, he became increasingly stubborn, succumbed to delirium, and eventually ended up in Esquirol's institution. The man met each of Esquirol's efforts to shift his emotional state with increased resistance; he reportedly refused food, would not leave his bed, and reacted with violence to the doctor's attempts to disrupt his senses with sprays of cold water to the face. The only tactic that seemed to make any impression involved Es-quirol's assignment of a new servant to the patient's quarters: a former soldier, like the man himself. The attendant reminisced with his new charge, talking to him about "war, the countryside, and military service."[40] Nostalgia and kindness distracted the patient from his frustration; he immediately began to eat and two weeks later regained his reason entirely. Esquirol claimed that recollecting shared wartime experiences with a stranger led to the replacement of a patholog-ical passion with something far more benign: in this instance, burgeoning com-radeship conquered self-destructive stubbornness. Furthermore, a bit of male bonding had encouraged the return of sanity, thereby solidifying the perceived connection between manliness and rationality that doctors both relied on and helped to perpetuate.

Women also responded to gendered treatments according to Esquirol, al-though the role of the family in the redirection of a woman's passions could be complex. All doctors agreed family life could aggravate the passions and that a return to the household too early might even inspire a relapse in an apparently healthy person, but the promise of going home could also inspire hope—an especially useful emotion—in melancholic patients. Since doctors believed women focused their emotional lives on their families, they took this predisposition into account when devising plans for emotional redirection. For instance, Esquirol cited the case of a woman who harbored intense love and devotion for her husband and children yet felt profoundly depressed. At first, she reacted positively to a stay in the asylum, but she soon became bored and the depression returned. Esquirol thought that surprise would prepare her mind for hopes of recovery, so he orchestrated a series of visits between the patient and her loved ones. These visits intensified the woman's desire to return home. But Esquirol refused to let her leave; he even cut off all communication between the patient and her family. Then, when she least expected it, he arranged for them to visit again. In toying with her emotions in this fashion, the alienist claimed to have his patient's best interests at heart. She supposedly became reasonable after this bit of theater and happily resumed her role as wife and mother.[41]

Assumptions about gender and family life likewise shaped the self-presentations of doctors, whose writings reveal as much about shifting meanings of professional manhood in postrevolutionary France as they do the process of psychiatric treatment. Early alienists such as Pinel envisioned asylums as temporary stand-ins for their patients' homes and, accordingly, imagined their own roles in paternal terms. "In a word," explained the founder of French psychiatry, "the general governance of the hospital resembled that of a great family, consisting of turbulent and impetuous individuals, who must be repressed but not exasperated."[42] The doctor himself oversaw this "great family," for only he possessed the wisdom and patience such responsibility demanded.

Pinel's own son, Scipion, expanded on this familial metaphor and insisted that working with mental patients required a very specific fatherly disposition. The asylum doctor must have "a special vocation to pass his life among the alienated, to attach himself to their unhappiness, to find charm in that existence, so seemingly empty and at the same time so full of great lessons. . . . He must identify fully with [his patients'] pain, their joys, and all their interests." The younger Pinel also claimed that when a doctor suited for asylum management saw his patients following a short absence, he would feel joy comparable to that brought on by a reunion with "family long separated." "This type of man," Pinel *fils* famously wrote, "is more than a doctor, he is a consoler and a father."[43] The prototypical version of the doctor-father was, in this case, the writer's actual father as well, which might help to explain why he found the similarities between the household and the asylum so salient. All early practitioners of the moral treatment, however, believed that patients—like children—required education, and that the success or failure of the educative process would depend not only on their instructors' methods but on their personalities as well. The key was to convince the patient-child that it was in their best interest to obey the doctor-father—to inspire each patients' filial respect and devotion through a variety of strategies, some gentler than others.

Doctors cultivated and constantly reaffirmed their personae through the process of social interaction. Like early psychiatric conceptions of mental illness itself, the therapeutic persona did not exist in a vacuum and depended on the validation of others to a great degree. The projection of authority was the most important aspect of the alienist's self-presentation and, simultaneously, the one most in need of outside affirmation. Pinel considered the ability to "exude authority" a necessary attribute for a doctor because there were certain patients who could only be cured if they were suitably impressed by medical power. [44] Esquirol also asserted "the physician should be invested with an authority from which no one is exempt."[45] He thought even the representatives of local governments should take care to aggrandize psychiatric power because social respect outside of the asylum would add to the doctor's authoritative mystique when dealing with patients.[46] Likewise, authority should never be divided between doctors and families, or among members of the asylum staff. Instead, "everything should be controlled by the *chef*."[47]

As shown, practitioners of the moral treatment believed each element of a patient's daily life should work in concert and contribute toward the goal of mental recovery. This included everything from the design of the room a patient inhabited, to the food he ate, to the diversions that filled his time. Yet the perception of control was nearly as important as its existence because both encouraged the patient's eventual submission. The creation of an authoritative persona would allow the doctor to foster dependence, which alienists believed would make patients compliant and eventually lead to their cure. Isolation from family helped to aggrandize medical authority because it proved to the patient that he was truly alone and had no one to turn to but the doctor. As Esquirol explained, "from that first moment when the madman is isolated, surprised, disconcerted, etc., he feels a precious relaxation . . . finding the patient without barriers, [the doctor] can more easily acquire his confidence."[48] Family visitations were discouraged in most cases so that patients would depend on their doctor for all their needs and see him as the sole source of the eventual improvement of their situation, as the above case of the young mother implies.[49] This train of thought extended to the activities of the asylum's staff, who were expected to model correct behavior for the patients. Esquirol argued that "the doctor must give impetus to everything" and employees "must give the example of deference" in order to "show the madman that resistance is in vain."[50]

The first asylum doctors apparently saw no conflict between feeling genuine compassion toward their patients and enacting domineering performances of medical authority (although, as we will see in the following chapter, there was much debate within the profession when doctors appeared to cross the line from treatment to abuse). Because each patient's treatment regimen was individualized, it is easy to imagine the doctor changing his persona like a mask from one patient to the next—or even doing so vis-à-vis the same patient at various points in the treatment process. Pinel was acutely aware of the performative dimensions of psychiatric power, noting that the "appearance of repression," usually in the form of trickery, was a necessary evil justified only when other methods had proven futile and when practiced without malicious intent on the part of the doctor.[51] As Jan Goldstein has conclusively demonstrated, doctors sought to "console" their patients, not simply intimidate or frighten them—which itself speaks to the transition from an authoritarian conception of family life to something more benevolent. The tack a doctor chose to pursue depended on the specifics of a given case and how readily he thought the patient might respond to a particular treatment scenario. Doctors nonetheless agreed certain personality traits were more conducive to cure than others, especially since they considered patients' respect for medical authority essential in every case.

Pinel addressed the traits embodied by the ideal asylum overseer by using his assistant, Pussin, as an example. Pussin had no specialized medical training, but he served as the superintendent of Bicêtre before Pinel arrived and continued to work under him thereafter. He eliminated physical restraints in that asylum, although the credit for this action has often been attributed to Pinel himself. The role played by gender in Pinel's discussion of Pussin is noteworthy and suggests that only a man could run an asylum in the therapeutic fashion promoted by psychiatry's founder. Some traits championed by Pinel could arguably be understood in gender-neutral terms; he writes, for example, that Pussin exhibited "alongside the most pure philanthropic morals . . . an indefatigable diligence in his [duties of] surveillance."[52] Yet Pinel soon transitioned to a list of characteristics associated more obviously with manliness, noting that the overseer's "unshakeable firmness [and] reasoned courage" helped him manage the asylum.[53] If it was unclear that such sure-mindedness and savoir-faire were personality traits that Pinel classified as masculine, he erased any doubt by linking them to physical features. Pinel even titled the relevant section of his treatise "The Physical and Moral Qualities Essential to the Surveillance of the Alienated," suggesting the asylum overseer's physicality was inseparable from his authoritative character. Pinel claimed Pussin's courage was "supported by physical qualities best suited to impose [his will upon patients]." Notable were his "well-proportioned body" and "limbs full of strength and vigor."[54] Furthermore, "in stormy moments his voice is thunderous, his attitude proud and intrepid."[55] When taken all together, the various traits Pinel associated with successful asylum management point to a conception of psychiatric authority that was masculine by definition.

This did not mean Pinel denied the possibility of a more feminine style of psychiatric self-presentation—a fact that points to the incompleteness of psychiatry's professionalization at this time. Pussin lived with and worked alongside his wife, Marguerite Jubline, when he managed Bicêtre. Although Pinel alluded to Jubline only in passing, it was always with admiration for her character and for the work she performed as the *surveillante.* As in his depiction of Pussin, Pinel described his wife as someone who used gender to her advantage when interacting with the asylum's patients. Pussin used his authoritative demeanor and physicality to encourage respect and obedience. Jubline, on the other hand, tended to appeal to her male patients' belief in feminine virtue and their desire to protect vulnerable women. Most of Pinel's descriptions of the *surveillante* appear in a section related to the art of "directing the mad, while appearing to assent to their imaginary ideas."[56] It should perhaps come as little surprise that it was Jubline who proved most adept at this particular tactic; a woman of the popular classes in a patriarchal society such as hers likely had considerable experience avoiding direct confrontation with men while seeking to get her way.

Pinel's version of Jubline used a combination of charm, flattery, and distraction to persuade patients to behave ways she found desirable. For example, one day a patient entered the asylum's kitchen, grabbed a knife, and threatened the cooks and servants. As they prepared to physically overpower him, Jubline interceded and asked "why prevent so strong a man from working with me?"[57] She then proceeded to instruct him on the proper way to chop vegetables, subtly taking the knife from his hands. She successfully pacified the patient by making him feel useful and manly. Pinel recounted another time when Jubline played on gender norms in the course of the treatment process, which resulted in a previously willful patient securing his release with her help. The patient arrived in the asylum with symptoms of depression and mania; he soon experienced a brief period of recovery, but then apparently started to doubt the desirability of his cure. At this point, the *surveillante* convinced him that she would be punished if he experienced a relapse; in order to protect the woman from harm, he remained "cured."[58] Both these examples suggest that the late eighteenth-century belief in gender complementarity in marriage extended to the workplace as well.[59] Pussin's wife used gender in her interactions with patients in a very different way than did her husband, but Pinel found both methods worthy of praise. There remained a possibility, albeit often unrealized and always contested, for women practitioners to play a part in the direction of asylums throughout the nineteenth century.

As his discussion of the Pussins indicated, Pinel's conception of psychiatric expertise was not class dependent. Pussin became Pinel's employee once the doctor took charge of Bicêtre, and the overseer's subordinate status within the asylum's occupational hierarchy despite his commanding persona would certainly have propped up the authority of his superior. Nonetheless, Pinel suggested he viewed Pussin as an equal despite his lack of a formal education, especially by presenting him as a model for students to emulate. It is also significant that Pinel stressed Pussin's physicality over his mental acuity when outlining his most admirable traits, although he also presented Pussin as very self-possessed. The emphasis on the physical prowess of the ideal asylum overseer would dissipate among those who followed in the founder's footsteps—men who resolutely sought to safeguard their professional interests and expand psychiatry's reach. Conveniently for them, alienists' own theories propped up cultural associations between rational self-control and bourgeois masculinity, thereby legitimating their profession's takeover as the guardians of the insane.

This tendency can be seen clearly in the writings of Scipion Pinel, the son of Philippe, one of the most vocal proponents for the construction of new asylums during the 1830s. The younger Pinel wrote extensively about the characteristics of the perfect asylum director and helped to spread the false assertion that his father freed the inmates of Bicêtre from their irons, thus giving credit to a bourgeois professional for actions actually initiated by a layman.[60] He parroted many of his father's descriptions of Pussin when describing the ideal asylum doctor by arguing he should possess a commanding physical presence, a strong constitution, a sense of dignity and calm under pressure, a deep voice, and a kind and well-meaning regard.[61] There was one major difference, though, and it pointed to the professionalization of psychiatry that had occurred between the pinnacle of the father's career and that of the son. Namely, Pinel *fils* noted that the alienist "by nature of his studies . . . [must] become the natural judge of all that happens in the asylum." Education, in other words, now preceded character.

This suggests that some of the integrative potential of the psychiatric enterprise began to deteriorate as early as the 1830s, at least with respect to the type of person alienists thought could successfully implement the moral treatment. This shift occurred as asylum doctors became increasingly preoccupied with safeguarding their professional prerogatives and eliminating rivals amid the oversupplied medical job market of the July Monarchy, which offered considerable opportunities for individual advancement but also increased competition. The senior Pinel's relative openness to lay expertise had not lasted long. Gender-based treatments in which all members of the asylum staff played a part, however, did not disappear—doctors merely began to argue more insistently that the orchestration of such scenes required the trappings of professionalization.

THE FOUNDING "FATHERS" of French psychiatry made use of widespread attitudes toward the family and its associated gender roles when identifying symptoms, designing treatment protocols, organizing institutional spaces, and crafting their personas. In so doing, they promulgated increasingly narrow definitions of sanity that reinforced sexist and classist structures of power from which they personally benefited. Yet, although historians have typically viewed the relationship between gender and psychiatry as inherently repressive, the way that doctors imagined their patients as capable of responding to gendered treatment processes indicates that the medicalization of mental illness—at its base—was about the possibility of patients' inclusion in French society rather than their segregation and stigmatization. The approach of early alienists toward gender and the family aligned with their stated belief in the universality of human emotions and the social experiences that inspired them, and there would remain a therapeutic space for gender inside asylums as long as doctors considered emotion an essential aspect of treatment and cure.

Doctors' attempts to put these ideas into practice nonetheless appear supremely hypocritical considering how thoroughly the nineteenth-century asylum system failed to live up to the expectations of its founders. Indeed, it is easy to ascribe self-interested motives to the first asylum doctors because they conveniently understood the values of their own class as those to which all French should conform. But their role in the perpetuation of bourgeois gender values—and therefore bourgeois class distinction—was always double-edged. Alienists unwittingly questioned the naturalness of middle-class gender norms in the very act of promoting them by pinpointing women and men's enactment of their familial roles as key sources of mental illness. The influential theory of familial isolation similarly hints at the threat posed by psychiatry to the image of the uniquely tranquil bourgeois home: early alienists never outright blamed well-meaning families for a patient's mental distress, but they nonetheless presented a less than peaceful portrait of family life by insisting that a mad person would only become madder when living at home. Even Pinel's discussion of the ideal psychiatric persona suggested that medical power could be wielded by a layman—or even a laywoman—thus posing a subtle yet meaningful challenge to the authority of all professional men.

There was always a tension between the ways in which the enactment of the moral treatment promoted notions of natural class and gender difference while simultaneously revealing their flexibility and constructedness. This essential contradiction did not necessarily undermine medical, masculine, or bourgeois power in the opening decades of the century—at least in part because the political situation did not yet fully support the expansion of the psychiatric enterprise. The implications of the moral treatment's gender dimensions remained relatively limited until the 1838 establishment of the national asylum system, despite the method's use in individual institutions well before that time. Practical consequences, however, soon emerged. As psychiatry's influence spread and various professional controversies took hold, doctors' contradictory relationship to bourgeois values would rise to the surface in ways that constrained the behaviors of doctors themselves, proving that medical men were as beholden to new gender expectations as were their patients.

CHAPTER 2

Medical Controversy and Honor among (Mad)Men

O N A SUNDAY AFTERNOON in late January 1839, a man named Alexis Bourgeois attempted to murder the doctor M. Bleynie.[1] Bleynie worked at Charenton, the large mental asylum on the outskirts of the capital, and spent several nights a week in an apartment in Paris. As the doctor entered his flat that fateful weekend, Bourgeois pursued him and forced his way into the study. The would-be murderer directed a pistol in Bleynie's direction, but in the course of a struggle it was forced from his hands. The attacker then produced another gun, hidden in his pants pocket, and fired several times. The noise stirred the neighbors, who entered the apartment as Bleynie restrained his attempted killer. When questioned as to why he would try to murder the asylum doctor, Bourgeois explained that Bleynie had subjected him "to cold baths that had been very harmful" many years earlier. From that point on, the patient plotted his murderous revenge. He planned to kill Bleynie, then two other doctors who had also performed the "cold shower" treatment. The police found multiple weapons when they searched his room later that day. Esprit Blanche, the director of a private asylum and critic of the aforementioned cold shower, would seize upon this incident and the press coverage it inspired as evidence that the violent expression of medical authority damaged psychiatry's honorable image.[2]

The timing of Bourgeois's rampage—a source of "lively gossip"—was indeed unfortunate for alienists, as it coincided with the recent passage of the law of 1838, the culmination of a nearly twenty-year campaign to persuade lawmakers to institute a nation-wide asylum system.[3] By this time, France had once again experienced revolution, and the comparatively liberal political atmosphere of Louis Philippe's constitutional monarchy—established in 1830—was more conducive to both asylum reform and the professional aspirations of alienists than the previous regime had been. The rising legislative influence of the Doctrinaires, proponents of a particularly conservative variant of liberalism most closely associated with the politician François Guizot, was especially auspicious for alienists seeking to transform their medical expertise into tangible social authority.[4] Furthermore, as Jo Burr Margadant argues, the July Monarchy tended to support the political and financial interests of the haute bourgeoisie, and the royal family itself embodied bourgeois family values (with the king visibly committed to the well-being of his children and the queen relegated to the domestic sphere).[5] "Bourgeois monarchy" proved a contradiction in terms, and Louis Philippe eventually abdicated in response to the Revolution of 1848. In the meantime, however, his government proved open to the implementation of psychiatric reforms that would, like the monarchy itself, reflect the cultural transition from authoritarian to more sentimental family values.

Legislators replaced what had previously consisted of a localized and somewhat haphazard process of institutionalization with a set of national regulations that called for the availability of one public asylum per department where patients could be treated by a trained doctor and his underlings. Lawmakers provided two paths for patient entrance into the new asylums, one instigated by the police and the other by families of the insane.[6] Both methods hinged on the opinion of psychiatric professionals. Discussions concerning the codification of the law amounted to what Jan Goldstein describes as a boundary dispute between doctors, the judiciary, and the clergy—with the alienists ultimately succeeding in the attempt to secure their positions as the rightful caretakers of those deemed mad.[7] The 1838 law represented a major turning point for the profession, for it increased the power held by individual doctors and the legitimacy of psychiatry as a whole. However, the new asylum regulations also opened the door for criticism of a newly formed professional group that had yet to earn the respect of the public at large, even if alienists had successfully convinced representatives of the state that they warranted patronage. Calls for reform of the law, which many French citizens claimed was open to abuse, lasted throughout the nineteenth century and often centered on the claim that doctors had not shown themselves deserving of this newly attained authority.[8] Incidents such as the attempted murder of Dr. Bleynie wounded psychiatry's fragile image and gave credence to those who criticized the overzealous enactment of medical power.

A debate erupted almost immediately following the bill's ratification between two eminent asylum doctors, François Leuret and Esprit Blanche, over the appropriateness and the efficacy of subjecting patients to a stream of cold water to the face in order to cure them of delusions.[9] At first glance Blanche and Leuret's disagreement appears to have stemmed from divergent conceptions of medical ethics or related questions of medical effectiveness.[10] Yet they also disagreed sharply over what constituted honorable behavior in a professional setting that provided unique challenges for bourgeois men: the insane asylum.

Honor in postrevolutionary France operated as a mechanism of inclusion and exclusion that propped up cultural associations between middle-class masculinity and worthiness for participation in the public sphere. Robert Nye has conclusively shown that bourgeois men in the nineteenth century adapted the early modern honor code as a form of conflict management because it allowed them to prove their personal distinction in a meritocratic society while simultaneously serving as a "collective warrant for certifying the superiority and exclusiveness of their class."[11] Honor worked in conjunction with rationality itself as the foundation of bourgeois masculine superiority, in that the possession of one of these attributes implied the presence of the other, and the appearance of either distinguished a professional man from less privileged members of the social order. As William Reddy has argued, honor proved central not only to men's self-perceptions and self-presentations in postrevolutionary France, but also to the very construction of masculine rationality as a gender ideal.[12] It could be possessed and defended, but it was supposedly not *felt*. This allowed men to conceive of the public sphere—where an "invisible" code of honor regulated interactions between them—as a space where logic rather than emotion determined all decision-making.

Contestations over honor during the cold shower debate, as well as related disagreements over how to best express psychiatric power, allow us to further test the degree to which French medical men embraced bourgeois gender ideals as they navigated the process of professionalization. As seen in the preceding chapter, psychiatric institutions featured interactions between men and women of various classes and degrees of psychological impairment. This, in itself, makes the asylum a revelatory entry point into the intricacies of the nineteenth-century gender performance. More significantly, asylum interactions also laid bare the very processes through which gender was made and unmade at this time because psychiatric discourse played an essential role in solidifying rational self-control as a central characteristic of masculinity during the pivotal decades following the French Revolution. The behaviors of doctors during the debate over the cold shower further indicate the transition away from a cultural conception of masculinity based primarily on physicality to one that foregrounded psychological self-mastery instead. This proved a fraught process, even within a profession whose members benefited from and helped to disseminate these increasingly influential gender expectations.

Psychiatric Paternalism and Professional Honor

Patients reported being subjected to the cold shower well into the late nineteenth century, although it is impossible to determine how often doctors carried out the "treatment."[13] Warm and cold baths had long been used in institutional settings to treat various symptoms related to madness. For example, eighteenth-century mad doctors suggested a cold bath might improve melancholy and a warm one could temper the effects of mania. What Pinel called the bath of surprise, and later asylum doctors referred to as the cold shower, had some proponents in the early years of the moral treatment era, but few asylum directors openly advocated its use by the mid-nineteenth century.[14] Nonetheless, many asylums were equipped to perform the practice, which certain doctors and their employees carried out in specially designed tubs that encapsulated the entire body save the head. The device rendered anyone sitting in the tub immobile with their face exposed. The treatment entailed spraying water onto the patient for as long as the doctor deemed necessary, supposedly between five and thirty seconds, in order to shock the senses and create a drowning sensation. The element of surprise inherent in the method paralleled that of "isolation" more generally. Just as doctors intended the patient's removal from the family home to disorient him or her, they likewise subjected patients to the cold shower to create a blank slate upon which to (re)inscribe a rehabilitated and rational personality. Its main proponent, François Leuret, at least made this claim.

Widespread discussion of the cold shower treatment did not begin in earnest until after the passage of the law of 1838, although Pinel had commented negatively on its use at the start of the century. After a brief survey of examples of the ineffectiveness of the cold shower, he concluded that "this method, however successful in some instances, might in others be extremely dangerous, and it can only be resorted to with propriety in almost helpless cases, and where other remedies are ineffectual."[15] Pinel's admittedly mild rebuke of the practice did not keep his intellectual descendant, Leuret, from exploring the possible therapeutic value of the cold shower approximately three decades later in an 1837 treatise on how to best treat delusions.[16] The author was one of several directors of the great Parisian public asylum Bicêtre, a position that Pinel himself had held before his death in 1826.

Leuret was born in 1897 in Nancy, where his mother encouraged his studies, but his father, a baker, expected the boy to follow in his footsteps. Leuret eventually moved to Paris to study medicine after years of paternal resistance and a stint in the army. In a life reminiscent of a nineteenth-century novel, he struggled to survive off a pittance sent to him by his devoted sisters as he forged connections with Parisian psychiatry's leading figures.[17] The young doctor eventually studied under Esquirol and worked for him at his private mental institution, proving himself a gifted alienist noteworthy for the powerful sway he held over his patients.[18] Firmly entrenched in Esquirol's circle, Leuret had in him an influential ally. Leuret's controversial opinions were sure to gain attention by virtue of his professional appointment at Bicêtre and his impressive academic lineage.

He did not consider the cold shower appropriate for every patient, just those who showed resistance to other, less traumatic forms of cure. In this way he sidestepped what might have seemed like a disagreement with the master, Pinel. Ideal candidates were those patients who held "false ideas" or delusions, but still retained some of their "intelligence" and a sense of their former, rational selves; this excluded those with chronic conditions such as dementia or "idiocy." Those who Leuret considered most suited for the cold shower were therefore stubborn but still curable. This population was different than that which typically faced physically repressive measures in asylums that purported to perform some variation of the moral treatment. Unlike the so-called furious mad whom asylum doctors sometimes put in strait jackets because they appeared to pose a danger, the patients Leuret subjected to the cold shower did not usually physically threaten others. Instead, they often insisted they were someone they were not—for example, the sons of Napoleon or Napoleon himself (Leuret had met twelve Napoleons in the course of his time at Bicêtre).[19] Leuret sought to eliminate what he considered dangerous thoughts, not violent behaviors, and he claimed the showers, or even the threat of their use, could help him in this task.

Another asylum doctor, Esprit Blanche, issued a scathing response after Leuret presented his opinions to colleagues at the Société Royale de Médecine and published his findings in their minutes. Unlike Leuret, Blanche operated a private asylum, the Maison Blanche, located in Montmartre. There he practiced a form of treatment called the *vie de famille*, which assumed mental illness stemmed from a patient's domestic situation and that exposure to and participation in a bourgeois household routine would help them reclaim their rationality. Blanche, his wife, and his children stood in for the patient's actual family, having dinners and socializing together as a group.[20] He thus took the concept of familial isolation to its logical extreme, quite literally replacing the patient's real family with his own in order to separate them from the milieu that had given rise to madness. He presented himself to his patients as a figure of authority and a provider of domestic comforts, very much playing the part of a strong but benevolent patriarch.

Blanche and Leuret's disagreement arose over how, not whether, to wield power over their patients. Each embraced the moral treatment as the best method of psychiatric care, although Leuret insisted that the "energetic moral treatment," a euphemism for the cold shower, was sometimes a necessary addition. They also both described the alienist's role as rooted in fatherly authority. Blanche often referred to "paternal kindness" as an important attribute, suggesting doctors should use their moral force to influence their patients' behaviors. Leuret additionally seized on the doctor's physical authority over the patient's person as a way to educate or instill discipline, and argued that the insane were like children whose upbringing depended on the strategic deployment of physical intimidation.[21] Leuret and Blanche debated the merits and deficiencies of each form of psychiatric paternalism in their analyses of the use and abuse of the cold shower, using the language of honor in the development and defense of what they considered the ideal self-presentation for men of their profession.

The controversy over the cold shower therefore provides a snapshot of normative masculinity in flux. It likewise highlights a tension between the goals of the psychiatric profession and shifting standards of bourgeois masculinity. According to Pinel, the purpose of the moral treatment was to console and ultimately heal the mad. But doctors were equally concerned with presenting psychiatry as an honorable, and therefore independent, profession worthy of increased responsibility and influence. The law of 1838 went far in propping up this image. Nonetheless, official support had been a long time coming, and the cultural authority of psychiatry was not firmly entrenched.[22] The midcentury "doctor glut" put alienists in a particularly precarious position in the years surrounding the law's passage.[23] Asylum doctors' connection to madness also likely compromised their ability to play the ideal bourgeois professional, who was a respected member of the public sphere by virtue of his own rationality as well as his association with other rational men.[24] Indeed, references to the madness *of* psychiatrists have existed nearly as long as the profession itself. For men such as Leuret and Blanche, behaving honorably in their professional and personal interactions constituted a necessary corrective to the various liabilities associated with psychiatric labor. One way to signal their status as men of honor was through the projection of authority vis-à-vis their patients and subordinates, and all asylum doctors agreed this power should be absolute. Yet in the course of its expression, some committed acts one could easily interpret as abuse, thereby undermining the very honor they sought to project.

Leuret used the case of a patient named Theodor as an example of the efficacy of the cold shower treatment, and Blanche eventually responded with an alternate interpretation emphasizing the dishonor inherent in his rival's methods.[25] Asylum overseers admitted Theodor to Bicêtre in 1831, shortly after the revolution that had toppled the reactionary monarchy of Charles X and brought the "bourgeois" monarch Louis-Philippe to power. Leuret himself arrived about six years later, so his patient had already lived in the asylum for some time before the controversial treatment began. The alienist described Theodor as a large, robust man, formerly employed as a clerk in the Ministry of Finance, whose symptoms involved uncontrollably wailing while working in the fields attached to the institution and talking to himself while indoors. He claimed to be Louis-Philippe's nephew and the secret husband of the Duchess of Berry, assiduously recording these delusions in a set of personal notebooks, and insisted that his political enemies had orchestrated his internment.

Leuret first approached Theodor with kindness and invited the man to dine with him personally. Theodor declined, claiming he did not want to be an imposition, so Leuret set about a new plan. He took the former clerk to the showers, where the patient became visibly frightened and began to cry. Leuret put him under the faucet and turned it on for thirty seconds, stopping only when Theodor quit insisting he was related to the royal family. When Leuret later caught the man writing his delusional thoughts down instead of muttering them out loud, he snatched the notebooks and again took Theodor to the baths. There Leuret threatened Theodor with the cold shower until the subdued patient let Leuret burn the pages in front of him. The doctor subjected Theodor to the cold shower once more the following day, but afterward warmed him with a fire and gave him a hot meal. The once recalcitrant patient apparently acted grateful, polite, and said "see you tomorrow" after the meal was finished.[26] After several more fits and starts, Leuret asked his patient to renounce his delusions in writing, which Theodor agreed to do. He also wrote that he felt "as if his flesh was being snatched with pliers at all times of the day"; Leuret disregarded this sentiment in his write-up of the case.[27] At this point, the doctor declared Theodor healed and his "education complete," suggesting he considered his patient a child who simply needed to learn how to behave.[28]

Leuret could not have made the perceived link between rationality and masculine adulthood more clear. Neither was this attitude confined to the outspoken advocate of the cold shower method, for virtually all asylum doctors rhetorically equated insane men with children. So too did French legislators, a sentiment first expressed through the Civil Code of 1804 and, again, with the law of 1838. Such laws essentially stripped institutionalized people of the rights of citizenship, thereby assuring that the infantilizing assumptions held and spread by doctors were backed by the full weight of the state. Despite the horrific consequences this situation created for Theodor and others in his position, the conceptual association between childishness and insanity also suggests that doctors in the first half of the nineteenth century still viewed madness as a psychological rather than a purely somatic condition. As such, they expected patients such as Theodor to learn (or relearn) the behavioral repertoires of masculine adulthood, for children were not irrational but rather prerational beings. Leuret insisted at the end of this story that the baths indeed constituted a psychological, not a physical treatment, and that fear could function as impetus for cure.[29] In this sense Leuret proved a true descendant of Pinel himself, who argued that fear was a particularly useful "passion" with which to combat a patient's distorted emotional state.

Although Leuret claimed Theodor and other patients should not be viewed as guilty, he clearly used punishment as part of his psychological tool kit—going so far as to assert that he provided "remedy and punishment" in equal measure and that "those words are sometimes equivalent."[30] The apparent incongruousness of this perspective rested at the heart of Blanche's critique of Leuret's methods. Blanche wondered how a delusional person could comprehend the purpose of punishment to begin with, which would deter only someone in possession of rationality. Since "a mad person is a thousand times more innocent than even a child," corporal treatment such as Leuret's shower method was ineffectual, not to mention inhumane.[31] Clearly, the two doctors disagreed over how to properly enact their paternal roles. Where Leuret fashioned himself as the disciplinarian, Blanche sought to treat his innocent "children" with fatherly kindness.

Blanche and Leuret's disagreements over the proper expression of psychiatric authority revealed longstanding contradictions at the center of doctors' self-presentations that rose to the surface and became more urgent as the profession grew in size and influence. Men such as Pinel and Esquirol viewed themselves as puppet masters of sorts, and many of their actions can easily be interpreted as manipulative or even cruel. Yet *douceur*, or gentleness, was also central to their conception of the moral treatment, particularly when it came to creating personal bonds with patients and convincing them that regaining reason was both possible and desirable. Part of enacting their fatherly role involved discipline, an issue that comes up forcefully in the Blanche-Leuret debate, but most doctors additionally focused on the paternal kindnesses expressed by psychiatric professionals. For example, Pinel emphasized the "paternal oversight" taken by the directors of asylums in provisioning for basic necessities, and his son, Scipion, later insisted that the asylum director is "more than a physician, he is a consoler and a father."[32] Like Rousseau's educator, the all-knowing, all-powerful alienist would mold the child-patient in order for him to become a rational individual capable of exercising the duties of citizenship.[33]

It made sense for alienists to make use of the language of fatherhood because it allowed them to capitalize on the cultural legibility of paternal power. Medical authority was more comprehensible when couched in familiar, familial terms. It also solidified the cultural linkage of masculine adulthood with rational self-possession at a time when professional, educated men sought to supplant traditional elites as society's most powerful constituents. Yet the doctor-father persona also required constant reinforcement and renegotiation at a historical moment in which all forms of authority—political, but also familial—were in transition. Middle-class fathers, in particular, exercised power over their wives and children in a less draconian fashion during the nineteenth century than had been the case for the typical father of the Old Regime. The legal status of fathers in the postrevolutionary period likewise indicates a tempering of the most authoritarian aspects of paternal power, even though fathers remained the most privileged members of French society. The Napoleonic Civil Code had inscribed the authority of husbands, and of men more generally, by limiting women's access to divorce and property, thereby codifying the gendered division of separate spheres.[34] However, while the code granted significant legal privileges to male heads of household, it also promoted the idea that the home was a woman's domain and that mothers were most responsible for raising children.

Thus, although the legal ascendancy of fathers remained securely in place, their cultural relevance had declined and there was arguably less acceptance of despotic paternal behavior within the family than there once had been.[35] Alienists had to keep this in mind when constructing their public image if they hoped to extend their professional gains, particularly because they explicitly contrasted their methods with those of the Old Regime. Many of the first asylum doctors, à la Pinel, modeled themselves on *pères de famille* who sought love and respect from those of their households even if the realities of both family and asylum life often failed to live up to these standards. Doctors such as Pinel, and later Blanche, seemed to understand that their profession both embodied and benefited from the more sentimental, bourgeois conception of fatherhood. Leuret was on shakier ground when he relied on the behavioral repertoire of authoritarian paternalism in the 1830s and 1840s.

Blanche highlighted these incongruities in his discussion of Leuret's treatment of the patient Theodor. He critiqued Leuret and his approach from multiple angles, noting there was no proof the man had been cured by the shower treatment or even that he had been cured at all. Blanche expressed particular ire at what he viewed as Leuret's misplaced willingness to turn to drastic measures before exhausting more typical forms of the moral treatment. Any "true practitioner" would have seen in Theodor a great candidate for cure, but instead Leuret subjected "this unfortunate and interesting patient" to the baths. Even though it did not work the first time, Leuret continued to torture Theodor with an "inquisitorial" passion. [36] Leuret interpreted Theodor's eventual submission as cure, but Blanche believed the patient had simply turned inward from fear of further punishment and that his delusions would eventually manifest as dementia. Whereas Blanche saw some value in psychological intimidation, he found physical intimidation counterintuitive and cruel, indicating with his reference to the inquisition that Leuret's methods had no place in a modern society. He advised fellow alienists to "present yourself to your patients with a grave exterior, a fixed regard, and words forcefully pronounced. The patient will believe that he has obtained your support, and his attitude towards you will pass easily from fascination to confidence, from confidence to respect, and from respect to blind submission." [37] In order for this to work, however, these sentiments should be combined with esteem. Force should only be used in the most extreme and necessary of circumstances, such as when confining a violent patient with a strait jacket.

Blanche's critique of the cold shower exhibited keen awareness of the unease produced by the postrevolutionary expansion of medical authority, and he implied that the cultivation of professional honor might serve as an effective shield against potential public criticism. The private asylum doctor condemned Leuret for his willingness to embrace brutality in the name of cure and felt the cold shower was tantamount to torture: a grave injustice in and of itself. Yet it was no coincidence that Blanche published his critique at the precise moment when the psychiatric community, after much debate and legislative pressure, persuaded the government to institute a national asylum system and to codify new processes of institutionalization into law. As of 1838, asylum doctors had become the key link in the process of confinement, acting sometimes as the allies of their patients' families, but also working against their wishes at times. Blanche's mention of patients' families, "already worried," point to his belief that doctors like Leuret—who irresponsibly pushed the boundary between treatment and punishment—were a liability to the profession because families might not deem them worthy of the responsibility legislators had given them. [38]

Asylum doctors risked undoing the professional gains they had so recently made if they failed to live by Pinel's enlightened principles. Blanche described the treatment of madness through corporal punishment as a "barbarous method" and one of "a number of dangerous and illogical doctrines" for which "the honor of medicine and the interest of humanity demand justice."[39] The asylum doctor's authority should never be questioned, but Blanche worried alienists would be perceived as abusers rather than healers if they resorted to the physical intimidation of their patients.[40] Blanche's concerns would be validated as time wore on, as a number of cases of asylum abuse and unjust internment came to light and a nascent anti-alienist movement gained steam by the 1860s. Critics accused asylum doctors of simply replacing one Bastille with another and creating a new form of confinement as repressive as the prerevolutionary system had been. At least one doctor anticipated the emergence of anti-alienism by highlighting the vulnerability of his profession at what, in hindsight, would appear to be the peak of its success.

The Medical Uses of Honor

Honor proved a double-edged sword for medical men. Abiding by standards of honorable behavior safeguarded the reputation of the psychiatric profession and assured the place of individual doctors within it. Furthermore, honor bonded members of their class, gender, and occupational group by excluding women and men unable to meet the code's standards for one reason or another (often their lack of cultural, educational, or financial capital).[41] As Blanche so clearly understood, honor had the potential to ensure the power of the psychiatric profession and the social standing of its individual members, but the consequences of dishonor could also prove steep.

Honor likewise played a complicated role in the fates of male mental patients during the July Monarchy. Doctors tried to manipulate patients' feelings toward honor and shame—and their sense of self more generally—during the treatment process, a tendency that had been present from the earliest incarnations of the French psychiatric enterprise. Honor's use in the enactment of psychiatric treatment became more pronounced in the years surrounding the passage of the 1838 law on asylum commitment. Although members of the profession had good reason to concern themselves over their own reputations at this time, the significance of honor to all French men increased as the relative social immobility of the Old Regime and Restoration was replaced by something far more fluid.[42] Paying attention to honor allowed a man to signal his deservedness for social belonging and to identify his equally honorable peers.

Yet it would be a mistake to consider honor's cultural import too mechanistically. The desire among men to protect their honor was profound, and this desire held an emotional valence as much as a social or economic one. This is precisely why it was useful to practitioners of the moral treatment. If the cultural influence of honor could simultaneously ensure and threaten the status of the psychiatric profession, it likewise held the capacity to inspire madness and its cure. Psychiatric writings suggest the pressures of living up to relatively strict standards of masculine behavior contributed to the proliferation of insanity among men. At the same time, the masculine culture of honor provided asylum doctors and their patients a powerful common language on which to base their interactions. Both major participants in the cold shower debate acknowledged that the need to preserve honor and dignity influenced the behaviors of their male patients, just as it did their own. Ultimately, expectations regarding masculinity shaped and constrained doctors' professional self-presentations, but they also offered a path toward the treatment of male patients that suggests the malleability of the honor code itself.[43]

Psychiatric case studies pertinent to the cold shower debate suggest honor held a great deal of integrative potential despite its role in the perpetuation of class and gender difference. Although historians have noted honor's democratization in the postrevolutionary era, they have additionally emphasized its role in excluding those thought of as outsiders. In truth, the honor code served as a method through which all male members of the community might be incorporated into a bourgeois, liberal social order that counted self-mastery as its price of entry. At least, the ways in which asylum doctors made use of honor in the course of patient treatment implied this was the case. Practitioners of the moral treatment assumed all men—no matter their mental health status or social standing—felt shame over a wounded sense of self or a damaged reputation. Doctors thus drew on the threat of shame and the desire to restore honor in order to bring male patients back to rationality.

Pinel himself argued that the maintenance of a patient's self-respect was essential to the successful implementation of the moral treatment. In his writings on madness during the French Revolution, he related the story of a man who had lost his fortune, became depressed, and eventually came to insist he was an Austrian general. Several decades later, Leuret would have considered the cold shower perfect for this type of patient and, in fact, a provincial asylum director did subject the man to the treatment in an attempt to force him to renounce his false identity before sending him to Pinel's facility. Pinel claimed the patient's "fury had redoubled" when he approached the showers because he perceived the treatment as unbefitting the "respect due his rank."[44] Conforming to what would become a familiar pattern in case studies involving men and the moral treatment, Pinel interpreted the man's reaction as proof that the *faux* general considered the cold shower a personal affront—that he perceived the "bath" as an insult to his dignity. The method entailed violence, to be sure, but to Pinel this was almost beside the point. The accompanying sting of disrespect made it ineffective and therefore unsuitable. Pinel took the man under his observation, ceased the cold shower treatment, and released the patient several months later.

As a man preoccupied with the construction and maintenance of psychiatry's professional honor, it should come as little surprise that Blanche was also attuned to the ways a patient's sense of honor could affect the success of the moral treatment. Like Pinel and Esquirol, the private asylum doctor insisted that each patient possessed specific personality traits irrespective of their mental state and that these characteristics could be useful when devising treatment regimens. It was a "fatal error," argued Blanche, to "see maniacs as incapable of holding sentiments other than those that suggest to them the habitual form of their delirium."[45] Doctors should study patients as unique individuals in order to understand their personalities, their tastes, and their "dominant sentiments." Ignoring these fundamental aspects of a patient's character—like the proud temperament of the aforementioned "general"—would "slow the process of the moral treatment while leading [doctors] to employ physical rigueur to achieve what could be obtained through more gentle means without pain."[46] Rather than resort to physical intimidation, he sought to return patients to a state of rationality through less forceful forms of manipulation. Paying close attention to each patient's idiosyncrasies allowed doctors to devise a cure before resorting to the violent methods that could bring dishonor to the profession and to their male patients.

Blanche defended his assertions through the presentation of several case histories, a typical strategy in nineteenth-century psychiatric treatises and journal articles.[47] The case history explained the patient's unique challenges and highlighted the doctor's chosen treatment, which in the first half of the nineteenth century involved a surprising level of individualization. Neither Blanche nor Leuret promoted a "one size fits all" approach even if they believed particular strategies could be useful in every situation. In this they were truly the heirs of Pinel and Esquirol, both of whom published myriad case histories highlighting the various pressures and dissimulations that might encourage a particular patient to regain his or her sanity. The specifics of the treatment depended on the contours of the patient's mental alienation and life history, including their emotional predispositions.

Always told from the doctor's perspective and sometimes long after the treatment itself took place, the case history is an incomplete and undeniably biased record of events. Still, the genre reveals much about how alienists envisioned their roles and how they might best articulate medical authority. Case histories are also remarkable in that they reveal the cultural values asylum doctors believed held sway in the minds of those they labeled insane. When Blanche closely observed the personality traits of his patients in order to determine the best curative strategy, he sought to use the cultural legibility of certain codes of conduct to his advantage, especially the relevance of honor to masculine self-perception.

Blanche found that even men in the midst of a mental breakdown retained the desire to uphold their honor, a fact he exploited in the name of rehabilitation when given the chance. A young male patient, described by the asylum's proprietor as consumed by shame, arrived at the Maison Blanche in 1832. He possessed a "vain character, but a superior intelligence and a distinguished education."[48] After losing much of his fortune in a failed industrial enterprise and feeling betrayed by those around him, he "fell into a state of melancholy that soon degenerated into a furious delirium, with a tendency towards suicide, which he attempted twice."[49] Blanche insisted the man's insanity was brought about not just by sadness or regret, but also through the "shame, especially, of knowing his name was compromised."[50] Before arriving at the Maison Blanche, the young industrialist had been housed in another asylum where he was subjected to the cold shower treatment and other "rigorous bodily repressions" following a furious episode. These treatments had done nothing but aggravate the man's symptoms, and Blanche decided to try a tactic more suited to the personality of this particular patient once he took over.

Because the patient already felt his honor compromised, Blanche wanted to avoid discouraging him further. The alienist immediately attempted to earn the young man's trust and assigned two servants to accompany him, "charged to exercise over him the most active surveillance, but to be free of all actions that might cause humiliation." By treating his patient with respect and by avoiding counterintuitive and humiliating forms of treatment, Blanche eventually earned his confidence and the man regained his reason. Blanche's knowledge of the patient's history and of his intense feelings of shame allowed the doctor to craft a method of treatment particularly suited to his needs. In this instance, the alienist used established gender assumptions to his and his patient's advantage.[51] Although the young man's self-worth was perhaps overly dependent upon the perceptions of others, his faith in the reestablishment of his personal honor eventually allowed him to exit the asylum and resume his life, according to Blanche.

Honor thus played a contradictory role in the life of this patient and, indeed, in the lives of all French men. It provided reassurance that interactions between them would be dictated through a supposedly logical and universally under-stood set of values rather than by chance or temperamental idiosyncrasies. At the same time, the pressure to defend one's honor amplified the stresses involved in navigating postrevolutionary social life, thereby bringing inner emotions up to the surface, sometimes in a form deemed pathological. Although adherence to the honor code required prioritizing rationality over emotion, shame—honor's counterpart—was undeniably a feeling, one to which middle-class men seemed especially (but not exclusively) attuned. In fact, the exacting standards of hon-orable behavior among the professional class in particular ensured that the po-tential for emotional distress inevitably bubbled beneath the cool, collected, and rational façade of the ideal Frenchman. Doctors recognized honor's emotional intensity, even if they did not all conceive of honor as a "passion" per se. Not only shame, but also pride, vanity, and fear could seamlessly transform into madness when men considered their honor—and thus their livelihoods—at stake.

It made sense for adherents of the moral treatment to focus on the curative potential of the honor code because of its omnipresence in the French cultural imagination. It represented a shorthand of sorts that was immediately legible to patients, doctors, and families alike. Thus, in addition to considering the emotional resonance of shame as a source of insanity, alienists also attempted to convince their more resistant patients to submit to treatment by appealing to a shared understanding of honorable behavior. For example, Blanche described a man treated by a colleague, one Doctor L. of Montpellier, the "maniac son of a former general, a young man of excessive pride and a fiery, irascible character."[52] Doctor L. decided bloodletting was a necessary course of action and notified his patient that it would occur the following day. The general's son, however, refused to submit. According to Blanche, "the doctor knew from experience that one concession in this circumstance would destroy the ascendance that [Doctor L.] had over [the patient], without which it would be impossible to put the brakes on his bizarre tastes and disorderly passions."[53] At a predetermined hour, the doctor entered the patient's room and had his employees restrain him completely.

But rather than letting the patient's blood without his consent, Doctor L. forcefully asserted his medical authority and called upon the young man's sense of honor instead. As the two guards physically subdued the patient, the doctor explained, "You see . . . that in all things I am the master . . . but you are a man of honor; give me your word that tomorrow you will not put up any opposition, and these two men will leave at this very instant."[54] The young man—"flattered by the appeal to his honor"—gave Doctor L. his word that he would submit to the procedure, which he did the following morning.[55] Blanche cited this case as evidence that corporal methods such as the cold shower were unnecessary and counterproductive. He implied Doctor L. had successfully navigated the tense relationship between personal honor and medical authority by appealing to the patient's attachment to his own honorable character, sentiments that existed independent of his mental alienation. Whereas Leuret dishonored the profession by actually committing acts of violence against his patients, Doctor L. supposedly maintained his authority and honor alike by merely threatening the general's son with physical harm.

Although Blanche criticized Leuret for dishonoring psychiatry, Leuret's actions often mirrored the very behaviors that Blanche celebrated in the case of Doctor. L. of Montpellier. Like Blanche, Leuret sought to craft an individualized treatment regimen for each patient, one that drew on shared conceptions of honorable and shameful behavior in men. The first case described by Leuret in his 1838 defense of the shower treatment involved manipulating a patient's concern over his reputation. He tells us that a twenty-six-year-old traveling hat seller named Vincent entered Bicêtre in February 1838 exhibiting signs of delusion. Vincent insisted he was sane but that numerous dark forces had recently conspired against him. According to the young peddler, he had many dangerous enemies. The people he lived with supposedly piled boxes on the stairs to make him trip and, even more menacingly, engineered a latrine pipe (an "infernal machine") that would spit fire when Vincent entered the bathroom.[56] Eventually Vincent took his various complaints to the police. They promptly sent him to the asylum.

Leuret listened attentively as Vincent told his life history and tried to convince the doctor he was not delusional, but rather persecuted by those around him. "He explained to me all these things," wrote Leuret, ". . . to justify the complaints he brought to the police and to demonstrate the culpability of his enemies."[57] Following Vincent's long explanation, Leuret turned toward several of his students accompanying him on his rounds and said, "Look here, sirs, it's one of those terrible types that the police send to us from time to time; a vagabond who counts on finding food here without being obliged to work for it."[58] Leuret made it clear to Vincent that he did not find him insane in the least and sent him to work in the fields. The following day, the doctor informed Vincent in a "cruel, mocking tone" that he would need to write a letter to his parents, asking them to come to the asylum and reclaim their son because "I did not want him to stay in a hospice where we receive only honest people."[59]

Up until this point, Leuret's approach toward Vincent's treatment had much in common with the methods of care promoted by Blanche. Leuret had set up an elaborate, personalized bit of theater meant to convince Vincent to disavow his delusions. The doctor refused to acknowledge the patient's ramblings at all, calling him a liar rather than a madman. Leuret counted on the likelihood that Vincent's desire to be perceived as an "honest" man was stronger than his emotional attachment to his hallucinations. The plan assumed the traveling salesman would feel no shame in being called insane, but that calling him a charlatan would prove unbearable. When Vincent refused to write the letter to his family, Leuret subjected him to the cold shower and demanded the patient "obey him" and explain his life story in rational terms. If Vincent's descriptions were not "perfectly reasonable," the doctor would "continue the shower as threatened, and would do so in this way each day" thereafter.[60] Within a month Vincent had stopped insisting upon the truth of his previous statements. Leuret and his attendants carried on the charade that Vincent was a liar, not a madman, throughout his time at Bicêtre.

According to Leuret, "I wanted to turn his attentions away from his delirious ideas, and let him believe that if he insisted upon his assertions, I would take him for a scoundrel." The charge of *friponnerie* served as "a happy mental diversion" that forced Vincent to focus his attentions on restoring his reputation instead of convincing his doctors that his delusions were true.[61] Leuret's accusations gravely wounded Vincent and he regained his reason in order to prove that "in reality, he was an honest man."[62] For Leuret, the threat and the actual use of the cold shower constituted forms of distraction, methods to convince an "indocile" patient to play his proper role in a treatment scenario centered on shared understandings of proper masculine comportment. Vincent's "cure" resulted from Leuret's manipulation of culturally dominant conceptions of masculinity combined with a violent projection of medical power.

The story of Vincent the hat seller begs the question: if the culture of honor held the potential to reincorporate those considered insane back into French society, did it do so for men of all class backgrounds, or merely the well-to-do? Blanche's patients were exclusively members of the elite, people whose families could afford to pay a premium for private care. His clientele consisted of intellectuals, professionals, and even wealthy aristocrats. Conversely, Leuret worked at the largest public institution in Paris dedicated to the psychiatric treatment of men.[63] Although a number of his patients were members of the middle classes who found their financial status on the decline for one reason or another, others—such as Vincent—belonged undeniably to the lower rungs of the social ladder. Vincent's experience at Bicêtre suggests Leuret considered working men just as sensitive to attacks on their sense of self as their upper- and middle-class counterparts and that the emotional valence of shame could be used productively in such cases.

Leuret nevertheless indicated there might be a limit to the applicability of these strategies to the treatment of non-elite men. This qualification is apparent in another case history presented in defense of the cold shower method, one in which he attempted to start a "quarrel" with a long-institutionalized man in the name of cure.[64] The patient was a frustrated middle-aged son of a baker who had exhibited signs of madness for about nineteen years. According to Leuret, he possessed a "lively and strong" sense of vanity, which led him to believe he was marshal of the French army and Napoleon's close relation.[65] Upon meeting the patient, Leuret manipulated his supposedly inflated ego and coaxed him into sharing his life history with "caressing and flattering words," slowly gaining the man's trust and waiting for the opportunity to confront his delusional ideas head-on. Leuret treated his patient with kindness and respect until he began relating his hallucinations, at which point the alienist threatened him with physical violence unless he renounced his claims.[66] The baker's son refused, and Leuret's assistants physically overpowered him. They restrained him and then subjected him to a forceful spray of cold water to the face. About to spray the patient again, Leuret explained "I want . . . to spare you the humiliation of the shower, of this punishment I inflict only on bad men, to liars and evil sorts. You, honest boy, good worker, will you expose yourself to this?"[67] The threat of further humiliation and pain eventually led the patient to disavow his beliefs. He even began to work in the asylum's bakery before gaining release, explaining to Leuret that "when he was idle, his head fluttered here and there (*papillonait*) . . . now that he had an occupation, that no longer happened, and he believed himself completely healed."[68]

Leuret's interactions with Napoleon's false relation represented an almost textbook performance of the moral treatment. Leuret first attempted to bolster his own credibility and inspire affection, molding his behavior in such a way as to anticipate his patient's reactions. Once he gained the patient's respect, he used the threat of violence and humiliation to coerce him into disowning his delusional beliefs. Underlying these various machinations was the doctor's assumption that certain codes of conduct were culturally legible even to the mad. By appealing to his patient's sense of respectability—calling him an "honest boy, a good worker"—and presenting himself as both authoritative and well-meaning, Leuret showed a rather nuanced understanding of the performative dimensions of both gender and profession, not to mention medical treatment.

Notably, Leuret never used the word "honor" in his description of this case, and the level of infantilization (literally calling the man a "boy") is striking. Instead, the doctor focused on his patient's desire to appear "honest" and considered the man's willing return to labor as proof of cure. In this way Leuret exposed the possible shortcomings of the honor code—not to mention the moral treatment—as a means of social inclusion by suggesting that the precise contours of this patient's restored reputation were quite distinct from his bourgeois counterparts'. Although this might indicate that Leuret considered lower-class men incapable of expressing honor, this interpretation is belied somewhat by the doctor's emphasis on the threat of shame, which he assumed a mad son of bread maker could feel as acutely as a bourgeois professional such as himself. Then again, Leuret too was a bread maker's son, which might explain his willingness to see such a patient as responsive to the same emotional cues as those of Blanche's more elite clientele.

As the case histories of the cold shower debate show, alienists persistently defined sanity in men as the ability to conform to masculine norms associated with the bourgeoisie. But they also implied that all men—those considered irrational, even if they were lower-class—were capable of responding to honor- and shame-based treatment scenarios. Asylum doctors' understanding of the behaviors and motivations of their male patients therefore undermined bourgeois class distinction in the very process of upholding its gender dimensions as the benchmark for sanity.

Concluding the Controversy

The outcome of the cold shower debate proved somewhat ambiguous, but medical opinion largely sided with the critic Blanche. Leuret still succeeded in promoting his methods to a wide audience; he remained a respected member of the medical community and published continuously until his death some ten years later. Leuret's mentor Esquirol—in a report co-presented with fellow asylum doctor Étienne Pariset—also defended him in print, describing the treatment process in heroic and dramatic terms. The mentally ill patient in the process of recovery at Bicêtre was like "a warship beaten in a tempest, piloted by an experienced captain who, by tossing baggage into the sea, returned [the ship] to port without ballast, but healthy and safe, and ready to leave on a happier voyage."[69] According to the report, Leuret was a uniquely experienced practitioner who could be trusted to carry out the treatment responsibly and only in the appropriate cases. He "deployed all the wisdom, perseverance, and mental resources imaginable," and his patients were the better for it.[70]

Esquirol and Pariset nonetheless remained cognizant of the dangers posed by the cold shower. While unwilling to criticize Leuret's actions directly, they conceded that the controversial treatment should be avoided by less skilled asylum doctors. The pair warned against adopting any system of care based on physical intimidation: "Badly understood by your auxiliaries and your students, this rigueur soon degenerates into barbarism. Violence escapes, and from that moment on, all connections are broken, and for the rebellious patient you become an object of distaste, aversion, and sometimes vengeance."[71] The incorporation of violence into the treatment process obviously contradicted Pinel's teachings and the overarching goals of the profession. Furthermore, Leuret's writings had "made a great commotion in the medical world."[72] Esquirol, as psychiatry's greatest spokesman, could hardly risk outright promotion of tactics that might tarnish the reputation of the profession. He therefore gave his seal of approval to the gentler methods promoted by Blanche while still publicly proclaiming his admiration for his close friend and protégé Leuret. Moreover, upon his death, Leuret's obituaries alluded to the high degree of criticism he faced for his promotion of the cold shower during his lifetime.[73]

Despite all this talk about the public image of the profession, the cold shower treatment generated little outrage beyond the medical community, and the few outside observers who commented at all tended to side with its proponent. In 1841, Leuret published yet another defense of his methods, this time in a substantial tome reviewed by various nonmedical publications. In this book, *Du Traitement moral de la folie*, Leuret focused on the merits of the moral treatment in general and the utility of the cold shower in particular cases. He painted his adversaries as stubborn somaticists, complaining that they disagreed with his tactics because they considered mental illness a physical condition, whereas he, like Pinel, believed madness was psychological. He argued that the elaborate treatment scenarios concocted by doctors during the moral treatment, including those that made use of the cold shower, addressed the mental bases of insanity and thus represented the best hope for cure.

This position proved convincing to the reviewers at the *Journal des débats* and *La Revue indépendante*, who described with admiration Leuret's commitment to his ideals despite the criticisms his peers. One review, signed A. Donné, claimed the cold shower posed a negligible risk to patients—after all, it only lasted a few seconds, and Doctor Leuret had even subjected himself and his students to the procedure, just in case.[74] Widespread attacks on the asylum system would eventually emerge over claims of patient abuse and unjust institutionalization, but this was less common during Leuret's lifetime, when alienists themselves proved the greatest proponents of asylum reform. If anything, reviewers suggested there was a certain honor in Leuret's consistent willingness to stand up for his anti-somaticist conception of insanity without regard to the professional consequences.

The historian Ian Dowbiggin likewise focuses on Leuret's psychological approach to patient treatment in his book about the professionalization of French psychiatry. He argues that Leuret's detractors sought to legitimize psychiatry by insisting on the physical origins of madness, thereby implying that only medical specialists such as themselves—as opposed to lay healers or clergy—could cure mental illness. The controversy Leuret aroused in the late 1830s and early 1840s therefore indicated that the psychiatric community had begun to reject the moral treatment in favor of pursuing chemical or surgical options instead.

The rise of a somatic interpretation of insanity did contribute to the professionalization of French psychiatry, and to critiques of Leuret in particular, but this was far from the only factor at play in the disagreement over the cold shower. For one, even alienists with the most overtly materialist interpretations of mental pathology—men such as Georget and Voisin—considered cultural attributes related to gender and class in their discussions of diagnosis and treatment during the first half of the nineteenth century. Furthermore, Esquirol, someone heavily influenced by Pinel's formulation of the moral treatment and the concomitant belief in the mental bases of insanity, criticized the cold shower for reasons that had nothing to do with whether madness constituted a mental or physical affliction. Finally, the critic Blanche practiced a variation of the moral treatment in his own institution even if he also made use of physical treatments such as purgatives and bloodletting.

Thus, although Leuret's medical theories might have undermined the purported uniqueness of psychiatric knowledge, the general condemnation of what one writer called the "cruel shower" represented more than a convenient tactic with which to silence a professional rival.[75] For Leuret's colleagues, friend and foe alike, the stain of dishonor was just as dangerous as the implication that the cure for insanity might not require an alienist at all. Honor represented an essential precondition to the consolidation and extension of professional independence, a goal shared by those who advanced a materialist conception of mental alienation and those who did not.

The cold shower debate undoubtedly shows how the performance of the moral treatment—especially the "energetic" version promoted by Leuret—complicated the cultivation of this honorable image. A doctor giving medication did not risk the appearance of abusiveness in the same way as did Leuret and his subordinates at Bicêtre, whose methods depended on the inculcation of emotional and sometimes physical distress. Furthermore, a somatic approach to mental illness did not require taking the patient's personality into account when devising treatment strategies, thereby avoiding the complex doctor-patient interactions that sometimes turned the treatment process into a battle of wills.

On first glance, the threat of dishonor seems not to have bothered Leuret as it did his colleague and rival because he never mentioned the negative effects the cold shower might have on his own reputation. But the director of Bicêtre did express concern over maintaining his honor. He simply did not see any contradiction between the violent expression of psychiatric authority and his ability to do so. Rather, for Leuret, coming across as weak was more damaging than dominating his patients to a potentially excessive degree. This fact supports a point made by Christopher Forth in his survey of masculinity in the modern West: "The changes generated by modernity and modernization processes have always been attended by resistance and ambiguity, not least because they threaten traditional institutions and habits while displacing people who are unable or unwilling to adapt."[76] I would add that even quintessentially modern institutions like the early asylum featured such ambiguities, and not only because they served to constrain the primal urges of men who worked and lived within them, thereby punishing those who could or would not change. Indeed, it was possible for men to embrace traditional elements of masculinity for intrinsically modern purposes. This was the case for Leuret, who championed the violent expression of medical power in a way that actually supported the democratization of honor.

A brief analysis of Leuret's conception of his own honor will elucidate this point. After Blanche first criticized Leuret's original treatise on the shower method, he felt the need to defend himself in print. He insisted that the physical risks, the various practical difficulties involved, and the patient's terror were all justified because of the method's curative possibilities. However, despite this sustained emphasis on the patient's potential for recovery, Leuret also highlighted the effects of his actions on his own image. In the most revealing example of this preoccupation, Leuret described his reaction to "untamable" madmen: "If the patient is too obstinate . . . because the moment of direction or the form of treatment was not well-chosen . . . I will interrupt the duration of the shower, without letting (the patient) believe that I am giving in, but instead saying that I don't want to waste my time or fatigue myself caring for someone who does not dignify my time."[77] Through this bit of deception, Leuret made it possible to try the shower treatment again or carry out some other method at a later date without having encouraged the patient's "... obstinacy through the memory of a first success."[78] Perhaps more important, Leuret had not admitted "his defeat." Therefore, his "honor is safe."[79]

In spite of his violent methods, this example indicates that Leuret's interactions with male patients proved remarkably consistent with the universalizing impulses of the moral treatment. The private asylum director Blanche mainly concerned himself with the medical utility of patients' feelings toward honor and the impact of negative press. Leuret additionally perceived each doctor-patient interaction as a crucial moment in the maintenance of his own personal honor. The elaboration of an honorable professional persona depended on his own actions, but it also depended on the reactions of those he sought to remold. Like his colleagues who judged the honor of the cold shower method via Leuret's public writings and speeches, his patients also had the authority to determine whether Leuret deserved to call himself an honorable man. He thereby acknowledged that mental patients, like their rational male counterparts outside asylum walls, participated in the continual give-and-take that constituted the mutual elaboration of the honor code. In other words, Leuret behaved as if patient treatment was a site of masculine contestation, proving that he thought of his male patients as *men* rather than simply as *mad*. Unfortunately, although he might have preferred to gain his patients' respect through more peaceable means, fear served as an adequate substitute.

A MAN'S INABILITY to control his behavior in a fashion deemed honorable represented straightforward evidence of insanity by the 1830s. Deficit in this regard brought shame not only to the patient, but to his family as well (which, much like an emergent profession, could be tarnished through its association with dishonorable individuals). Families of "madmen" sought to intern them in private rather than public institutions whenever possible because secrecy safeguarded their relatives' already embattled social status and protected the honor of the family as a whole. Nonetheless, mid-nineteenth-century asylum doctors did not assume a man's dishonor to be permanent. Throughout the debate over the cold shower, both Blanche and Leuret acknowledged that any man would desire his honor to be restored and used this assumption when trying to persuade patients to behave rationally. Although families might have felt shame over their loved ones' irrational behaviors, shame itself offered a path toward sanity's return, and therefore the return of once-compromised honor. With a circular logic, honor had come to function as a proxy for rationality and thus, for manliness itself.

The history of the cold shower indicates this particular gender formulation structured and mediated intra-psychiatric disputes that arose along the path toward professionalization. Alienists such as Blanche constructed their professional identities through gender, modeling asylums on the familial relations practiced within the *maison bourgeoise* and using "paternal kindness" to instill obedience in patients. They suggested that their behavior *as men* made them modern and therefore worthy of trust, because the type of man they were said something about the treatment they would give. Leuret likewise tied his professional role to his manliness, suggesting that the perpetuation of psychiatric power relied on the strength of will and the threat of force.

Although these two representatives of the profession had different ideas as to what constituted appropriate behavior, each doctor's gender performance entailed attempting to navigate the honor code. Doing so successfully would prove psychiatry worthy of public influence and authority, but required the skillful manipulation of a gender ideology that remained unsettled. Honor itself transformed at this time by adapting to values more representative of the middle classes than to those of the aristocracy. Conflicts within psychiatry reflected and increasingly played a part in this process—as evidenced by the widespread acceptance of Blanche's definition of honor and the general condemnation of Leuret's among members of the profession.

In certain respects, the spread of new masculine values proved a boon for alienists. Even in the midst of controversy and uncertainty, all asylum doctors benefited from the development of cultural associations between honor and sanity, for such men literally defined the meaning of madness and presented themselves as the guardians of rationality writ large. As of 1838, the gender assumptions undergirding psychiatric medicine not only informed the cultural expectations that delimited participation in the public sphere, but they provided the legal definition of citizenship as well. Yet despite all this, doctors exposed the fiction of innate masculine rationality in the very act of naturalizing it and promulgating it as a gender ideal. Time and time again, alienists like Leuret and Blanche bore witness to the inability of many French men—worker and bourgeois alike—to live up to the postrevolutionary definition of what it meant to be a man. Perhaps more surprisingly, psychiatric attitudes and practices concerning feminine domesticity also posed a challenge to bourgeois notions of class and gender difference.

CHAPTER 3

Domesticating Madness in the Family Asylum

P UBLISHED IN 1866, DR. Alexandre Brierre de Boismont's *De l'Utilité de la vie de famille dans le traitement de l'aliénation mentale* immediately set a unique tone among psychiatric writings by featuring a photograph of the author's wife on the book's first page. The doctor dedicated the work to his "dear companion" of many years, to whom he believed he owed both his domestic happiness and his professional success.[1] Little is known of Athalie Brierre de Boismont (née Maillard) beyond what her husband and, later, her daughter wrote about her role in the family business.[2] She was born in Paris, where she reportedly met her husband in 1825; although it is not certain, she seems to have come from a humbler background than Dr. Brierre de Boismont, as his father supposedly cut him off financially because of his decision to marry her.[3]

This choice eventually served the young doctor well, for he insisted that he was able to publish extensively on various forms of mental alienation only because of his wife's talent for medical observation ("daily and long-term") and their many fruitful discussions.[4] He was grateful for the role she played throughout his long career and argued that their institution could scarcely function without her, writing that private asylum care only succeeded "with the help of a wife capable of supporting a heavy load."[5] The couple would eventually raise a daughter, Marie Rivet (née Brierre de Boismont), who operated a similar institution of her own. Both Rivet and her father published extensively on the workings of their asylums. In the process, they shed light on the contradictory relationship between gender, the family, and the psychiatric profession that had emerged by midcentury. Women like Rivet and her mother simultaneously upheld and undermined prevailing notions about domesticity and femininity, insisting on the curative value of bourgeois family values while choosing not to embody those values themselves. Their life histories shed light on the gender dimensions of the moral treatment from a novel perspective—that of women practitioners rather than women patients.

Public asylums offered few opportunities for women to take on authoritative positions before medical schools began to accept women students in the 1860s, and even then women were not allowed to take the exams required of hospital interns. Private asylums, on the other hand, regularly featured the involvement of women, not only in subordinate roles as maids or guards—as was the case in public facilities with female patient populations—but as *directices* as well. In particular, institutions like those of the Brierre de Boismonts, in which patients lived alongside the doctor and his family, provided women with the chance to take on unexpectedly prominent roles in the treatment of both male and female patients. As we have already seen, doctors' theories regarding women and madness perpetuated widespread cultural associations between femininity and irrationality, and their diagnoses of women patients often pathologized the behaviors of those who did not conform to the tenets of bourgeois domesticity. At the same time, psychiatric attitudes toward femininity also empowered elite women working in private institutions. Such women served as exemplars of ideal womanhood while laying bare the artificiality of a gender construct that insisted on women's irrational nature. Their interactions with patients often showed that the cultural elevation of masculine self-control as gender ideal had the potential to shift power dynamics in women's favor under certain circumstances.

Histories of the psychiatric profession rarely mention these *directrices*, in large part owing to the scholarly emphasis placed on public, as opposed to private, asylum psychiatry.[6] A bourgeois woman's lack of a formal education in mental medicine would have blocked her employment at a public institution, and even if it had been possible it would have compromised her reputation. Neither of these barriers existed in the case of private *maisons de santé*, for although men owned most private institutions, their wives also took part in the day-to-day administration.[7] Women even directed some private asylums on their own, always with a male doctor serving as the *médecin attaché à l'asile*. These facts have received little historical attention owing to a paucity of source material and the much larger scale of public asylum operations. Still, their presence reveals certain possibilities for feminine self-fashioning that existed within the legal and cultural constraints imposed by French family law and middle-class gender ideology.

On the surface, psychiatry's relationship to femininity appears far less problematic than its relationship to masculinity, in large measure because of the comparative stability of the feminine ideal versus the masculine one. While alienists tended to support a benevolent yet authoritative expression of masculinity that they associated with rationality and self-possession, French men never fully rejected more aggressive iterations of masculine comportment (as evidenced by the public support expressed for the controversial proponent of the cold shower, Leuret). Conversely, the bourgeois values of domestic motherhood and feminine virtue were embraced much more readily as a means of class and sex differentiation—certainly among men, but also among many women. Yet like the deployment of masculine honor in the context of doctor-patient interactions, psychiatric conceptions of ideal femininity and its use in the course of patient treatment reveal the fragility of nineteenth-century understandings of both gender and reason. Far from assuring the naturalness of woman's subordination based on her inherent lack of rational capacity, the practice of private asylum psychiatry suggested that rational women might be the most suitable overseers of irrational men. This contradiction was not enough to overturn the inequities of the French legal code as they pertained to women, of course, and numerous women patients suffered because of the persistent assumption they belonged to the less rational sex. It did, however, open the door for certain women to take on authoritative roles within the psychiatric community itself, thereby undermining the class-based notions of gender and family life that even women asylum directors claimed to support.

The family history of the Brierre de Boismonts is an ideal prism through which to view the unexpected uses of bourgeois femininity in the nineteenth-century asylum, especially because they opened their first institution in the 1830s and their last did not change hands until at least 1888. Most of the source material related to the inner workings of the Brierre de Boismont asylums comes from members of the family. While their descriptions should be evaluated with some skepticism, they also provide invaluable insight into each author's contribution to the creation of a family myth. Indeed, their writings reveal the face of private psychiatry they wanted the world to see, allowing us entrée into what can best be described as a multilayered performance of domestic life, one that took place both on the page and within asylum walls.

Domesticity and the "vie de famille"

Most operators of private asylums left behind little published or archival material. However, some private asylum directors shared educational and professional ties with those working in the public sector and thus were more likely to have left a written record, as was the case for Dr. Brierre de Boismont. As a young man he moved from Rouen to Paris in 1821, where he earned his doctorate in medicine in 1825 and attached himself to the intellectual circle surrounding the famed asylum doctor Jean-Étienne-Dominique Esquirol. His career in mental medicine began as the physician for a private institution in Sainte-Colombe; after failing to secure a position in a public institution, he moved permanently into private asylum psychiatry in the mid-1830s. An outspoken Catholic and spiritualist, Dr. Brierre de Boismont became well-known for his work on such topics as hallucinations, suicide, and the construction of model asylums.[8] He served as president of the Société Médico-Psychologiques and was a prodigious contributor to the preeminent French journal dedicated to psychiatric science, the *Annales médico-psychologiques*.[9]

As the owner of an elite institution that utilized the *vie de famille* method, Dr. Brierre de Boismont relied on his wife and children to an extent that would have been unrecognizable to his colleagues operating public asylums. He incorporated patients into the household routine and members of his family likewise took part in the treatment process. Other asylums divided patients into numerous sections strictly segregated by sex and by the form and perceived degree of mental alienation, whereas Dr. Brierre de Boismont removed physical barriers between individuals and encouraged them to live as a family of sorts. As he explained, his asylum avoided the "appearance of a cloister" and was instead "closer to the bourgeois home."[10]

Over the course of his career Dr. Brierre de Boismont operated two such institutions, one located in the Parisian quarter of the Panthéon and the other in the Faubourg Saint-Antoine. The only surviving promotional pamphlet derives from the earlier phase of his career at the Panthéon facility, which his family founded in the mid-1830s after Dr. Brierre de Boismont had gained considerable experience working in asylums owned by others. Several elements of the advertisement made it clear that they geared the institution toward an elite clientele. The asylum offered a number of amenities, including a prime location in one of the most healthful parts of the city, a lush garden shaded by beautiful trees, well-heated conversation and game rooms, bathing facilities, and abundant high quality food.[11] Only someone from a family of means would be able to afford a stay in this *maison de santé*, although its proprietor carefully noted that the price—never mentioned explicitly—was a bargain for the level of treatment provided. If it were not already clear that Dr. Brierre de Boismont intended his institution for wealthy patients alone, the inclusion of a list of necessary items to be provisioned by each patient's family also assured that they came from an elevated social class. Few working-class men, for example, owned three sheets, six shirts, six handkerchiefs, two neckties, three pairs of socks, six napkins, two pairs of shoes, and a hat.[12] A contemporary account mentioned that Dr. Brierre de Boismont charged from 800–1200 francs per year per patient.[13]

The privacy afforded within *maisons de santé* appealed to many wealthy families who sought to discreetly commit relatives. Source materials related to such settings are exceedingly rare, however, and it is impossible to determine how many private asylum directors promoted any particular form of treatment. According to a report by the Inspectors-General Constans, Lunier, and Dumesnil, there were twenty-five private institutions in France dedicated exclusively to the treatment of insanity in 1874 with 1,632 patients in total; roughly half of these facilities were located in Paris or its environs.[14] Numerous editions of the *Annuaire Statistique de la France* confirm these figures, which remained static until at least the turn of the century, when the *Annuaire* stopped recording the names and locations of each individual asylum. It is more difficult to obtain information for earlier in the century, but the 1842 edition of the *Almanach Bottin* mentioned fourteen private asylums in Paris and the 1862 volume listed eleven.[15] Of these, at least four promoted methods related to family life. Two belonged to the Brierre de Boismonts and two to the Blanche family, whose example had initially inspired the Brierre de Boismonts to open their first family life facility.[16] It is likely that these four *maisons de santé* had some influence on the rest because of the elevated professional status enjoyed by their operators. The fact that *veuves*, or widows, owned several of the institutions listed in the almanacs further indicates that it was not uncommon for private asylums to be run as family businesses.

This put the gender dynamics of such institutions at odds with those typical of many nineteenth-century work and living spaces, precisely because men and women simultaneously lived *and* worked within them. Because Dr. Brierre de Boismont sold an explicitly domestic vision of psychiatric treatment, it was in his financial interest to highlight how the family life method replicated the gender values of the French middle classes by presenting Athalie Brierre de Boismont as a bourgeois matron *par excellence*. Promotional material for the asylum advertised her contributions, noting, "the interior administration is entrusted to Madame Brierre de Boismont, who presides over all the details, and lavishes the most attentive care on the patients of her sex."[17] Like other married women of her class, the doctor's wife supervised servants, cared for children, kept up her personal appearance and that of the home's interior, and frequently entertained guests.[18] Perhaps more surprising, she also hosted a salon attended by nonviolent patients of both sexes.[19] Her daughter, Marie Rivet, described the salon with admiration in her only published work, explaining, "Although the conversations made there were quite disconnected, this simulation of a salon sweetened for some [of the patients] their sequestration."[20] The foyer fit approximately thirty closely supervised individuals whose "confusion of discourse" reminded the young Rivet of the Tower of Babel.[21] The family nonetheless considered participation in this salon an opportunity for patients to experience the sociability of domestic life, which, according to Dr. Brierre de Boismont, was the key to their eventual recovery.[22]

Athalie Brierre de Boismont's performance of her wifely duties was thus essential to the mode of treatment carried out in the asylum-home. At the same time, the very act of monetary exchange situated the institution in the public realm of market competition rather than the supposedly private and enclosed domain of the family. By focusing so heavily on the participation of Athalie Brierre de Boismont, her husband revealed the extent to which the gender roles enacted within his own household differed from those familiar to most other bourgeois families. In the midst of the political turmoil and economic upheaval characteristic of postrevolutionary France, the middle classes situated the home as a refuge from the public world of politics, commerce, and, in time, the various social problems associated with industrialization. Women sought to organize the household so as to rehabilitate their husbands' sense of calm after long days at work and to prepare their (male) children to embark on careers and to fulfill the duties of citizenship. Moreover, as a symbol of her husband's wealth and respectability, the wife played a vital role in establishing and maintaining her family's reputation. She accomplished this in great measure by removing herself from the labor market. Indeed, if a wife needed to work, her family could scarcely consider itself bourgeois or middle class at all. The elevation of this domestic model and a decline in women's participation in family-run firms occurred at the same time.[23] The Civil Code of 1804, which restricted married women's property rights, further discouraged their involvement in the commercial sphere.[24]

The boundaries between public and private life were always porous despite these legal and cultural disincentives, particularly when women made use the cachet of domesticity to justify their activities in the public sphere. For example, participation in philanthropic causes geared toward bettering the living conditions of lower-class women and children afforded elite women opportunities for public engagement by expanding their orbit of motherly influence.[25] The value placed on motherhood similarly sanctioned the involvement of an upper-class woman like Athalie Brierre de Boismont in the direction of a *maison de santé*. That said, while it could be argued that Athalie Brierre de Boismont devoted herself selflessly to the needs of her patients, her actions were advertised in the interest of private financial gain. Not only was a bourgeois woman working for money contrary to the domestic ideal but the French also expressed considerable unease regarding entrepreneurialism itself, particularly during the July Monarchy.[26] One might assume that marketing the "angel in the house" in a promotional brochure would prove controversial in a postrevolutionary society trying to balance a newfound commitment to meritocracy with a traditional distrust of self-interestedness. Yet nothing in his writings suggests that Dr. Brierre de Boismont thought this to be the case.

To understand why, it makes sense to remind ourselves of the particularities of alienism's relationship to the family in the opening decades of the nineteenth century. All asylum directors aimed to rehabilitate patients' disrupted sense of domestic harmony by interrupting their daily routines and (re)educating them in proper behavior. While the resources available to public and private asylum operators differed with respect to accomplishing this end, each insisted that separation from family and friends constituted an essential first step in the process. Legislators embedded the concept of isolation into the 1838 law on asylum commitment; this legal innovation augmented the authority of doctors, whose process of professionalization occurred at the expense of familial control over those considered insane.[27] Patients' isolation from their own families also made the subsequent creation of a simulated family within the institution possible. In the case of private asylums, this new "family" included stand-ins for patients' female relatives, who would help to cultivate a rehabilitative atmosphere.

Like Pinel and Esquirol, but in even more forthright terms, Dr. Brierre de Boismont argued, "The family, in effect, is the point of departure for a considerable number of mental illnesses."[28] He believed that incurability often resulted when relatives refused to bring their family members in for treatment or removed them from the *maison de santé* earlier than needed.[29] For Dr. Brierre de Boismont, family life contributed to the mental alienation of some of his patients, and the familiarity of the family home for those who never sought outside intervention made the possibility of successful treatment unlikely.[30] One could not expect a patient whose "intellectual and moral faculties improved themselves in a notable manner through a prolonged stay in the *maison*" to experience the same type of recovery in the very situation in which their illness initially took root.[31] The *vie de famille* method could therefore only be carried out under the strict supervision of a medical professional and with the help of the replacement family that came into being within a private institution.

Dr. Brierre de Boismont's desire to simulate family life might have paved the way for his wife's involvement in the treatment process, but her assumption of an authoritative role vis-à-vis bourgeois male patients also relied on and perpetuated widely held associations between madness and childhood. Doctors' tendency to imagine patients as children and themselves as father figures legitimated women's authority as much as the related concept of familial isolation. Legislation also imposed familial hierarchies upon the asylum space by granting patients a legal status virtually identical to that of minors. Once institutionalized, mentally ill adults depended on doctors and relatives to decide their eventual release date and lost control of their estates until that time.

Dr. Brierre de Boismont used an extended discussion of the commonalities between childhood development and the treatment of insanity in order to justify his methods, noting that "We [asylum doctors] wrote long ago: the alienated are children; we should have added: spoiled children."[32] He believed that tutors and involved parents were best suited to successfully instill character and encourage children to develop "that interior force called a conscience."[33] Individualized attention supposedly served to moderate their faults and kept them from succumbing to weaknesses later in life. According to Dr. Brierre de Boismont, "this familial influence" had the same effect on mental patients. In their case, however, the educative process was far more difficult and their successful upbringing took "extreme patience, a spirit of justice and firmness, a great equality of humor, a perfect moderation of sentiments, inexhaustible kindness, and an enlightened [sense of] religion."[34] These qualities, particularly in a wife, would help to assure domestic happiness in any bourgeois home, but they were even more critical in the private asylum.[35]

By indicating that women's maternal natures could encourage the insane to embrace rationality, Dr. Brierre de Boismont echoed Rousseau's idealized descriptions of domestic motherhood—a concept which the philosophe and his intellectual descendants invested with the great responsibility of molding citizens capable of exhibiting self-control.[36] In so doing, Dr. Brierre de Boismont brought the infantilization of mentally ill adults to its logical conclusion when many of his colleagues did not. For if mad men and women were essentially children, then it was culturally acceptable or even "natural" for bourgeois wives to play a part in their rehabilitation.

The patriarch of the Brierre de Boismont family found the influence of a nurturing woman proved most beneficial for those patients whose depression was aggravated by the gaiety and distraction of the asylum salon. He believed it often helped to converse with and console such patients on a more individual basis, noting that "little by little, the ice melts" if there was someone available "to cry with those who suffer."[37] The asylum doctor admitted this intense form of interaction was not his forte, and that his wife deserved most of the credit when it resulted in cure.[38] Men like himself were supposedly unaccustomed to submitting to the sort of "slavery"[39] required in listening to the unending complaints of the most depressed patients, especially because he claimed their diatribes often included malicious lies and slanderous accusations. Conversely, he suggested that women's characteristic patience and desire to nurture (not to mention their apparent capacity to endure verbal abuse) made them better suited to deal with these frustrations. For this reason he advised his fellow alienists that they should take great care in choosing a wife.[40]

While Dr. Brierre de Boismont relied on his wife as a caregiver and encouraged her to embrace the maternal aspects of bourgeois femininity to aid in the treatment process, women's display of expected gendered behavior within his institution also operated in more subtle ways. We can see this in a treatise written by his daughter, Marie Rivet, in which she describes her childhood in her parents' asylum. Specifically, Rivet noted that when she was a child she often convinced patients to submit to treatment more readily than her parents could. Those diagnosed with "persecution mania" (whose worry over their doctors' intentions was considered a symptom of their madness) supposedly trusted that Rivet was too young to wrong them. Her childlike cajoling convinced her fathers' patients to eat and drink when they had previously refused. Rivet, however, became less comfortable in her role as "the years added themselves to years, and the influence of the woman substituted itself for that of the child."[41] Some men confused the adolescent Rivet with their wives or lovers while in hallucinatory states, and she occasionally went so far as to insert feeding tubes and to secure them in straitjackets by taking advantage of their affections. Yet because Rivet used her patients' feelings for her in a way that seemed to produce results, she "did not have the courage to deplore the drawbacks of this education that strongly taught *coquettishness* while prematurely revealing to the young girl the powers of the woman."[42]

This complaint, one of the few specific negative aspects of her upbringing Rivet mentioned, points to some challenges brought forth by the *vie de famille* method. While women's manipulation of family and gender values within private asylums could conceivably convince patients to embrace rationality and conform to the behavioral expectations of French society, this tactic also entailed some danger because it drew attention to womanliness in a way that might be interpreted as dishonorable. As Michèle Plott explains when comparing nineteenth-century French attitudes regarding women's sexual natures with those of Britain and the United States, "French women simply could not rely on more general ideas about women's asexuality to support their reputations as respectable women."[43] Rivet's unease with her own "coquettishness" suggests that women's sexual power over men was taken for granted.

Doctors often interpreted women's sexuality as pathological if it was expressed in manner they deemed overly explicit, as indicated by the institutionalization of women for a variety of sex-related mental "disorders."[44] Rivet herself came to associate overt expressions of female sexuality—particularly lesbianism—with madness, noting that hysterical patients required "incessant surveillance" for this very reason.[45] Allusions to the adolescent discovery of her own sexual desirability must be understood in this wider context, for the same class-based standards of honor and virtue that constrained women patients limited Rivet's behavior as well. She thus risked bringing dishonor to herself and her family by using her sexual influence over the men in her care, even if the outcome was positive, at least from the perspective of an asylum director. Notably, the manipulative aspect of Rivet's behavior did not concern her. It was rather the premature education in flirtation—and the nascent female sexuality it brought attention to—that she ultimately deemed improper. Nonetheless, this example demonstrates the usefulness of Rivet's womanliness in a setting where irrational men seemed more inclined to trust an adolescent girl than a male doctor.

Dr. Brierre de Boismont likewise indicated that his wife's behavior had a positive effect on their male patients, particularly those who retained their understanding of proper gender comportment despite having lost many of the traits commonly associated with middle-class manhood (most notably their rationality, but also their ability to maintain a household or hold onto a professional position).[46] As an ever-present and idealized example of bourgeois womanhood, Athalie Brierre de Boismont played a special role in convincing such patients to act in a normative fashion by encouraging them to again behave like men. Furthermore, she did not risk dishonoring herself as her adolescent daughter had precisely because she was already a married woman.

Dr. Brierre de Boismont's recollections of his wife's interactions with an army officer who arrived at the asylum exhibiting signs of profound melancholy and "violent grief" were a case in point.[47] The man had supposedly sat mute for many days in a corner of Athalie Brierre de Boismont's salon until he gradually began to participate in the conversations and diversions surrounding him. He even consented to go on walks with the *directrice* in the Bois de Boulogne, where, one day, he stopped brusquely and asked her if she was afraid to be alone with him; after all, he could kill her if he pleased. She replied that such a thought had never entered her mind, for "I am a woman, you are a soldier, don't I have your protection?"[48] The officer agreed and shortly thereafter he left the asylum cured, never again mentioning their conversation that took place in the grand park in western Paris. In recounting the army officer's recovery process, Dr. Brierre de Boismont emphasized the curative influence of his wife's presence, giving her complete credit for pulling the patient out of his depressive state. While it is possible the doctor exaggerated the details of the episode for dramatic effect, he did so in a way that legitimated the familial atmosphere cultivated within his institution. Moreover, he presented Athalie Brierre de Boismont's involvement in the treatment process in profoundly unthreatening terms, for it was only through her display of a traditionally feminine attribute (i.e., her vulnerability) that she convinced the soldier to embrace middle-class notions of honorable, protective, and rational manhood.

The life of Athalie Brierre de Boismont exemplifies historian Jennifer Popiel's assertion that the eighteenth- and nineteenth-century celebration of the role of women in the home "established domestic nurturing as a high calling."[49] For not only did she hold real authority within the domestic sphere, but the parameters of the Brierre de Boismont household were capacious enough to include numerous individuals who would not have been present in a typical family home. The cultural elevation of domesticity, when combined with various assumptions embedded in mid-century psychiatric practice, encouraged Athalie Brierre de Boismont to play an active role in the family business without raising objections from her contemporaries. More unexpectedly, she also exerted a considerable amount of power over men of her class, which would have likely been difficult without the partnership of her husband. His presence as a university-educated physician, a celebrated and frequently published member of the greater psychiatric community, and the official director of their *maison de santé* made his wife's role in the asylum's operation culturally palatable. By working as the comparatively silent partner in a joint enterprise, male alienists had no reason to consider Athalie Brierre de Boismont a threat to their own advancement. Further analysis of her eldest daughter's relationship to the psychiatric profession, however, will throw the limits of domestic ideology as a source of women's authority into sharp relief.

Marie Rivet: The Woman as Expert

Born in Paris's fourth arrondisement in 1829, Marie Rivet was the first of several children.[50] She came of age in the family-operated asylum owned by her father, where the Brierre de Boismonts lived alongside their patients and incorporated them into the routines of the household. She was named *directrice* of her father's institution in 1848[51] and married Arthur Jean Baptiste Rivet in 1850 at the age of twenty-one.[52] Approximately ten years later she opened a *maison de santé* in Saint Mandé, a commune located on the eastern outskirts of Paris, after running another institution in the same neighborhood as Athalie and Alexandre Brierre de Boismont (on the Rue Neuve-Sainte-Geneviève) since 1850.[53] Neither of her facilities precisely emulated the family life method of her parents, as all her patients were women. Furthermore, Rivet's husband did not play an active role in the institutions' operations, although her daughter and niece did. Despite these differences, she attested that her attitudes towards the treatment of insanity were heavily influenced by her childhood spent living "amidst the mad."[54] The "Maison de Santé de Mme. Rivet," as the Sainte-Mandé institution was called in promotional materials, housed anywhere from twenty-five to sixty patients at a time according to Rivet's own calculations and to the *Annuaire Statistique*.[55] Rivet catered to a wealthy clientele and charged an average of 1,100 francs per year per patient in 1859.[56]

As mentioned above, women operated a small but not insignificant number of mental health facilities in Paris during the first half of the nineteenth century; for example, women proprietors owned three out of the twelve private asylums that catered exclusively to the "alienated" in 1842, in addition to five *maisons de santé* open to patients experiencing mental or physical ailments.[57] Furthermore, judging from the writings of male private asylum operators like Dr. Brierre de Boismont and Esprit Blanche, their wives often took part in day-to-day operations even when official records failed to reflect their participation in a formal capacity. These women rarely recorded their experiences in their own words. The substantial treatise entitled *Les Aliénés dans la famille et dans la maison de santé,* which Rivet published in 1875 after twenty-seven years directing private asylums, is therefore quite exceptional.

While her mother's life history points to the elasticity of domestic ideology and its ability to sanction women's empowerment in certain settings, Rivet's memoir additionally reveals the contradictions that emerged when a woman used bourgeois gender values as a justification for her expert status. Athalie Brierre de Boismont had expanded an essentially domestic role in an unexpected direction. Rivet, on the other hand, sought a greater level of professional independence by taking on the traditionally paternal role of asylum owner-operator. Her writings therefore shed light not only the role of women in private asylum operations but also on the ways that gender tied into psychiatry's process of professionalization. Ultimately, Rivet's memoir presents an image of womanly expertise that simultaneously conformed to middle-class gender norms and threatened male asylum directors' assumptions regarding the inviolability of their own scientific knowledge.

Like her father, who published his treatise on the *vie de famille* twelve years earlier, Rivet began her only published work with a dedication to a member of the family: Dr. Brierre de Boismont himself. While she praised her mother—who had died unexpectedly in 1873 in the presence of her patients—for her inexhaustible patience and diagnostic expertise, she reserved her most effusive thanks for the wisdom passed down by her father. Rivet noted gratefully that "madness was no longer one of God's mysteries that he kept to himself" owing to the esteemed asylum doctor's "knowledge and precious teachings."[58] What stands out in Rivet's descriptions of Dr. Brierre de Boismont's influence, however, is an emphasis on the difficulties her unique upbringing had wrought. While she claimed not to regret her "sorrowful apprenticeship in mental alienation" and to be thankful for the opportunity to "utilize with profit some of the knowledge I acquired," she also referred to her life as "a bit sad."[59] Her participation in the workings of the Brierre de Boismont asylum during her youth helped to simulate an ideal family life for her parents' many patients, yet it kept Rivet and her siblings from experiencing "normal" childhoods themselves. Indeed, while the institution was designed to celebrate the curative potential of bourgeois family values, the roles played by women and children in the treatment process differentiated the Brierre de Boismont's lifestyle from that of others of their class—to the extent that Rivet's childhood was defined by her exposure to individuals who interacted with their own families in a manner deemed pathological.

Her somewhat backhanded dedication to her father the eminent alienist also points to some contradictions at the heart of Rivet's self-presentation, particularly with respect to the performance required to manage her dual identities as a woman taking on the traditionally masculine occupation of asylum director. Despite expressing a certain amount of justifiable pride for all she had accomplished—a fact that comes across later in the text—Rivet began her book by framing her professional existence in terms of her father's success and with a considerable dose of feigned reluctance.

Considering the social condemnation and institutional obstruction experienced by women practitioners who sought employment in public facilities, her decision to downplay her ambitions made a great deal of sense. The Paris medical faculty opened its doors to women in 1868 and some women—mostly foreign-born—had begun entering the medical professions by the time Rivet published her memoir in 1875.[60] At that point, however, she was nearly fifty years old and had been running her own institution for decades. Furthermore, women's acceptance into the echelons of higher education was a long time com-ing and the first women doctors often faced the scorn and ridicule of their male colleagues.[61] The feminist-socialist physician Madeleine Pelletier was the first woman allowed to sit for the exams required of doctors interested in interning in public mental asylums. This occurred in 1902 and required both a forceful press campaign and the reversal of long-standing practices and regulations, and even then Pelletier never directed a public asylum.[62]

Rivet, on the other hand, managed to carve out a professional space within the domestic sphere and move beyond it in certain respects without inspiring much controversy. Her institution was well-regarded and even famous. Guidebooks occasionally mentioned it,[63] and her social circle included various literary types. Philoxène Boyer, the poet and contemporary of Baudelaire, held his marriage breakfast at Rivet's *maison de santé* in 1857[64] and even dedicated a poem to her.[65] The playwright and editor of the *Féerie Illustre*, Marc Fournier, lived with Rivet as a guest for some time before his death in 1879.[66] The daughter of Victor Hugo, Adèle, was undoubtedly Rivet's most notable patient, and she resided at the *maison de santé* for many years. After living in squalor in the Caribbean, estranged from her family throughout much of the 1860s, Adèle returned to France in 1872 following the cessation of her father's exile. Her increasingly erratic behavior and her insistence that she heard voices led Hugo to reluctantly send his "poor child" to a *maison de santé*: "the best possible," according to his diary.[67]

For Rivet to have achieved this level of notoriety was quite a coup, and it involved adeptly manipulating cultural attitudes about women, work, and au-thority. Nonetheless, her contemporaries seem to have viewed her as a special case rather than as a woman to be emulated, and historians have neglected her story almost entirely. Like any woman with professional aspirations in mid-nine-teenth-century France, Rivet experienced a double bind. If she broke free of the constraints of acceptable femininity and unabashedly pursued her ambitions, she would lose the virtuous image so essential to her success. Yet reliance on the tropes of bourgeois domesticity necessarily limited the impact she might have.[68]

She never mentioned it outright, but Rivet seemed aware of the contradictory nature of her position. While she clearly sought to present herself as an authority in mental medicine—the publication of her work is a testament to this fact—she carefully limited her claims to ideas, practices, and people that fell within the do-mestic orbit. Rivet maintained that she directed her insights to everyday people, not necessarily the scientific community, and almost all her advice hinged on in-timate knowledge of her patients and their families.[69] In so doing she presented herself as a selfless and long-suffering caregiver, a good *bourgeoise*, rather than a medical expert. Nonetheless, she undermined her professed modesty throughout the book by slipping into medical language, citing the work of male asylum doctors, and weighing in on contemporary debates over controversial psychiatric practices. Although many of Rivet's attempts to prove her respectability involved highlighting the ways in which she conformed to bourgeois gender norms, they can also be interpreted as claims for the superiority of lay expertise.

For example, Rivet took pains to establish her credentials by continually making reference to her unique upbringing. She immediately set herself apart from formally educated psychiatrists, arguing that she possessed a specialized form of knowledge inaccessible to those entering the profession in adulthood. She noted that scientific authorities "confine themselves to treating madness from a purely medical point of view, but a scientific book appeals only to professionals."[70] She instead directed her book to the *gens du monde*—which she contrasted to *gens de métier*—using a new form of psychiatric writing in which she gathered together all her "memories" and "observations" in order to teach people how to recognize the signs of insanity and know what to do if they noticed symptoms in a relative.[71] Because "madness has that sad property of being appreciable to everyone," then "an intimate work" should be written and read.[72] In this way, Rivet depicted herself as a particularly familial, and thus womanly, sort of medical expert.

Despite emphasizing the distinctiveness of her background, many of Rivet's opinions tended toward the conventional. For the most part, her case studies reveal attitudes one might expect from a woman of her status with respect to both class and gender values, such as when she conflated hysteria with lesbianism and other manifestations of female sexuality. She likewise expressed shock towards the religious, familial, and political values of female supporters of the revolutionary Paris Commune, suggesting she saw herself as profoundly typical in these respects despite her own unconventional lifestyle.[73] Yet even when repeating some of the prejudices commonly associated with her class and profession, Rivet set herself apart from other psychiatric practitioners by critiquing the bourgeois family to a degree that went well beyond the observations previously set forth by Pinel, Esquirol, and even her father—who claimed that mental illness took root in the home, but was not the result of pathological family relations. Her willingness to impugn the family was particularly apparent in discussions of the onset and manifestation of insanity. Jan Goldstein notes that Rivet's book was the earliest she discovered that situated familial interactions as the source of mental illness, for Rivet pointed out that jealousy between adolescent girls and their mothers sometimes contributed to insanity's onset.[74]

One poignant example of Rivet's critical stance toward the family involved a fifteen-year-old boy whose parents asked Rivet to examine him because they noticed his mental and physical health slowly breaking down. Upon inspection, she concluded that the adolescent's "solitary habits" had provoked madness: a euphemistic suggestion that excessive masturbation had driven the boy insane. This assertion was very much in line with middle-class beliefs that stigmatized nonreproductive sexuality. In the words of Robert Nye, the ability to engender children was an essential aspect of a bourgeois Frenchman's identity and all forms of sexual expression that did not achieve this result were considered "parasitic."[75] Doctors gave scientific credence to this belief, going so far as to suggest that ejaculation depleted a man's life force and, by extension, his masculine honor. Medical interest in the social and mental effects of masturbation (in addition to impotence and homosexuality) increased throughout the century in response to the changes in daily life brought about by industrialization and, eventually, the widespread perception of demographic crisis.[76] Rivet reproduced the assumptions of bourgeois medical men in pinpointing onanism as the source of the adolescent's mental and physical state.

Nonetheless, her interpretation of this particular case also exhibited a subtle critique of those who sought to keep women ignorant of all things sexual. Rivet immediately questioned the boy's family when called in for assistance and expressed shock and disappointment when she discovered that the mother, a woman in her thirties, had never considered "the vice of childhood" as the source of her son's illness.[77] While one might consider her ignorance of sexual behavior a mark of respectability "in a century such as ours," Rivet nonetheless argued, "the mother of the family had assisted, worried but unaware, in the mental and physical deterioration of her child, without power to stop it."[78] She expressed further disappointment that "the health of the child was sacrificed to the delicacies of the mother."[79] Rivet thus critiqued the sexual mores of the bourgeoisie in a fashion unique among pre-Freudian mental health practitioners, even as her negative attitude toward nonreproductive sexual activity served to legitimize and compound them.

The purposes for which Rivet infantilized her patients likewise appeared to conform to the attitudes expressed by male alienists, but ultimately served to distinguish her approach from theirs—justifying, in the end, her cultivation of a different sort of rehabilitative atmosphere. She often likened her patients to children, as had her father. For example, in a chapter called "On the Childish and Destructive Habits of the Alienated," she characterized the misdeeds of certain patients in order to present a tableau of asylum life and document what she considered the most effective methods of treatment. One anecdote involved the family pet, a Great Pyrenees who never left Rivet's daughter's side. As the girl made her daily rounds, visiting with the patients, the dog followed her and begged for food along the way. One day, he did not come when he was called. The family finally found him in a patient's bedroom, so "completely shaved that large flakes of white fur formed a veritable carpet on the floor."[80] Rivet did not attribute her patient's actions to any sort of malice. Instead, the woman had been seized by an "eccentric idea" and reacted like "a child who, left alone, becomes unsettled" and breaks something.[81]

As already shown, most doctors emphasized the supposedly childlike natures of their patients in order to tout the curative potential of their particular brand of psychiatric care. Just as Leuret invoked the childishness of patients to justify punitive methods of treatment, so Dr. Brierre de Boismont highlighted the supposed congruities between children and the mad to argue in favor of the educative and reformist elements of the *vie de famille*. Conversely, Rivet's attention to the character traits supposedly shared by children and mental patients revealed a particularly modern approach to both the treatment of insanity and the raising of children.[82] For the *directrice*, patients were not "spoiled," and she emphasized the importance of treating "childish" behaviors with humor and compassion. While those on the outside might wonder why she did not institute strict procedures that would help avoid "degradations" (like the occasional dog-shaving), Rivet called on the metaphor of familial order to argue for leniency. She compared private asylum directors to parents who submit themselves to "small sacrifices" in the best interests of their children and she tolerated certain inconveniences in order to ensure what she called the "relative happiness of the alienated."[83]

In choosing not to punish patients who occasionally caused disorder, Rivet behaved in a fashion at odds with the practice of some of her male colleagues. She made this comparison explicit, but with caution. Rivet never criticized the public asylum system or its proponents outright, explaining, "whatever we [in private institutions] permit, it is impossible to do so in the great public establishments in which order and harmony must be the rule."[84] The need to regiment and regulate patient behavior in public institutions presumably involved their much larger patient population and its primarily working-class composition. Moreover, she also noted that the appearance of order in public asylums also helped to sustain France's *amour-propre* because foreign observers so often visited them in order to spur medical innovation in their own countries.

As the operator of a private institution, Rivet did not have to worry about how her actions reflected on French national esteem, for the doors of her asylum opened to regulatory authorities and to the families of the mad alone. She implied that her independence from the state allowed her to more fully establish the familial atmosphere required for effective patient treatment, writing:

> Our patients are ours.
>
> They are not the alienated of such and such department, they do not belong to such and such establishment, they are not submissive to any experience, to any attempt outside of those done to heal them. . . . They are patients treated by the doctor, they are not the *subject* of medicine.[85]

Rivet thus described her patients as part of the family instead of as cases to be explored in a disinterested or purely scientific manner. And while she avoided openly criticizing the methods of her male counterparts, she not-so-subtly suggested that the interests of doctors and those of their patients were not necessarily the same. She claimed that operators of public asylums treated patients as subjects, not people, and she believed that those individuals who rarely caused disturbance were especially "tyrannized" in large facilities. Rivet denied arguing that public asylum operators mistreated the mentally ill, but nonetheless expressed concern over the level of control exercised over each patient's individual actions, claiming that the constant regulation of a patient's interior life caused unhappiness that might be avoided if he was able to "give himself up to his fantasies" to a certain degree.[86] This attitude could not be further from those of her contemporaries, many of whom insisted that any expression of irrationality must be countered with forceful, albeit usually nonviolent, efforts at reformation.[87]

Rivet therefore combined attributes associated with both femininity and masculinity when constructing her relationship to her patients, and she implied that this very mixture was what made her successful. She exercised the authority of a male asylum director when weighing her patients' freedom against the orderliness of her institution and when determining whether an incident called for leniency or punishment. Yet she argued that it was her motherly concern, her womanly intuition, and her lifelong experiential training that allowed her to cultivate and project this authority in the first place.

A Mixed Reception

While critics lauded Rivet's book for providing insight into topics often neglected in accounts written by medical men (most notably private asylum operations and the relationship between family life and mental illness), most reviewers tended to focus their attention on Rivet's sex more than on her ideas. For example, the reviewer for the *Chicago Journal of Mental and Nervous Disease* consistently highlighted the fact that Rivet was a woman in his assessment of *Les Aliénés dans la famille et dans la maison de santé*, always as one of the work's virtues, writing that "The book deserves success for the spirit in which it is written; it is the first contribution to literature of the author, an amiable woman who has struck out in a new line for her sex."[88] Still, in the span of a paragraph the reviewer referred to Rivet's work as "little" three times, despite the book spanning several hundred pages. One can only suppose that the adjective applied more to the assumed diminutive stature of the author or the perceived weight of her observations than it did to the length of her work. Another reviewer, who signed his piece in the *Union médicale* with the initials M. L., went so far as to insist that books have a sex, and that this one was "absolutely female (*féminin*) from one end to the other, from the first page to the last."[89] He then offered his impression of Rivet's personality (it "produced a singular effect, and was not without charm") and ended by calling himself "her devoted servant" after apologizing (ad nauseam) for having unchivalrously made a "lady" wait for the publication of his reflections.[90]

Other reviews were more substantial. Her father actually wrote a lengthy piece for the *Annales d'hygiène* recounting Rivet's myriad talents as an asylum director and the pride he felt as her parent, pointing out that he neither read nor discussed the book with her as she wrote so as to avoid unduly influencing its character.[91] He found Rivet's analysis of the role of the "passions" in the onset of mental illness especially exciting, and he discussed at length the sad case of a young mother whose husband interned her at Rivet's asylum after he refused to end an affair with one of their household servants. The woman arrived profoundly malnourished and soon died in the asylum. Her fate—which seems, to modern eyes, so clearly linked to her experience living in a society that ascribed one set of sexual standards to men and another to women—made a lasting impression on Dr. Brierre de Boismont and his daughter, who had reportedly expressed a great deal of compassion for the wife and had roundly condemned the actions of the husband. While Rivet never blamed gender inequality for her patient's breakdown, her sympathy for a woman driven mad by her spouse's infidelity can be interpreted as another subtle critique of bourgeois family values. It is worth noting that Dr. Brierre de Boismont failed to make this connection in his review, and that he instead emphasized the ways this case merely exhibited the potentially deleterious effects of the passions on the development of mental alienation.

Even more significant for her father was Rivet's defense of the psychiatric profession, a goal she explicitly set forth in her preface. A noticeable uptick in

the numbers of accusations of arbitrary asylum sequestration occurred in the
1860s and 1870s. During this period, novels and plays, not to mention press reports, accumulated on the subject of collusion between asylum directors and
unscrupulous families hoping to rid themselves of inconvenient relations, as we
shall see in the following chapter. By the time Rivet published her book, legislators had begun to investigate the possibility of revising the 1838 law on asylum
internments, whose passage had been a key moment in the professionalization
of French psychiatry.[92] Asylum directors like the Brierre de Boismonts considered their livelihoods under threat, and Rivet's book constituted a much-needed
defense of their profession. As Dr. Brierre de Boismont wrote, the best way to
clamp down on the public's fear of asylum psychiatry, perpetuated "by the enemies of alienists," was to "open completely these so-called *basses-fosses*," just as
Rivet had done.[93] Her father's review can thus be read as another contribution
to the creation of a family myth, one which positioned the Brierre de Boismonts
not only as devoted caregivers to their patients and members of an ideal bourgeois household but now as the saviors of French psychiatry as well.

Not all members of the French medical community were convinced Rivet's
work helped their cause, as one can see in the review published by the *Gazette
hebdomadaire de médecine et de chirurgie*, a weekly journal geared toward medical professionals of all subfields. As the only review that challenged any of Rivet's
claims, it is worth examining in detail. The journal critiqued Rivet's book as part
of a larger piece on a handful of major contemporaneous works including those
by such eminent figures as the British Henry Maudsley and the Austro-Prussian
Richard von Krafft-Ebing. Also reviewed alongside *Les Aliénés dans la famille
et dans la maison de santé* was a recent book by Jules Dagron, the director of
Ville-Évrard, a departmental asylum. Written as a firsthand account of asylum
operations over the course of several years, Dagron's book painted a detailed
picture of life in public asylums much as Rivet had done for private facilities.
Comparing the *directrice* to such illustrious company strongly suggests that her
expertise was acknowledged by at least some of her male contemporaries.

The reviewer Aimé-Jean Linas, a Paris-based physician who regularly published on mental health and other medical topics, praised Rivet for producing a
work that shed light on an aspect of the profession that rarely received attention,
particularly from a woman's perspective. He also accorded her a certain level of
professional respect, describing Rivet as the "daughter of an eminent alienist,
and an alienist herself."[94] Rivet's work was both informative and "charming,"
two traits that Linas seemed to hold in equal esteem. The book represented "an
intimate study of madness" and he believed that Rivet "loves her patients . . .

(and) treats them as much with the concern of a mother as with the devotion of a sister." Thus, for at least one reviewer, it was possible for a woman to take on the traditionally masculine role of asylum overseer precisely because the private asylum was a familial space, or at least a simulation thereof. Her domestic qualities—motherly concern, sisterly devotion—were useful in a professional context which called for the re-creation of family dynamics but required the absence of actual family members. Her lack of formal training did not disqualify her from this occupation and her specifically feminine form of expertise could even be construed as an asset.

However, Rivet's situation was undeniably unique. Her path toward becoming an active member of the profession could not be emulated by other women. Furthermore, despite his initial praise, Linas also pointed to the dangers of allowing someone like Rivet to fashion herself as a psychiatric authority, particularly because Rivet did not direct her insights toward the medical community alone. Her stated goal was to give the families of potential patients the tools to recognize the signs of mental alienation so they could seek help as soon as possible. Rivet and Linas agreed that the successful treatment of mental illness depended upon the patient entering an institution early. However, Linas took umbrage with Rivet's assertion that "[m]adness has that sad quality of being appreciable to everyone," as opposed to other illnesses that could only be diagnosed by a doctor. He expressed shock that the daughter of Dr. Brierre de Boismont would say such a thing and found it particularly regretful that "these words are placed on the first page of a work directed at *gens du monde*; this book should be written to enlighten their ignorance, and not to encourage and exalt their presumptuousness on the matter of madness."[95] He also skeptically took note of Rivet's assertion that she learned how to tell the difference between madness and sanity at a young age. Despite the uniqueness of Rivet's personal situation, Linas worried that she would spread the idea that psychiatric knowledge was accessible to those not trained in the traditional manner. This attitude propped up Rivet's own authority, but undermined that of her male colleagues. Linas seemed to recognize this and crafted his review accordingly.

In certain respects, Linas's critical approach to Rivet's ideas indicated that he respected her as a fellow medical professional. Her work was not simply an amusing diversion, but worthy of debate. That said, his specific complaints had everything to do with her status as a lay practitioner. His greatest bone of contention related to the way Rivet contrasted the atmosphere of her asylum to those of the great public asylums run by men. As already noted, she had taken care not to criticize the operators of public asylums, explaining that it would be unfeasible

and even undesirable for such emblems of national prestige to be run in a disorderly fashion. Linas, however, was not pacified by Rivet's attempts to avoid
controversy and instead latched onto her assertion that the patients in her institution were treated by the doctor but "were not the subject of medicine."[96] Linas
defensively declared Rivet had forgotten the role played by public asylums in the
education of alienists and in the establishment of the honor of mental medicine
(although she had indeed pointed this out). He wrote in grandiose terms that
"these public establishments of which she speaks were the cradle (*berceau*) and
the home (*foyer*) of ... psychiatric study."[97] Rivet thus forsook the legacy of "the
immortal works of Pinel (and) Esquirol" by criticizing "the great schools where
these celebrated masters were taught and had practiced."[98] Critiquing the public
asylum, even by implication, was practically unforgivable, all the more so at a
time when the psychiatric profession felt itself under siege.[99]

Thus, while the reviewer from the *Gazette hebdomadaire* respected Rivet's
ideas enough to debate her in a public forum, he did so in such a way as to undermine the very "intimate expertise" he had initially praised. Linas emphasized
the fact that Rivet had not been educated within the walls of the great asylums
whose operations she dared to critique, writing that the public asylum system
served as "the nursery (*pépinière*)" for "the most eminent psychiatrists of our
epoch."[100] He implied that Rivet, as someone who had not worked in one, could
never rank among psychiatry's leading figures. And while he did not state outright that Rivet's sex disqualified her opinions, his insistence that studying in a
public asylum was the most valuable form of psychiatric training necessarily excluded all women from reaching what he considered the heights of professional
expertise because it required both university training and the completion of an
internship exam unavailable to them. He thereby called into question Rivet's
right to enter into psychiatric debates as an equal even in the course of reviewing
her work alongside that of her male contemporaries.

Linas's use of household terminology in the course of his review subtly revealed his sense of unease. Usually, when doctors discussed asylums in familial
terms, they did so in ways that positioned themselves as father figures inside
the "home" of the asylum. Linas, however, flipped this metaphor on its head
when discussing public institutions, positioning young male doctors as children
coming of age in the course of their training. He referred to the public asylum
system as a "cradle," a "hearth," and a "nursery" in his passionate explanation of
its role in the education of future asylum directors. While it might be tempting
to dismiss Linas's domestic references as rhetorical flourishes, their use exposes
his underlying anxiety regarding Rivet's particular form of psychiatric expertise.

In other words, it took a great deal of intellectual maneuvering for Linas to claim that the *public* asylum was the "cradle" of psychiatric learning when the Brierre de Boismont children had actually been raised in a mental institution. For Rivet, the asylum-home was no metaphor, which gave her the authority to speak to those like Linas on her own terms.

Rivet's reviewers tended to agree that her medical opinions held merit. Yet framing her expertise as "intimate" had restricted her ability to convince medical men that she was their peer. Her self-presentation as an expert not just in madness but also in its familial contexts set her apart from other practitioners, particularly those who ran public asylums. However, it did so in a way that reinforced doctors' expectations of gendered behavior. Only one reviewer concluded that Rivet's promotion of her own abilities undermined the authority of the profession. This reviewer was also the one who took her ideas most seriously, for he at least considered the implications of her work. Ironically, the generally uncritical reception of *Les Aliénés dans la famille et la maison de santé* suggests that the power Rivet held within the asylum was largely limited to that space. Rivet's strategic focus upon the domestic attributes of her own expertise ultimately condemned her to remain on the outside the psychiatric profession looking in. Or, perhaps more accurately, it kept her on the inside, looking out.

Rivet persisted in her attempts at self-fashioning to the last. She passed away in 1895 after nearly thirty years spent running the institution in Saint-Mandé, leaving some of her fortune to the Academie des Sciences so that a bust of the professor and expert in forensic psychology, Ambroise Tardieu (1818–1879), could be constructed in her name.[101] Like Rivet and her father before her, Tardieu had identified the family as both a potential source of danger and as society's bulwark, in his case controversially writing about the sexual abuse of children and its effects.[102] Thus, in her final paradoxical act, Rivet recommitted herself to the concerns of the domestic sphere, but in an undeniably public manner. Moreover, she linked herself to official medicine in spite of the ways her own career exemplified the richness of lay expertise, thereby insisting, once again, that a woman with no formal training had something to offer the psychiatric profession.

THE FAMILY MYTHOLOGY presented by the Brierre de Boismonts often reinforced conventional attitudes towards both psychiatry and the cult of domesticity, with the women of the house quite literally serving as the gatekeepers of rationality and, therefore, of French society itself. The cultural elevation of motherhood made this possible, but so too did the medicalization of mental illness and the cultural elevation of rational self-control as a central component of bourgeois masculinity. Private asylum *directrices* supervised people considered unsuited for participation in the public sphere by virtue of their perceived madness who were nonetheless expected and often forced to leave their own homes. Even when the ultimate goal (in the case of male patients) was to inspire them to embrace stereotypically masculine attributes and reenter the public world of work and sociability, their institutionalization marginalized them further, and many patients who entered asylums never left. The Brierre de Boismont women perpetuated this system and benefited from it, for it was only through the general devaluation of those considered insane that their opportunities for empowerment arose at all.

At the same time, the very existence of women like Marie Rivet and Athalie Brierre de Boismont called attention to the artificiality of nineteenth-century gender norms and the medical beliefs that perpetuated them. When Rivet and her mother played the roles of exemplary bourgeois women—both in the course of patient treatment and in the act of self-promotion—they certainly drew on and reinforced the cultural potency of separate spheres ideology. However, by doing so in an environment so unlike the typical family home, they also highlighted the performative dimensions of bourgeois womanhood.

This not only served to expose the constructed nature of nineteenth-century gender values, but the theatricality of sanity itself. Rivet acknowledged this, albeit without self-reflection, when discussing the behavioral repertoire of hysterical women, writing that, "Madness brusquely unties the strings of the mask that cultivation (*éducation*) has affixed."[103] A madwoman was simply one who no longer behaved in the way she had been taught to, whether she drank alcohol excessively; mixed with those beneath her station; or had otherwise transformed herself from an "honest woman" into a "shameless pleasure-seeker (*viveuse éhontée*)." [104] Rivet, of course, also wore a mask, one designed to make her appear eminently qualified to retie those that her patients seemed determined to rip away. Yet in the process of carefully constructing her identity as a woman who had long been able to differentiate the dividing line between lucidity and madness, she revealed her own class-based and gender-based notions of rationality to be a facade.

As someone who established her professional independence on the basis of her ability to police the behavior of other women, Rivet's actions often appear self-serving if not downright hypocritical. Nonetheless, in teasing out her various claims and self-justifications, it becomes clear that Rivet's seemingly strange life story sheds light on innumerable contradictions inherent in the bourgeois, postrevolutionary worldview. The history of *asiles privés*, especially those run by women, reveals the tendency among nineteenth-century elites to construct and then reify boundaries between the home and the outside world; the masculine and the feminine; the scientific and the emotional; the respectable and the disreputable; and, most important, the sane and the insane. The tales Dr. Brierre de Boismont and his daughter told about their family and about the psychiatric profession were meant to reassure people that these binaries remained stable and that irrationality could be contained to the asylum space. Instead, they exposed the instability of all these supposedly natural divisions. As we will see, patients began to use psychiatric understandings of gender and family life against the very professionals who sought to intern them, directly challenging French psychiatry and the various assumptions it took for granted.

CHAPTER 4

Scandalous Asylum Commitments and Patriarchal Power

I N 1840, AN ANONYMOUS AUTHOR published a play condemning the
institutionalization of sane people. Called *The Madhouse Supplier*, its plot
involved a scheming doctor who conspired with the relatives of potential
patients in order to turn a profit. In exchange for their payment, patients' families could commit their inconvenient relations and hold onto family fortunes
themselves. The play's most sympathetic character was Mademoiselle Varlon,
a young woman who hoped to marry an impoverished student much to her
wealthy father's chagrin. He brought her to the asylum several days before she
reached the age of majority, and the doctor diagnosed her with monomania—
supposedly sick with love, her insistence that her feelings were reasonable merely
reinforced the doctor's claim that she suffered from an unhealthy obsession. In
the end, the clever young woman took part in an escape, and agents of the state
put a stop to the illegal machinations of the asylum doctor. As for Mademoiselle
Varlon, she agreed to marry her betrothed on the condition that he become a
lawyer sworn to defend the unjustly interned against "religious, domestic, and
especially medical" inquisitions.[1]

Family conflicts surrounding the commitment process provided plenty of
ammunition for critics of medical power, and the writer of *The Madhouse Supplier* was hardly the only voice railing against the misuse of psychiatric authority
in nineteenth-century France. A full-fledged anti-alienist movement evolved by
the 1860s, focusing on the plights of men and women committed to institutions
against their will.[2] Asylum doctors had worried about their professional reputations before the rise of anti-alienism, as evidenced by the cold shower debate
of the 1840s. However, these concerns intensified and became more justifiable
under shifting political circumstances.

Alienists typically benefited from their association with the state. This was
certainly the case in the Revolutionary era and, again, during Louis-Philippe's
constitutional monarchy, whose government's promotion of bourgeois class
interests had much in common ideologically with the efforts of psychiatric

professionals despite the regime's extremely limited franchise. Yet the July Monarchy ended abruptly in 1848 when liberal and radical members of the middle and working classes rebelled against the elitist government in the name of increased political rights and, in some cases, economic opportunity. The revolution succeeded in bringing about a Second Republic, but it did not last long: the nephew of Napoleon Bonaparte, Louis-Napoleon, was elected president in 1848 and declared himself Emperor in 1852, thereby severely curtailing citizens' ability to openly dissent from the government for nearly two decades. In this context, critics expressed their dissatisfaction with the regime by publicizing abuses committed by the state-sponsored psychiatric system. Accusations of medical maltreatment continued after the 1870 inauguration of the Third Republic, when the denial of patients' liberty appeared especially incongruous with the stated values of a republican government.

While the asylum's critics did not succeed in overturning the law of 1838, their press campaigns represented the beginning of the end for the moral treatment. Critics vocally opposed the hypocrisy of a system that stripped innocent people of their independence under the guise of rehabilitation, calling the asylum a "modern Bastille" that benefited doctors but hurt their patients. Allegations of unjust commitment proved a liability to the psychiatric profession, and doctors regularly attempted to combat negative stereotypes about themselves and their institutions during the last several decades of the century. That said, many charges of unwilling institutionalization focused on the financial motives of patients' families and depicted doctors as convenient coconspirators or even dupes.[3] In this sense the asylum system provided a dangerous backdrop for the enactment of "inquisitions" whose origins resided in the domestic realm.

Representations of these medical dramas reveal a great deal about postrevolutionary family dynamics, especially the contested but steady transition from an authoritarian family ideal to something more sentimental and even egalitarian. We have seen how asylum doctors helped elaborate these family ideals by implying men should wield authority—within the home and society—by virtue of their rationality rather than their sex alone. However, as in the fictional case presented in *The Madhouse Supplier*, fathers who resisted the gradual leveling of familial hierarchies could also use the asylum system to discipline children who failed to display appropriate deference. Psychiatry thus helped to maintain authoritarian family relations despite the profession's intellectual commitment to bourgeois gender and family values. Press attention to cases of unwilling asylum commitment nevertheless often condemned dictatorial conduct within families, and controversial instances of the sequestration of male heads of household indicate that the medico-legal system actually threatened the powers of some fathers in the starkest of terms.

The writings of asylum inmates, in particular, provide evocative snapshots of evolving attitudes towards familial authority and its relationship to mental medicine. While psychiatric and legal discourses greatly circumscribed the options available to the interned when it came to mounting their own defense, the victims of unjust asylum commitment sought to expose their plights to the public whenever possible. Patient voices presented compelling counternarratives to those constructed by the psychiatric community and by family members using the asylum system for their own purposes.[4] The elaboration of these counternarratives, however, depended on each patient's ability to ascertain and manipulate cultural norms, particularly those located at the ever-shifting nexus of psychological disability, gender, and class. Publicizing their circumstances in a way that drew attention and sympathy required the navigation of a cultural landscape seemingly designed to thwart all their efforts. Some managed to do so, while others found themselves trapped—both physically and rhetorically—by the powerful alliance of medicine, the family, and the state.[5]

Despite working at cross purposes, the writings of mental patients featured a number of similarities with those published by doctors, in that patients consistently made use of normative values informed by psychiatry against the psychiatric establishment itself. Tropes associated with the sentimental family—domesticity, benevolent paternalism, personal and familial honor—provided male patients a powerful defense strategy, even if the spread of these same norms narrowed the range of gendered behaviors considered rational and, thus, acceptable. Scandalous asylum commitments drew attention to the constructed and performative dimensions of gender and rationality, undermining both asylum psychiatry and the family ideal it sought to naturalize. Against all odds, gender in nineteenth-century France constituted more than a prop for medical and patriarchal authority (the paired "inquisitions" central to the plot of *The Madhouse Supplier*): it was also a tool with which to challenge these very structures. Tragically, for most patients ensnared by the psychiatric system at the request of their families, this made for a hollow victory.

Asylum Psychiatry and the Legal Foundations of Patriarchal Power

The revolutionary origins of French psychiatry shaped the profession's self-image, as well as its practical role in a society newly rooted in class-based conceptions of merit rather than the legal privileges of the Old Regime. Psychiatric attempts to inculcate bourgeois gender norms in patients as proof of cure, and thereby reify such values, propped up associations between manliness and rationality in a way that aligned perfectly with postrevolutionary understandings of citizenship and economic participation. As we have seen, psychiatry stood for a new kind of freedom, but only for some—like political liberalism itself, the actions and attitudes of asylum doctors simultaneously challenged authoritarian sensibilities and enshrined new limitations. The specialty's connection to the French state likewise reflected this duality, in that laws pertaining to asylum sequestration reinforced the development of anti-authoritarian—but by no means equitable—family relations by curtailing the ability of relatives to imprison one another without medical cause. Such laws, however, were open to manipulation by men hoping to control their children and wives in ways that struck many observers as out of step with modern sensibilities. In spite of the profession's nominally progressive stance, critics leveled accusations of cruelty and corruption against asylum doctors as their legal and cultural influence grew.

In order to fully appreciate the tactics used by unwilling mental patients and their relatives, we must first understand the precise legal codes that regulated familial order during and after the French Revolution, specifically those statutes related to the expression of authority between parents and children and between husbands and wives. The emergence of sentimental family values among bourgeois families can be traced to the eighteenth century. It nonetheless took the intervention of Revolutionary and Napoleonic legislators to connect this way of life to the legal structures of the French state, legitimating it and further fueling its spread. In this way, postrevolutionary legal changes propelled the subtle but persistent shift from an authoritarian to a bourgeois family ideal while providing a new context through which families attempted to settle marital and intergenerational conflicts. The laws most relevant to cases of scandalous asylum commitment involved inheritance, property rights, and marital separation. Equally important was the law of 1838 regulating asylum admissions, although historians have largely neglected this law in discussions of postrevolutionary family legislation.[6] Aside from this addition, the legal status of the French family remained essentially static in the period between the elaboration of the Civil Code in 1804 and the passage of various policies related to child welfare, divorce, and paternity during the early decades of the Third Republic.

While Revolutionary family law and even the more moderate Civil Code created a situation that tempered paternal authority, the law of 1838 served to reestablish a method through which families could control relatives who behaved in a fashion they considered dishonorable, irrational, or financially risky.

This was not the intent of men like Jean-Étienne Dominique Esquirol, the prime force within the psychiatric community who pushed for the law's passage. As indicated during the debate over the cold shower, most asylum doctors considered the creation of a national asylum system a key moment in the profession's attainment of social and cultural authority, and they feared the mistreatment of patients would hurt their fragile reputations. Esquirol and his colleagues nevertheless opened the door for familial abuse of the new regulations. While he believed governmental intervention would secure the humane treatment of insane people and keep sane ones from ending up in asylums, it actually provided a legal means for family members to sequester inconvenient relations for an indeterminate amount of time, now with the state's official seal of approval.

In this respect, the law of 1838 could function as a replacement for the Old Regime *lettre de cachet*.[7] The king issued the *lettre de cachet*, literally a sealed letter, at the request of a family member—most often a male head of household, although there were notable exceptions—to imprison a wife, child, or other relative without trial. This process served to solidify the link between patriarchal and monarchical power and highlighted the interdependence between familial and governmental order. Dissatisfaction with this state of affairs revealed itself in the *cahiers de doléances*, petitions collected throughout France expressing various grievances against the state that the National Assembly took under consideration in 1789. A number of the *cahiers* pointed to the perceived injustice of the *lettre de cachet*,[8] and its abolition was one of many momentous alterations in family law that occurred during the Revolutionary period and shortly thereafter.

Fatherly authority, like kingly authority, was theoretically absolute in the eighteenth century, and when people began to question the legitimacy of the king, they likewise questioned the justness of hierarchical relations within the "small state" of the French household.[9] The *lettre de cachet* established the most obvious link between these two mutually reinforcing forms of domination and blatantly exposed the pernicious influence of arbitrary power on the expression of individual liberty, especially with regard to marriage choice. On the eve of the Revolution, children could control their property once they reached majority and marriage technically required the consent of both husband and wife. However, because of the *lettre de cachet*, parents—particularly fathers—continued to wield significant influence over a child's selection of a spouse, even when that child was an adult man.[10] The National Assembly's speedy abolition of the *lettre de cachet* in 1789 and the release of all those interned through the process who had not been found guilty of a crime attests to the widespread questioning of patriarchal power that occurred in the opening months of the Revolution. Unlike other provisions of family law enacted during the early years of the Revolution, later governments never reversed the abolition of the *lettre de cachet*, thereby striking a definitive blow against the Old Regime household.[11]

Inheritance law likewise underwent profound transformations during the Revolutionary and Napoleonic eras.[12] The first notable change involved the elimination of primogeniture in March 1790. The ability of parents to choose one successor among their children was eventually replaced by a requirement to divide family property evenly among them. By November 1793, the right of children to inherit equally also included illegitimate sons and daughters. Lawmakers ultimately reversed some of the most radical innovations in inheritance law in an effort to re-stabilize paternal authority within the family. Thus, the 1804 Civil Code did not require equal inheritance among legitimate and illegitimate children. In fact, as Suzanne Desan has shown, "natural" children could no longer become heirs at all, merely creditors of their fathers' estates and only if the deceased had explicitly included them in his will.[13] This reaffirmed the power of fathers, giving them more authority to dispense of their property in a manner of their choosing. Nonetheless, the Code maintained that all legitimate children had a right to a portion of the estate even as it also specified that an extra portion could be passed along in whatever way a father saw fit.[14] Few legal channels existed for someone who hoped to disinherit his legally recognized offspring. Some nineteenth-century families, however, eventually maneuvered around this restriction by using the law on asylum commitments.

In the decades following the Revolution but preceding the passage of the 1838 law, it was not uncommon for family members to deliver their purportedly insane relatives for treatment in private asylums. The government provided little oversight of this process and it required merely the support of an asylum director and the payment of boarding fees by the patient's family. The new law stipulated that the directors of public and private institutions could accept "voluntary" patients only with conclusive proof of an individual's deteriorating mental state.[15] Any person seeking the commitment of a relative had to present a doctor's certificate that outlined the particulars of the individual's illness and attested to the necessity of psychiatric treatment. Following placement in an asylum, the prefect of police (in Paris) or the prefect or mayor (in the provinces) would appoint at least one additional doctor to inspect and diagnose the interned individual, who would then be released as soon as doctors declared them cured.[16] Any person who found him- or herself in an asylum through *placement volontaire* could also secure release based on the request of whomever sought to have them interned in the first place.[17] The prefect might demand any patient's immediate discharge as well, and patients could appeal their commitment through the local court unless they had lost their civil status through interdiction.[18]

The second method of sequestration outlined in the law of 1838 did not involve the patient's family, at least not in theory. Patients interned through *placements d'office* found themselves in asylums at the request of governmental authorities. According to the law, the prefect of police could mandate that any person "whose state of mental disturbance might compromise public order or the safety of persons" be committed to a public or private asylum for an indeterminate amount of time.[19] Like family members, prefects needed to outline the circumstances leading up to the initiation of commitment proceedings, and a doctor had to certify the patient's mental instability.[20] The director of the institution subsequently delivered a report on the patient's mental state to the prefect twice a year.[21] If the doctor believed a patient cured, the law required him to immediately inform the prefect, who then determined whether the patient should be set free. The implementation of a *placement d'office* required cooperative interaction between governmental and medical authorities, the two groups specifically mentioned in the 1838 law. In practice, however, the patient's family often brought their relative's condition to police attention.

One final relevant aspect of the law on asylum commitments involved patients' finances. Almost all instances of unjust internment involved money in one way or another. Once put in an asylum, a patient lost the right to freely control their property. Instead, the courts appointed a provisional financial administrator who would see to the patient's best interests.[22] Sometimes the administrator was an employee of the institution or a notary appointed by the court.[23] More often, it was a member of the family—a rather opportune situation for someone wanting to curb the spending habits of a supposedly insane relative. The administrator would pay the patient's debts, collect their revenue, and even represent their interests in legal actions.

The law of 1838 included safeguards meant to protect patients from the financial manipulation of provisional administrators. For example, an impartial judge selected the overseer and their appointment required judicial renewal every three years.[24] Furthermore, a patient could request the additional appointment of a personal curator meant to guarantee that "the income of the insane person is used to improve his lot and hasten his cure" and that "said individual shall be restored to the free exercise of his rights as soon as the situation permits."[25] While the presence of such an advocate made it difficult for relatives to spend a patient's money indiscriminately, relatives still had the option to request a patient's interdiction (i.e., the loss of civil status) on grounds of mental incompetence. If the courts granted the interdiction, the patient's guardian effectively gained control over his or her assets. In sum, the law of 1838 created a new legal context within which to settle family disputes, or at least prolong them indefinitely: it filled the vacuum left by the *lettre de cachet*, replacing the king's seal with the medical certificate.

Institutionalized Sons and the Persistence of Fatherly Authority

One of the first instances of scandalous asylum sequestration occurred shortly after the passage of the 1838 law and involved a father with traditional ideas about paternal authority using the medico-legal system to keep a wayward son from inheriting his fortune. François-Joseph Mistral, a prominent businessman from the South of France, was livid when he discovered that his twenty-two year old son, Jean, had married a young Polish woman without his consent.[26] As a legitimate heir, Jean would inherit his father's property regardless, and Mistral *père* decided to orchestrate his son's internment in order to keep the family wealth out of the young couple's hands. Jean returned to his natal region for medical care following a brief sojourn in Paris, where he had contracted a chest ailment. Once he arrived home his father immediately sent him to the asylum and forced his new wife into the streets. The elder Mistral secured an interdiction shortly after committing Jean against his will, thereby gaining the power to have his son's marriage annulled.[27]

The sequestration of Jean Mistral—who came to be known as the "fou aux soixante millions"—gained notoriety shortly after his internment, when the writer Adolphe Dumas wrote a series of articles in the young man's defense.[28] Dumas presented the *père de famille* as a conniving and money-hungry man whose understanding of the rights and responsibilities of fatherhood flew in the face of modern values. The writer argued "twelve good fathers" should assess François-Joseph Mistral's behavior, implying that a jury of the man's peers would judge him harshly. Conversely, François-Joseph insisted that his actions toward his son actually proved he was a good father. In several letters to the editor published by the local newspaper, he presented himself as an honorable man looking out for the best interests of his family, including his wayward son, whom he hoped to protect from the manipulations of a scheming foreign woman of ill repute.[29] He claimed the institutionalization of the young man fell within his fatherly prerogatives and complained that Dumas's depiction of his personal, family issue constituted an affront to his good name and a threat to his "rights as a father."[30] In time, Dumas abandoned Jean's cause after determining that his

Polish wife was not the virtuous girl he had initially imagined; the local press subsequently ceased to pay attention.

Despite some questioning of François-Joseph's behavior, the outcome of the case suggests that the rhetoric of paternal authority still held a great deal of currency at midcentury, particularly when the father in question was a respected member of the community and his son had a reputation for disobedience and irrationality (often viewed as one and the same). The father Mistral had followed the letter of the law in pursuit of his family's financial interests, which he argued that his son had betrayed by marrying irresponsibly. In this way, the tragic life of Jean Mistral reveals not only the halting nature of authoritarian paternalism's legal and cultural decline but also a fundamental tension within the bourgeois family ideal.

The nineteenth-century family was supposedly built on sentimental foundations; love bonded husbands to wives, parents to children, and brothers to sisters. The legal code supported an individual's right to make his or her own choice regarding the pursuit of marital happiness, thereby perpetuating the sentimental ideal across generations by encouraging ties of affection within each grown child's nuclear segment of the extended family. At the same time, the middle classes celebrated affective family relations at least in part because they helped preserve and expand family wealth in an economically tumultuous society that lacked the protections of primogeniture.[31] Conflict arose when a child's actions appeared to contradict this essential goal by threatening the fortunes of the family as a whole. François-Joseph Mistral effectively argued this was the case when Jean sought to marry a woman he deemed inappropriate: Mistral *père* was merely protecting the family's interests, albeit at the expense of his son. The fact that Jean's support in the press evaporated when his fiancé's apparently sordid past came to light suggests that despotic fatherly behavior was still largely accepted, even within bourgeois families. Jean Mistral would remain locked away for the next forty years, all but forgotten until his father's death.[32]

The case of a middle-aged man named Ernest Faligan had similar overtones but a happier outcome. Relatively few scandalous commitments gained enough public attention to result in wide coverage in the nonmedical press, so it can be difficult to make claims about changing attitudes over time, even when two examples share a number of salient features. A brief comparison of the predicaments faced by Jean Mistral and Ernest Faligan, however, speaks to the persistence of dictatorial family dynamics in the nineteenth century and their ready accommodation within the so-called sentimental family. Faligan's institutionalization occurred in the early 1870s, several decades after the passage of the

1838 law, at a time when many French viewed the psychiatric profession with suspicion. Authoritarian family relations likewise became more controversial as the century wore on, especially after the establishment of the Third Republic.[33] That said, Faligan regained his freedom only when his father gave his blessing, on the condition that his son recoup from his purported illness at the family estate, and not because of any backlash from the press.

Faligan's parents interned him against his will twice in 1873, first in a provincial private institution for several days and later in the Parisian public asylum Charenton for almost nine months.[34] In 1879, one year after his father's death and the subsequent discovery of papers detailing the events surrounding his incarceration, Faligan sent petitions to the Chamber of Deputies and the Senate charging the police with unlawful arrest and sequestration. The publication of two narrative descriptions and a document collection relating his ordeal represented part of the unwilling patient's effort to persuade the government to open an investigation into his treatment.[35] These reports roundly condemned the alliance between state, family, and medical authorities. As in the case of Jean Mistral, Faligan's situation revealed inconsistencies inherent in postrevolutionary family law, not to mention the middle-class family ideal, when it came to the expression of paternal power.

The purported motivations behind the commitments of Faligan and Mistral represented two sides of the same coin, each reflective of parental desires to control a son's marriage choices in order to secure family property. Like most bourgeois parents, Faligan's mother and father aimed to keep family properties intact, and they attempted to force their son into an unwanted marriage to his cousin by threatening him with indefinite internment in an asylum if he did not comply (at least this was Faligan's claim). The would-be patient recalled a tumultuous upbringing marked by near-constant disagreement between himself and his family.[36] As a young man he dreamed of cutting family ties, while his mother and father hoped to ensure his continued dependence. Age forty at the time of his arrest in Paris, he had maintained only irregular contact with most of his relatives during the sixteen years since his arrival in the capital.

The events leading up to Faligan's commitment were complicated and, according to him, required a multiperson conspiracy. He worked in the acquisitions department of the French National Library when his father initiated the commitment plot, although he was also a novelist and a trained doctor of medicine (a fact displayed prominently on the frontispiece of each petition to the legislature). In 1872, he began to suspect his parents of meddling in his personal and professional affairs, and he reluctantly decided to visit them in Angers to

investigate the situation. He soon determined that they aimed to marry him
to his cousin, Louise, to whom he had been promised since childhood, and he
decided to flee. The police arrested the wayward son at the local train station
and sent him to an institution. He was later released thanks to the entreaties
of a friend.

The plot against Faligan escalated upon his return to Paris in late January
1873. With his family's urging and financial backing, several colleagues approached the prefecture of police in Passy with suspicions that their coworker's
behavior had recently become erratic and dangerous. They expressed concern
that he would attempt to burn down the library, persuading the prefect to bring
him in for questioning and an evaluation of his mental state in an effort to trigger
a *placement d'office*. According to Faligan, someone drugged him on the way to
the police station, and he appeared out of sorts when taken to Paris' Sainte-Anne
asylum, where all the city's mental patients went for processing before being
dispatched to other public institutions. Shortly thereafter the authorities transferred Faligan to Charenton, where the asylum director, Doctor Constans, and
his colleague Henri Legrand du Saulle certified his insanity with a diagnosis of
délire de persecution (persecution mania).[37] Faligan's father finally agreed to his
release eight months later on the assurance that his son would return to live in
the family home. Faligan moved back to Paris less than a year after that, at which
point the now unemployed librarian claimed he faced considerable harassment
from his cousins and their various agents within the government. Faligan relocated to Angers between the November 1878 death of his mother and that of his
father almost one year later, and the two men seem to have reached an accord
during this period if not before. He nonetheless expressed fears of another confinement, now at the instigation of his cousins, in writings published six years
after his institutionalization.

It is impossible to determine what is true and what is false in Faligan's narrative. From an outsider's perspective, nothing especially conspiratorial stands out
in the letters discovered and later published by Faligan after his father's death;
while the son saw proof of collusion in his parents' correspondence, their behavior could also reflect genuine concern. In Faligan's case, unlike that of Jean
Mistral, there seems to have been little public pushback against his relatives' and
doctors' claims that he had been institutionalized for his own good, despite his
publication of a vigorous self-defense. If a child exhibited signs of insanity, even
in middle age, his father had every right to step in. The persistence of this idea,
in and of itself, indicates how easily a sentimental family might be confused for
an authoritarian one. The rationale behind the expression of paternal power

might have changed, but many French—certainly those who had influence in the medical, legal, and political realms—maintained the belief that fathers had every right to control their sons under certain circumstances.

Faligan's experience reveals more than the persistence of parental control over children in the nineteenth century, or even the great liability of being perceived as insane at this time. Although we cannot discover the "truth" of his predicament, Faligan's presentation of his story reveals the strategies a man accused of insanity might use to best press his case, no matter the motivations of those behind his sequestration. Faligan's tale was convoluted, but he presented it in a relatively dispassionate and straightforward manner, strategically emphasizing his rationality and trustworthiness. He made evidentiary use of his adversaries' writings by publishing a trove of letters among his parents, his cousins, his doctors, and even people he had once thought of as colleagues and friends. These letters, and the narrative as a whole, underscore the role played by gendered notions of reputation in the tactics of unwilling mental patients and their families.

By virtue of his commitment at Charenton, Faligan found himself in the unenviable position of defending his sanity against some of the most respected and influential alienists of his day. Henri Legrand du Saulle was the preeminent French authority on *délire de persecution,* a common and exceedingly convenient diagnosis for patients who resisted treatment. He famously argued that a significant proportion of Communards suffered from the malady and even used it to their advantage in the months when all of Paris had purportedly "gone mad."[38] Faligan, like most individuals who later published accounts of their internments, sought to present himself as rational by poking holes in Legrand du Saulle's interpretation of his behavior and contesting the terms of his diagnosis. Faligan argued, for example, that people who actually suffered from *délire de persecution* thought the entire world was out to get them, whereas he concerned himself with a very specific group of people who would all benefit financially from his sequestration.[39]

Faligan thus sought to prove his sanity by engaging with alienists in their own language. Although this strategy was not likely to sway the men who initially diagnosed him, Faligan hoped to convince outside observers that he was a rational man struggling to assert his rights within an insane medico-legal system. This did not work very well, since the publication of his lengthy story—especially his numerous diatribes against government officials he called "shadowy" and "occult"—could itself be construed as a symptom of persecution mania, as the legislative tribunal seemed to conclude.[40] The deaths of Faligan's parents probably ensured his continued freedom, but the Senate rejected his call for an investigation into police conduct.

As a corrective against the accusations of his doctors, Faligan regularly highlighted his social connections to men whose own performances of bourgeois, rational manhood proved beyond reproach: old friends and mentors who happened to be doctors themselves. He had trained in medicine before leaving his home province for Paris in his mid-twenties and had worked in a hospital before changing careers. A friend from university named Doctor Combes rushed to Faligan's aid when he learned of his initial sequestration at the private asylum in Saint-Gemmes. Combes vouched for his former classmate's soundness of mind, secured his release, and delivered him to the train station for his trip back to Paris. In this way, Faligan undermined the family plot against him and briefly regained his independence before being rearrested and eventually sent to Charenton. Faligan also stressed his reputation among other medical men when he made his case to the legislature some years later, specifically citing his status as a titular member of the Société du Médecine of Angers at the invitation of his mentor, Doctor Farges. He went so far as to republish the letter from the medical society first announcing his membership in the document collection relating the events of 1873. While his induction occurred long after his initial confinement, Faligan pointed out that Farges had also helped orchestrate his release from Charenton.

Faligan's attempt to combat his diagnosis through his acquaintance with other professional men suggests that the definition of madness was not so much objectively fixed as agreed upon communally through an informal process of perception, judgment, and consensus. Alienists had long claimed this role for themselves, but despite the stamp of professional legitimacy conferred by the law of 1838, the authority to determine who was and was not sane never confined itself to the psychiatric community. The cultural project of demarcating lucidity from madness was profoundly gendered, both in terms of its conclusions and the individuals who had a say in establishing them. Faligan's case revolved around decisions made by bourgeois men about who should be considered sane and, therefore, accepted as an equal and a peer.

Asylum doctors, the Angers medical society, judges, legislators, and a large cast of assorted colleagues and friends—what they all shared, aside from their influence over Faligan's fate, was their class and gender. The frustrated patient seemed well aware of this fact and planned his self-presentation accordingly, trying to convince his readers of his personal honor by linking himself to other honorable men. He might not have succeeded in having his case reopened, but he almost certainly safeguarded his freedom when he became a member of the medical society in Angers. If Legrand du Saulles's diagnosis had first certified Faligan's insanity, then his inclusion in a professional society signaled the opposite.

The sequestrations of Jean Mistral and Ernest Faligan took place several decades apart, but the legal apparatus stayed constant throughout this time. The divergent outcomes speak more to personality differences between the major players than a changing legislative context. Nonetheless, had Jean Mistral's father committed him in the 1870s rather than the 1840s, his unfortunate son's fate might have been very different. When the story of the "fou au soixante millions" came to light in 1886 the public reacted with widespread horror, leading to the prisoner's immediate release (although Mistral died shortly after leaving the asylum).

Despite this apparent change in values, many individuals continued to face forced sequestration in the final decades of the nineteenth century, even after the establishment of the Third Republic and the election of legislators presumably more critical of the most anti-democratic aspects of the asylum system. It still required social connections, luck, and a knack for self-presentation—all advantages possessed by Ernest Faligan—for the unwillingly interned to push back against those who sought to commit them. If anything, the cases of Jean Mistral and Ernest Faligan each show continuities between the Old Regime and the nineteenth century in that bourgeois family dynamics appeared to readily accommodate oppressive treatment by fathers toward their sons when accusations of insanity were thrown into the mix. Asylum doctors' own self-fashioning as sentimental father figures who nonetheless insisted on absolute psychiatric authority indicates much the same. Disappointed, angry, or merely worried heads of household, however, were not the only people institutionalizing their relatives in nineteenth-century France—sometimes they were the ones locked away.

Irrational Husbands in an Age of Reason

French family law encouraged the misuse of the asylum system by unscrupulous relatives by allowing parents who resented the newfound freedoms of children a chance to maintain hierarchical family dynamics, and some fathers, like François-Joseph Mistral, faced criticism for using the medico-legal system to keep children from exercising their rights. Republican polemics describing asylums as modern Bastilles, places more suited to the political atmosphere of the absolutist monarchy than that of a modern nation-state, likewise indicated discomfort with the way medical and familial collusion might undermine the freedoms conferred by citizenship. These critiques point to fears of a return to a prerevolutionary past, a time when individual happiness was subsumed by the demands of family and monarchy in both a cultural and legal sense. However, representations of madness and family strife also suggest that psychiatry had a less expected and seemingly contradictory effect on nineteenth-century family and gender values. If the experiences of Jean Mistral or Ernest Faligan reveal continuities between the Old Regime and the postrevolutionary family, the institutionalization of heads of household reveals an aspect of psychiatry far less accommodating to the maintenance of patriarchal authority.

Honoré de Balzac recognized that new attitudes toward rationality and madness had the potential to undermine fatherly power. He presented this perspective in one of his lesser-known entries of *The Human Comedy*, titled *L'Interdiction* in reference to the legal process through which an individual might lose their civil status.[41] The action unfolds over several days in 1828, making the Civil Code rather than the asylum law of 1838 the most relevant legal context. Like other works by Balzac, *L'Interdiction*, first published in 1836, bemoans the superficiality and acquisitiveness that supposedly defined postrevolutionary family life. The plot revolves around the plight of the Marquis d'Espard, a father and husband whose wife, the Marquise, attempts to have him declared incompetent by the state. A fair-minded judge, Popinot, is put in charge of the investigation, and the reader slowly learns the details of the case through his eyes. It is clear from the start that we are not to trust the Marquise, who we first meet in a discussion between the lawyer and social-climber Eugène de Rastignac and his friend, the doctor Bianchon. Honest Bianchon describes the Marquise as a "woman of fashion," and, like others of her ilk, she "is no longer a woman: she is neither mother, nor spouse, nor lover."[42] She supposedly "has more head than heart" and is prepared to sacrifice both her friends and her so-called "true passions" if it means achieving her social and financial ambitions.[43] Balzac depicts the Marquise as self-interest personified: an expert in deception, not to mention ruthlessly rational.

By the time the plot of *L'Interdiction* begins, the Marquis and the Marquise have been separated for over a decade; they married in 1812 and had two children before parting ways in 1815. The couple live independent of one another, the husband controlling his family wealth while the Marquise lives off her dowry. The Marquise proffers a diverse array of evidence in her attempt to prove that her husband is insane. Most damningly, he is slowly but surely giving away his fortune (to an unattractive woman, at that). But he also keeps his wife from seeing her children, pays undue respect to those beneath his station, and is profoundly obsessed with the history and culture of China.

In the end the reader discovers a logical explanation for each of these charges. The Marquise supposedly lacks maternal instinct and her boys prefer spending time with their father, a man of generous spirit; as judge Popinot notes, the only madness he sees in this situation is that "the children are a little crazy for their father and he a little crazy for them."[44] As for giving away his money, this too stems from generosity. It turns out that the Espard fortune derived from the seizure of Protestant lands after the revocation of the Edict of Nantes. The poor woman receiving payments from the Marquis is the descendant of the original landowners, and Espard sees himself as righting a historical injustice by returning the money to her. Making the political implications of this setup clear, Balzac likens this Protestant family to the noble *émigrés* whose lands were seized during the Revolution. Perhaps most amusingly, the Marquis's fixation on China also contains a none-too-subtle critique of Revolutionary France—he admires the Chinese Empire because it is "a place where revolution is not possible."[45] Popinot rejects the scheming wife's interpretation of events, noting that "an interdiction can only be granted when a man's actions are devoid of reason," while those of the Marquis are "based on the most sacred and honorable of motives."[46] In a last-minute twist, the Marquise uses her significant influence in high society to go above the judge's head, and it is implied she will get her way.

For Balzac, the interdiction process offered an ideal scenario through which to explore common themes within *The Human Comedy*. The Napoleonic Code's treatment of madness and money sets the stage for his evisceration of postrevolutionary values writ large. Balzac's France is a topsy-turvy world in which vice is masked as virtue and surface appearances count as truth. The perspective put forth in the novel is not necessarily opposed to the process of interdiction itself, but to its openness to manipulation by a greedy woman in a corrupt society. The unsupported charge of insanity against a loving, aristocratic *père de famille* gives credence to Balzac's belief that postrevolutionary France is itself a world gone mad. The misogynistic portrayal of the Marquise, in particular, supports his contention that the family had become an institution built on financial expediency rather than ties of affection or respect. Here, the noble father embodies the sentimental family ideal, while his wife merely pretends to do so.

Balzac's critique contained a great deal of misplaced nostalgia, in that the *lettre de cachet* had likewise facilitated the summary incarceration of inconvenient relatives during the Old Regime (interdiction itself was a holdover from the previous century which, unlike the *lettre de cachet*, at least involved a lengthy and expensive legal inquiry).[47] Nonetheless, his depiction of the postrevolutionary family held more than a kernel of truth. The Revolution's attack on paternal authority—at the level of the state and that of the household—combined with newly emerging psychiatric practices in a fashion that did, in fact, undermine the traditional prerogatives of fathers.

This involved a subtle shift in the basis of paternal authority despite the patriarchal agenda embedded in the Civil Code. After the Revolution, both the law and the medical establishment legitimated the father's preeminence within the home on the basis of his supposedly natural rational capacities. As shown, the first asylum doctors played a significant role in the creation and perpetuation of gender-based definitions of rationality: for example, by suggesting that women who did not conform to the ideals of bourgeois domesticity were insane or that women's biology made them especially susceptible to madness. These notions clearly hurt women and aggrandized the power of men, in that the conceptual link between femininity and irrationality justified women's subordination in both the family and the polity. The flip side to this, however, was that charges of madness could now be used against husbands and fathers who did not seem to embody the new requirements of masculine comportment, like Balzac's Marquis d'Espard.

Accusations of insanity against husbands and fathers were not confined to the realm of fiction. Men and women found themselves committed to French asylums in equal numbers until at least the 1860s, according to Aude Fauvel.[48] This suggests the perpetuation of rational masculinity as a gender ideal could be dangerous for men whose behaviors fell outside the bounds of this new standard in one way or another, even if the assumed connection between manliness and rationality proved a boon for men as a whole (and for professional men in particular). Furthermore, while institutionalization threatened men who rebelled against the bourgeois family ideal in some way—through homosexual activity or libertinage, to name just two examples—men who conformed to middle-class expectations regarding family life also risked commitment under certain circumstances, and not only when their decisions contradicted the desires of their parents, as in the cases of Jean Mistral and Ernest Faligan.

To appear mad during the nineteenth century proved such a liability that not even the privileges of normative masculinity could entirely shield an individual from its consequences. At the same time, husbands and fathers committed against their will also constituted the subsection of the patient population most able to mobilize gender ideology to their advantage. Tellingly, while Balzac depicts the calculating rationality of the Marquise as both unwomanly and unnatural, he takes great pains to characterize the aristocratic Marquis d'Espard as a benevolent, kindhearted father figure—and it is this that wins the judge to his side.

Real-life examples of scandalous asylum commitment expose in full color what literary examples only hint at and what psychiatric case notes tend to obscure. By virtue of their notoriety, such cases were distinct from the vast majority in which patients faced the coalition of medical, familial, and state power in relative obscurity. First-person accounts nonetheless allow uncommon insight into the self-presentation strategies embodied by patients in their attempts to gain release. One particular case exhibited how the new rational masculine ideal could pose a danger to fathers, especially aging ones. Hippolyte Delas, who claimed his daughters and his sons-in-law orchestrated his asylum commitment, initially published his recollections anonymously in 1870, seven years after the fact, under the title *Histoire d'une maladie*.[49] Over the next two decades this first protestation against injustice would turn into a full-fledged crusade, as he took his desire for vengeance to the republican press. He wrote many articles under his own name for *L'Union républicaine* and eventually published a collection of anti-alienist writings in 1886 called *Les Bastilles modernes: nécessité de leur destruction*.[50]

Some who published accounts of their asylum experiences tried to present themselves as rational, insisting they did not deserve to be treated like asylum patients because they were not actually insane. This father, however, admitted that he experienced bouts of dementia and had not felt like himself in the weeks that led up to his eventual commitment in a private mental institution. Even the title of Delas's first book—*The Story of an Illness*—indicates a surprising level of forthrightness concerning his condition. Delas insisted that his daughters and sons-in-law arranged for his internment in 1863 at a moment of mental fragility, persuading other members of his extended family to go along with their nefarious plot in order to hasten his death and speed up the collection of their inheritance. Rather than proclaim his sanity, he decried the laws and attitudes that could result in the confinement of *any* individual—rational or not. "I did not know," wrote the unwilling patient, "that to be ill was the greatest of crimes, punished with the most frightening of punishments."[51] It was bad enough to be frightened of imaginary dangers, but commitment to an asylum justified his paranoia, making his subconscious fears "effectively real and the most frightening of all."[52]

Delas's personal experience showed him that collusion between alienists and patients' families undermined both the values of bourgeois domesticity and the

purported goals of the medical profession. He consistently contrasted his experiences inside the asylum to the peacefulness of the domestic ideal and showed
how his engagement with the psychiatric system polluted his family life. For
example, in *Histoire d'une maladie*, he criticized his sons-in-law for viewing the
family as a source of potential profit rather than a source of affection. Of one
son-in-law he wrote: "[I had] given my daughter [to him] believing he was an
honest man," only to have him become "the executor of my incarceration in
a place comparable to hell."[53] By conspiring with medical authorities, Delas's
sons-in-law spread this corrupted image of domestic life to the family as a whole.
His daughters turned against the father who raised them, his mother was too
feeble to defend him, and his wife ("as violent and troubled" as himself) was
afraid she would be committed to the asylum too.[54]

The unwilling patient also emphasized that asylum employees collected him
in his father's home—a place he insisted should be safe from intrusion. He asked,
"Was it possible for me to predict that because I went to take refuge at my father's
house under the vague impression that I was menaced by a danger, I would be
abandoned by him in such a way, after having committed no sin but to go to
embrace him?"[55] The family home, in theory closed to the dangers of the outside
world, led the distraught Delas to the asylum. There he faced a litany of horrific
experiences, including confinement in straitjackets, subjection to the notorious
cold shower, isolation in a cell, and the chaining of his neck and arms to his bed.

Delas's spell in the asylum led to the permanent severing of family ties. The
entire family had worked to arrange for his internment; although some relatives
might have believed it to be in his best interests, he understandably interpreted
their actions as a personal betrayal.[56] In the end, his wife regained her composure
and felt strong enough to demand his release. Yet it was impossible for Delas
to truly go home again. As he explained, "The victim who survives becomes a
frightening specter to the guilty."[57] Furthermore, his sons-in-law were no longer
welcome in his company, particularly if he ever experienced another period of
irrationality. They had proven they could not be trusted. Even if his family's
intentions were honest, another trip to the asylum would be unforgivable. "My
illness," concluded Delas, "had been caused by my imagination alone, but they
[his sons-in-law] were no less culpable; because, instead of trying heal me, they
tried only to make me incurable!"[58] He charged his family and the psychiatric
establishment with joining forces in the internment of a devoted husband and
father, irreparably destroying the tranquility of the household in the process.

Interest in cases of scandalous commitment intensified during the final decade of the Second Empire and continued to gain steam throughout the 1870s

and 1880s, when the image of the unjustly interned husband proved especially sensational. In November 1871, a mere six months after the fall of the Paris Commune, a play called *La Baronne* opened at the famous Odéon theater. The plot revolved around the machinations of the eponymous baroness, Edith, who sets her sights on marrying an elderly French aristocrat. Having already lost one fortune in an inheritance dispute and now the mistress of a penniless doctor, Edith wants to have her cake and eat it too—she will marry the old man, wait for him to die, then reunite with her true love as a rich widow. The physical health of Edith's new husband, however, proves hardier than she had hoped, and she soon orchestrates his internment in a psychiatric institution. She is on the verge of convincing the courts to grant her control of the patient's finances when he escapes the asylum and strangles his duplicitous wife with her own necklace—a visually disarming piece of jewelry that looks like a snake wrapped around the neck, a gift from her lover the doctor.

The playwrights, Edouard Foussier and Charles Edmond, were well aware that family drama lie at the heart of most unjust commitment scandals. Cases like that of the elderly Hippolyte Delas, however, did not serve as *La Baronne*'s primary source of inspiration, for the well-received play paid little attention to the issue of intergenerational conflict. In fact, the baron's daughter, played by a young Sarah Bernhardt, was the most sympathetic character and the only person interested in securing her father's best interests rather than a share of his considerable estate. Instead, like Balzac, Foussier and Edmond focused on the role played by a plotting wife in her husband's eventual downfall. *La Baronne* thus capitalized on the legitimate fear of unjust asylum commitment alongside a well-known nineteenth-century bogeyman: the overtly sexual, not to mention heartless and logical, woman.

The gender politics of *La Baronne* were profoundly conservative, and the play's conclusion represented a fantasy of masculine authority in an era of intense instability. Yet its plot also shared some uncanny similarities with a notable, real-life commitment scandal known as the "Puyparlier Affair." The case had recently gained widespread attention after an asylum inmate named Auguste Fault du Puyparlier, a former soldier in the North African campaign and an inductee of the Legion of Honor, spectacularly and mysteriously escaped from the Tribunal of Paris while present for an appeal hearing.[59] Like other victims of involuntary asylum confinement, Puyparlier began publishing refutations of his supposed insanity. The main similarity between *La Baronne* and the Puyparlier Affair was the role of the patient's wife in the commitment plot. The characters in the play were significantly wealthier than Puyparlier and his wife, but the timing of its production suggests that actual events inspired it. Observers like the satirist "Crispino" linked the two, grouping Puyparlier, the writers of *La Baronne*, and even the once exiled champion of the oppressed, Victor Hugo, in an imagined meeting of the fictional "Society for the Protection of the Alienated," published in Bertall's *La Revue comique* in 1871.[60] Puyparlier himself referred to another incident of unjust internment that occurred nearly simultaneously, involving a man sent to an institution by his wife and her lover, the asylum's director, with which the creators of *La Baronne* might also have been acquainted.[61]

Police arrested Puyparlier in his hometown of Beauvais, located approximately eighty kilometers north of Paris, in 1869. They accused him of acting erratically (he had been seen without his pants in public), and his wife claimed that he could no longer be trusted with their finances.[62] As in several other instances of unjust internment, Puyparlier argued he had been drugged before his confrontation with the police.[63] He wrote of a vast conspiracy involving his wife, members of her family, asylum doctors, and even household servants. Supposedly poisoned during a long lunch when the prefect of police searched his home, Puyparlier lost consciousness only to wake up inside the imposing Parisian asylum Charenton. He immediately began writing letters to his lawyer and other possible allies, including journalists and newspaper editors, in hopes that his sequestration could be legally challenged.[64] After successfully persuading the Tribunal of Paris to hear his case, he managed to flee from the courthouse through a private stairwell.[65] According to his obituary (he died in 1875), Puyparlier settled in England after this daring escape but returned to France following the fall of the empire and the death of his wife.

Like others in his position, Puyparlier forcefully argued that his commitment to an asylum was unwarranted. Involuntary asylum internment did not benefit his mental health; it merely aided his wife's pocketbook. After learning of her death he returned to France for the funeral and even wrote her epitaph:

> Ci-git ma femme! Oh! Qu'elle est bien,
> Pour son repose et pour le mien![66]

> (Here lies my wife! Oh! That she is well,
> For her rest and for mine!)

Clearly in good spirits, Puyparlier had the last laugh. Yet his published descriptions of his commitment and the events preceding it were far more serious in tone and offer an insightful perspective on the historical relationship between marital discord and psychiatric authority. Puyparlier cited "conjugal rebellion" as the root of his painful situation, writing in dramatic terms about his wife's premeditated manipulation of all the resources at her disposal in her efforts to secure his sequestration.[67] Her collusion with psychiatric authorities—whom the aging soldier called "a horde of foreign rascals" (because they resided in Paris, but sometimes collected patients in the provinces) and "undignified public functionaries"—was particularly loathsome for Puyparlier.[68] He wrote his "cry against injustice" in order to expose the ways a "rebel wife" could "counter all human and divine laws" to intern her husband in an insane asylum against his will.[69]

Puyparlier adeptly presented an image of his life and his marriage that served to vilify his wife without emasculating himself in the process. He was the perpetually abused but always loyal husband. He described his fate in dramatic and even heroic terms, highlighting his personal courage and resilience in the "battle" against those who sought to institutionalize him. He wrote of the "blood in (his) veins" that inspired the publication of his story and his disinclination toward scandal and "noise."[70] Puyparlier also depicted himself as a victim of what he called "feminine hate."[71] He and his wife had been married for sixteen years before his arrest and institutionalization. In a document produced by Puyparlier in order to prove his "moral sense," he spoke at length of their strained interactions. His wife tried to undermine his authority and control their finances, living in so-called "open rebellion" for much of their time together.[72] Against the advice of his priest and others acquainted with the couple, the aggrieved husband refused to keep a close eye on his spouse or attempt to regulate her actions or choices. Throughout their tense marriage, he defended her against the accusations of others and refused to take a mistress despite their estrangement. Puyparlier did all this, he said, because it was his duty and because he was a "gallant man."[73]

Like disagreements over inheritance, marital conflicts also played out within a specific legislative context. That most relevant to the Puyparlier Affair concerned the 1816 abolition of divorce following its brief legalization during the Revolutionary era. The re-legalization of divorce had long been a rallying cry and a goal of republicans, albeit one that often took a back seat to what they considered more pressing political concerns. During the Second Empire hopes for reform remained largely silent due to press censorship. The question of divorce came to the fore, however, during the 1870s and early 1880s, as republicans gradually secured control of the government and gained the ability to change the status quo. Numerous French people began voicing their discontents over their inability to legally and permanently sever marital ties, including the frustrated mental patient Puyparlier.

In many ways, and despite certain passages that carry a potentially misogynistic tone (notably his preoccupation with "feminine hate"), Puyparlier viewed himself as rather enlightened when it came to the question of marital and gender relations. He never promoted a return to more authoritarian conception of familial order; he did not, for example, hint that his wife owed him complete obedience by virtue of her sex or their marital status. His solution to marital unhappiness was both simple and forward-looking. Rather than harking back to a time in which the right of husbands to control their wives was taken for granted, the elderly veteran called for the right to divorce. It was "the object of ardent dreams for all honest hearts" and the "only moral counterweight to imprudent agreements."[74]

If he and his wife could legally and amicably separate, he never would have ended up in an asylum against his will. He could have divorced her before it came to that or she could have divorced him. Thus, Puyparlier took his critique of the asylum one step further than his contemporary, Delas. Not only did he present his mistreatment at the hands of the medical establishment as a perversion of bourgeois domestic values but he insisted that the middle-class cult of marriage was itself part of the problem. Or, perhaps more accurately, Puyparlier suggested that the only way to ensure the sanctity of companionate marriage was to allow incompatible couples to separate legally. Not surprisingly, the writers of *La Baronne* chose not to capitalize on this aspect of Puyparlier's story and instead focused on the cruel machinations of a money-hungry femme fatale.

Fictional portrayals of "mad" husbands exposed the gender anxieties of their time. Balzac regretted the passing of eighteenth-century family relations, showing with characteristic astuteness that the cultural and legal prioritization of rationality led to a potential rebalancing of power within the household. *La Baronne* picked up on a similar theme much later in the century and in more sensational fashion, as concerns over women's involvement in the public sphere began to escalate in the early Third Republic. Both stories feature a woman character whose rationality is presented as simultaneously cool and cruel. In this sense, *L'Interdiction* and *La Baronne* each relied on a stereotype—the logical woman as unnatural aberration—that alienists reified and helped to create, even if both works critiqued the pernicious influence of psychiatric authority.

Patient writings, on the other hand, exhibited a more subtle understanding of the nineteenth-century domestic ideal. Delas and Puyparlier understood the liability of madness in a rational age, yet neither man seemed to desire a return to more despotic gender and family relations. Delas attempted to use the behavioral repertoire of sentimental fatherhood to attack the psychiatric claim that institutionalization constituted the only valid response to mental distress. For his part, Puyparlier insisted that affective ties held meaning only if spouses had the right to dissolve them. In other words, neither man looked nostalgically to a prerevolutionary past and both, in one way or another, questioned widespread cultural assumptions concerning gender and psychiatric disability. That they were able do so points to the power of bourgeois masculinity in spite of the frightful prospects faced by men who did not meet its standards. Ironically, in rare lucky cases, men deemed insane successfully argued against their treatment at the hands of the psychiatric profession because doctors themselves had so effectively naturalized cultural assumptions regarding the ingrained rational capacities of middle-class men.

AT FIRST GLANCE, the history of the asylum and its relation to men's household authority might appear to support a continuity thesis rather than one centered on rupture and change. Like fathers and husbands of the Old Regime, those of the postrevolutionary era held considerable power over the lives of their wives and children by virtue of the Civil Code and the 1838 asylum law. Patriarchy—defined as a social and legal system where fathers hold power over women and younger men—spanned the eighteenth and nineteenth centuries and helped structure relations of gender and generation within "authoritarian" and "sentimental" families alike. Yet, as cases of scandalous asylum commitment show, the power dynamics of the nineteenth-century home were defined by a new sort of fatherly authority—one based more on men's purported rationality than their sexual virility or physical strength.

Cases of contested asylum commitment indicate that the postrevolutionary conflation of rationality and rights had a profound impact on the history of the French family, particularly with respect to the move away from the authoritarian family relations of the eighteenth century to the affective bourgeois ones of the nineteenth. Furthermore, highlighting the stories of unwillingly incarcerated men situates the nineteenth century as a transitional moment between the dictatorial family structure of the Old Regime and today's modern family. It becomes clear from this vantage point that gender and psychiatry were not only intertwined by virtue of their disciplining effects on nineteenth-century women, but also, ironically, through their long-term contribution to the emergence of more egalitarian family relations. By insisting that an individual's rationality conferred their autonomy, doctors suggested that rational women might deserve equal rights in the home and beyond. Here, as in the case of our women private asylum *directrices* from the preceding chapter, the actions of alienists subtly eroded the naturalization of gender difference.

As Balzac sensed, the postrevolutionary emphasis on rationality as the defining trait of personhood held the potential to undermine patriarchal authority within the home, as it had already undermined the concept of absolutist monarchy outside of it. While he was critical of this change, others saw it as an opportunity to rid themselves of inconvenient relatives. The nineteenth-century family might have been sentimental, but it could also be vicious—and it is really no wonder, considering the stakes. The cultural elevation of the rational individual combined with the particulars of French family law to create a perfect storm, in which representatives of the state, the psychiatric community, and the family might conspire against individuals accused of insanity in order to secure family property. As the century progressed, voices protesting against the psychiatric profession and the domestic conflicts it engendered continued to accumulate. Eventually, doctors themselves would begin to seriously question the value of the asylum as a curative space for the first time since the French Revolution, a tendency exacerbated by the national crises of the Franco-Prussian War and the Paris Commune.

CHAPTER 5

Rehabilitating a Profession under Siege

H ENRI BONNET, THE ALIENIST and director of the provincial Roche-
Gandon asylum, made an unusual decision after returning home from
a trip to Paris: he wrote a theater review. Bonnet had recently attended
a performance of the popular melodrama *La Baronne* and left concerned by its
depiction of the psychiatric profession. As shown, the play exploited contemporary fears over the unjust confinement of individuals in mental institutions by
focusing on the attempts of a greedy femme fatale to sequester her rich husband
with the help of an asylum doctor. Bonnet published his take in the *Annales
médico-psychologiques* for an audience of his peers, many of whom had already
expressed worry over well-publicized attacks on their reputations, noting the
play could open the profession "to scandal and lead to the discrediting of alienists."[1] Like many an asylum doctor before him, Bonnet decried the so-called
"war declared against alienists" that had, at this point, been a source of concern
for at least a decade.[2]

While doctors like Bonnet persisted in representing the profession as un-
fairly attacked by the critics of arbitrary confinement, clashes of a less meta-
phorical variety had recently overshadowed such public relations battles. France
experienced invasion, siege, and civil war between the fall of 1870 and the
spring of 1871. The Franco-Prussian War had as much to do with Otto von Bismarck's calculated march toward German national unification as it did with
any deep-seated conflict between the two European powers. France's devastat-
ing and embarrassing loss nonetheless had profound consequences for French
politics and national self-esteem. The war began in July 1870 and resulted in
regime change by early September. Some 80,000 French soldiers, along with the
emperor Louis-Napoleon himself, surrendered to Prussian forces at the Battle
of Sedan, and a coalition of politicians—liberal, conservative, and even mon-
archist—soon declared a republic in his absence. Unlike the governments of
1789 and 1848, what came to be known as the Third Republic was more the

product of political expediency than popular revolution. The new regime faced considerable challenges in both the short and long term as the war continued despite the changed political circumstances. Paris suffered under siege for five long months and the government, relocated to Bordeaux and later Versailles, finally capitulated in February 1871 to the dismay of many citizens of the capital. Fault lines soon become apparent between the conservatives of the national government and the popular classes of Paris, with Parisians declaring home rule in March 1871. The Third Republic subsequently massacred, exiled, and imprisoned thousands of revolutionary supporters of the Paris Commune in May of that same year.

The impact of these events stretched the limits of a chronically underfunded and already precarious asylum system. In certain respects, the period of turmoil wounded the image of the all-powerful doctor-father that alienists had attempted to project since the time of Pinel. Public and private asylum operators faced unprecedented challenges when it came to "consoling," let alone curing, their patients. Those who ran asylums located in Paris and its environs, where doctors had no choice but to rely on the goodwill of others for the maintenance of their institutions, were in especially insecure positions. However, the tumult also provided uncommon opportunities for doctors to promote a positive vision of the psychiatric community at a particularly low point for their public reputations. As the unwillingly institutionalized critic of the asylum system, Hippolyte Delas, had recently charged, doctors' power and status relied on appearances: in presenting themselves with "perfect propriety on the *outside*," they maintained the illusion that "The craft that they practiced could only be an honest one because they have such an honest air!"[3] The crises of 1870–1871 afforded doctors the chance to reassert this honest image, both on the spot and after the fact.

Medical men struggled through the Franco-Prussian War and the Paris Commune alongside their patients, and several chose to publish their interpretations of the events in the months that followed. Some of these writings took the form of personal narratives, while others were professional assessments of the impact of war and political trauma on cases of mental illness (and vice versa). These publications proved powerful tools in doctors' efforts to reshape their public personae. Like the unjustly interned patients of the previous chapter, doctors made use of the gender norms their own medical theories and practices had served to consolidate as they built their reputations and made their assessments. In some cases, they were satisfied to simply remind audiences of admirable actions undertaken by members of the profession during troubled times, often by drawing attention to doctors' exhibition of long-standing attributes of masculine self-presentation. Others narrated the experiences of the psychiatric community in ways that linked the profession with the forces of order. In these accounts, doctors presented themselves as bourgeois men dedicated to the values of the nascent Third Republic. Most obviously, they did so through their diagnoses of Communards and the equation of revolution with madness, but they accomplished something similar through less sensational explanations of the day-to-day functioning of institutional spaces during the siege.

Doctors aligned themselves with the Third Republic in ways both subtle and direct, constructing their gendered self-presentations as individuals and professionals but also as members of their class and nation. The republican press had often supported anti-alienist positions during the 1860s, in part because critiquing the psychiatric system allowed them to attack Louis-Napoleon by proxy while avoiding the ire of governmental censors.[4] But the actions of alienists also seemed to genuinely contradict republican principles. Doctors would need to win the new government to their side following the fall of the Empire if they wanted to maintain their cultural authority or even their livelihoods: that they largely succeeded speaks both to the astuteness of their self-presentation strategies and to the relative conservatism of the Third Republic (which did not set up a constitutional structure until 1875 and was, even then, dominated by monarchists and conservatives until the 1880s). Opposition to workers' rights was a consistent if contested aspect of French government policy throughout the late nineteenth century, a stance legitimated by the pronouncements of much of the psychiatric community in the aftermath of the events of 1870–1871.[5]

Alienists' personal reputations and that of the profession writ large looked better after the war and the Commune than they had in some time, despite concerns expressed by those like Bonnet. Psychiatry's public relations successes would, in turn, further strengthen the profession's position against critics. Observers continued to critique the asylum system well past the fall of the Second Empire, but alienists managed to aggrandize their influence throughout the early Third Republic in spite of continued backlash from the unjustly interned and their allies.[6] Indeed, medical involvement in judicial and legislative affairs precipitously increased in the decades preceding the First World War. The period of 1870–1871 therefore represents a crucial moment in the history of the profession, one whose success relied yet again on alienists' ability to cultivate gender- and class-based self-presentations well suited to their political context.

The Profession as Savior

French asylum doctors' descriptions of the *événements* provide a great deal of information about the functioning of institutional spaces during the period of crisis, in addition to underlining the continued relevance of now familiar aspects of psychiatric masculinity. Reports from Parisian bureaucrats emphasized the independence and self-reliance of the psychiatric profession by de-emphasizing the impact of war on asylum operations and consistently giving credit to doctors alone for the survival of their institutions. The Parisian private asylum operator Alexandre Brierre de Boismont highlighted another key aspect of the doctorly persona by presenting himself as a self-sacrificing father figure to his patients, even at times of profound distress. Both these narratives served to promote the psychiatric profession by showing its resilience against great odds. Critics had accused doctors of abusing their power, which was nearly absolute inside the walls of their institutions. Having that power taken from them through circumstances well beyond their control gave alienists a chance to convince people that they deserved to wield such authority after all.

Doctors in the Department of the Seine faced exceedingly trying circumstances during the Franco-Prussian War. City officials of all stripes sensed the oncoming disruption of their normal operations following the military disasters of Sedan and Metz, and the inhabitants of the capital prepared for the invasion of the Prussian army in the opening days of September 1870. Institutions inside the city of Paris were in an especially alarming position once the siege began: without food entering the city, there was no guarantee that patients could be properly fed. Malnutrition left them vulnerable to disease, not to mention the physical threat and emotional strain caused by Prussian bombardment. Asylums in the occupied territories were no better off. The directors of asylums just outside the city were left to their own devices, attempting to procure necessities and ensure the operation of their institutions without aid or communication from central authorities. Even public institutions in unoccupied zones faced difficulties because they were forced to operate without customary direction from the capital.

The organization of patient admissions in the department had been recently revamped as part of Baron Haussmann's efforts to streamline city administration in the 1860s. The first step in the admissions process involved an examination at the prefecture of police, often on the request of the patient's family, after which the potential internee was driven by coach to the Sainte-Anne asylum. There doctors performed a second examination and determined whether institutionalization was necessary. The next step depended largely on the patient's household income. Doctors sent patients who could afford it to Charenton, which accepted only those who could pay 900–1,500 francs per year. Patients designated as the most severely afflicted went to Bicêtre (for men) and the Salpêtrière (for women), both of which were located within Paris proper. The rest either remained at Sainte-Anne or entered one of two facilities located in the Seine-et-Oise, the department neighboring Paris. These asylums, Vaucluse and Ville-Evrard, had only recently opened when war broke out. Both were built on great expanses of land where patients, including "aliénés" and "idiots valides," did agricultural and other forms of manual labor as a form of treatment and source of funding.[7]

The Assistance Publique, the government agency under whose umbrella these various asylums fell, began to reorganize admissions processes when it became clear the Prussian army would make its way to Paris. In Louis Gustave Bouchereau and Valentin Magnan's *Statistique des malades entrés en 1870 et en 1871 au bureau d'admission des aliénés de la Seine,* they describe the modifications made in order to maintain services. Like other narratives written by public asylum doctors about Paris under siege, Bouchereau and Magnan's report is largely descriptive in tone while subtly glorifying the actions of the psychiatric community. The two doctors worked together at Paris's largest mental institution, the central entrance location for all the department's public asylums.[8] Sainte-Anne was under siege during the Franco-Prussian War, at times even in the line of fire, but the institution continued operations throughout the troubles. Bouchereau and Magnan consistently minimized the significance of alterations in patient services, claiming that the doctor-administrators of Paris's asylums kept their institutions running much as they had before the war. They explained that although the Service des Aliénés was "placed in a very exceptional situation in 1870 and 1871, the admission of patients was not interrupted, even on the most agitated of days."[9] Despite the ravages faced by the residents of Paris, the asylum's staff continued to "provide for all needs, with the aid of a few modifications of little importance."[10]

The "importance" of these "few modifications" was certainly a matter of perspective. Bouchereau and Magnan conceded that among the department's six public mental institutions, Sainte-Anne alone accepted new patients once the siege began. This remained possible because administrators transferred a number of patients as the Prussian army approached, thus leaving beds open for the projected influx during what would eventually turn into a five-month-long siege. Bicêtre and the Salpêtrière, also under siege, evacuated some patients and ceased to receive new ones, as did Charenton. Prussian armies cut off the suburban asylums Ville-Evrard and Vaucluse from Paris entirely.

While Bouchereau and Magnan presented the maintenance of Saint-Anne as evidence of the fortitude and self-reliance of the psychiatric establishment, it had just as much to do with their reliance on others. Specifically, only by sending patients to pensioners' homes in the provinces or, later, returning them to their families were the administrators of Sainte-Anne able to accept new patients or feed those they already had. As of September 10, 1870, doctors had transferred four hundred eighty patients to the provinces, leaving a total of one hundred thirty-eight residing in the institution. By January 20, 1871, toward the end of the war, the total number of patients had risen to six hundred thirteen.[11] Doctors made the decision shortly thereafter to return another one hundred eight "uncured" patients to their families in the city, leaving four hundred ninety-one patients in total after accounting for recent deaths.[12] Bouchereau and Magnan rightly noted that patients transferred early on "escaped the emotions of the siege, the dangers of the bombardment, and especially the deprivations and all the pernicious influences that caused such great mortality among our patients" in Paris, but they hardly acknowledged the efforts made by non-alienists in keeping these patients safe.[13]

The inspector general of the Service des Aliénés, Doctor Ludgar Lunier, similarly emphasized the resilience of French psychiatry as opposed to community efforts in a series of articles describing the effects of the events of 1870–1871 on the nation's mental health. Lunier's concerns as a high-ranking bureaucrat both before and after the events tended to reflect those of the administration, and he presented his observations in a dispassionate manner. Yet Lunier's air of objectivity was itself an element of his professional self-presentation, one that masked opinions as facts and thereby gave his interpretations the weight of truth. Like those of his colleagues from Saint-Anne, Lunier's depictions of mental medicine during the war and the Commune presented a chaotic picture of the challenges faced by alienists while giving doctors credit for maintaining patient services. He thus upheld the image of professional independence that had historically served to secure the honor of French psychiatry.

Lunier claimed the period of crisis created 1,400–1,500 new instances of mental illness.[14] Despite these cases, the rate of institutionalization throughout France had slowed significantly when compared with previous years. In fact, total admissions decreased by 1,412 individuals from fall 1870 to summer 1871, whereas the number of patients had steadily increased by approximately 1,000 annually in the ten years preceding the Prussian invasion.[15] This drop surprised the Inspector General, particularly because many of his fellow alienists argued that war and political perturbations aggravated mental illness, as had supposedly been the case during the first French Revolution and the revolution of 1848.[16]

Furthermore, scores of bourgeois critics described the Paris Commune in terms of "collective madness" at this very time.[17] In a moment when all of society was said to have gone insane, it seemed perplexing to Lunier that asylum admissions had actually gone down.

Lunier gave several potential causes for this decline, none of which faulted the psychiatric community in any way. One can hardly blame him, considering the circumstances. Much like Bouchereau and Magnan, he dismissed the efforts of other community members to keep asylums operational. The most convincing explanation for the reduction in patient numbers was certainly the chaos caused by advancing armies. Lunier explained that "the invasion brought about a great disruption in the administrative functioning of a certain number of our departments" and communication between provincial asylums, departmental processing centers, and the central administration in Paris was "brusquely interrupted" as a consequence.[18] French administrators did not reestablish communications in many locales until at least February 1871, when the siege of Paris finally came to an end. Many potential asylum occupants, even those outside the capital, thus remained with their families or in general hospitals for the duration of the events, and a number of them were either dead or otherwise no longer in need of services by the time institutional admissions began to function as usual.

Both these options—admitting patients to a general hospital or simply keeping them with their families—were actions alienists ordinarily sought to avoid. Doctors had long attempted to legitimate their intervention in the lives of the mentally ill on the grounds that the presence of their families could be harmful. They had also tried to distinguish themselves from other medical professionals, claiming that their specialized knowledge uniquely qualified them for their roles as the caretakers and overseers of the insane. The asylum supposedly provided a home away from home over which the doctor alone presided, a place conveniently and purposefully separated from familial and societal sources of mental illness. However, when many French citizens acutely needed mental health services, alienists found themselves incapable of meeting demand and relied quite heavily on the very groups they had long treated as rivals.

This dependence had the potential to undermine the authoritative image of French psychiatry doctors had cultivated throughout the nineteenth century, and Lunier played down the importance of administrative disruptions (warning his readers not to "attribute to these circumstances more importance than is right").[19] Instead, he argued that the decline in patient numbers mainly reflected the instability of household economies. Families were supposedly reluctant to pay to intern their relations when their own futures were so uncertain. In this framing, patients' relatives had neglected their familial duties, whereas doctors were still able and willing to pick up the slack. Lunier's accompanying tables do indicate that the numbers of paying patients in public and private asylums decreased by a larger percentage than did the number of indigent patients during the events, lending some support to his interpretation.[20] These figures might also suggest that families with other options decided it made little sense to deliver their loved ones to psychiatric institutions—places that often proved traumatizing in the best of times—when the asylum system was in such a state of disarray.[21]

The decision among public asylum administrators to put a positive spin on their experiences of 1870–1871 made sense, especially in light of recent unjust commitment scandals. It also reflected doctors' long-standing tendency to present themselves as protective and consoling father figures to their childlike patients. Alexandre Brierre de Boismont, the aging owner of a private "family life" facility, made the doctor's role as a provider of safety and domestic comforts explicit in his description of the siege. Brierre de Boismont faced challenges similar to those confronted by his contemporaries employed by the public asylum system. However, the private nature of his medical practice led him to approach the months of deprivation in different ways and narrate those experiences to different effect. Brierre de Boismont could not rely on public resources (i.e., the provincial pensioners' homes that absorbed the patients Sainte-Anne could no longer accommodate) as his colleagues had. He also could not easily send his patients to live with their families because they were paying customers rather than wards of the state. Because of these limitations, the private asylum doctor eventually called upon an international network of medical professionals—his friends and fellow alienists in London—to help provision his institution.

When comparing Brierre de Boismont's account of his experiences to those of Bouchereau, Magnan, and Lunier, his comparative willingness to give credit to others for the survival of his asylum is noteworthy. Brierre de Boismont published "A Lunatic Asylum during the Siege of Paris" in February 1871 in the British medical journal *The Lancet*. His hope was to "illustrate, on a small scale, the painful scenes of a family life in a *maison de santé* during the siege" and thank his far-flung colleagues for their help. He immediately positioned himself as the head of an asylum-household, describing the social relationships within his institution in familial terms and noting the disruption to "family life" brought on by the crisis. His word choice was fitting, considering that the doctor lived in the same building as many of his patients, located on a 12,000-square-meter complex at the edge of the Faubourg Sainte-Antoine. The rest of the account can be read as the tale of a desperate but unwavering father's struggle to provide for his "family" in trying times.[22]

There were 200 patients residing in his institution during the months of the siege, sixty-two of whom had formerly lived at a private residential facility operated by his daughter, Marie Rivet. Their transfer to the Faubourg Saint-Antoine, brought about because their rest home had recently been damaged in the defense of the capital, added stress to an already difficult situation. Brierre de Boismont's most pressing concerns included the acquisition of food and sources of heat. He discussed the lack of food in particular, emphasizing the impact of shortages on patient comfort. "In the early part of October," he wrote, "the supply of milk ceased. Those who know Paris will readily believe the privations my patients suffered from the absence of café au lait, this beverage being one of the principal items of the breakfast table."[23]

Circumstances eventually became far more dire as other basic foodstuffs experienced rapid price inflation or disappeared entirely. The availability of meat was a particularly poignant concern. By the end of October fresh pork had become unavailable and "the butcher's stalls, governed by municipal authority, now substituted horseflesh for beef, mutton, and veal."[24] Shortly thereafter the daily allotment of horsemeat per person fell to just thirty grams. Brierre de Boismont explained, "Consequences of a very grave nature would have ensued from this insufficient supply of nourishment had not my constant care for my patients impelled me to search for food in places where I thought it might be concealed."[25] He was able to purchase mule and horse meat from various underground sources and slaughtered several of his own animals to feed the patients; some amount of meat was therefore available for all but two days of the siege. Nonetheless, a number of elderly patients died who might have lived longer had milk, fish, and vegetables been available. Brierre de Boismont noted that mortality was high during the frigid months of November and December especially. Some patients "died just as a lamp burns out for want of oil."[26]

Unlike the operators of public institutions, who insisted on the continued efficiency of asylum administration throughout the crisis, Brierre de Boismont readily supplied evidence of his powerlessness. The doctor was forced to rely on his own ingenuity and his personal fortune in order to maintain the operation of his facility during the siege because he could not count on assistance from the state. He drew attention to the desperation of the asylum's inhabitants to great effect; in so doing, Brierre de Boismont fashioned himself as a self-sacrificing father figure, even describing his narrative as an illustration of "the painful scenes of a family life."[27] His tale was replete with moments of paternal devotion, from his multiple requests that the municipal authority provide the asylum with coal to his seemingly endless search for food throughout the city (impelled, he explained, by "my constant care for my patients").[28] He and his staff foraged for firewood in the city parks, bought horse meat on the black market, and chopped down trees on the asylum grounds. Even so, Brierre de Boismont was unable to provide sufficient food and fuel through these methods alone. He found himself profoundly malnourished after eating only horseflesh and black, gritty bread for four long months, noting that he and his patients were all pushed to a state of exhaustion. Many died prematurely and experienced "extreme emaciation, profound debility, disordered respiration, and sleeplessness."[29]

Brierre de Boismont's vulnerability in the face of catastrophe ultimately provided an opportunity to strengthen professional ties and elevate the reputation of the psychiatry as a whole.[30] To his great relief, the harried asylum doctor received the generous aid of international colleagues during this time of need. His account of the siege was published in dedication to his English peer, friend, and benefactor Dr. Forbes Winslow.[31] The French alienist addressed himself to "my dear *confrère*," again displaying his predilection for familial language, and explained that he sent his report "the more willingly as you have for so many years given me such abundant proofs of your friendship and devotion."[32] The provision of necessities at the end of the siege ranked highest among these "abundant proofs." Brierre de Boismont claimed he was on the verge of death when care packages began to arrive from London once the siege was lifted. If his personal sacrifices were not enough to save his patients, the devotion of the psychiatric profession would fill the void. The supplies—cheese, various meats, milk, potatoes, tea, biscuits, soap—did not begin to arrive until February, but "the food thus obtained may be said to have been the means of saving my own life, as well as the lives of several of my patients."[33]

While this statement could be interpreted as hyperbole, a way to strengthen professional bonds through excessive thanks, it is significant that Brierre de Boismont emphasized the benevolent strength of the psychiatric profession at his moment of personal frailty. He refused to take full credit for the asylum's survival, but he still positioned *psychiatry* as his patients' ultimate savior. Brierre de Boismont and the public asylum doctors therefore reached similar conclusions despite their distinct vantage points. Doctors who wrote accounts of the war and the siege sought to establish and maintain a resolute, competent, and dignified image of the psychiatric profession—at others' expense, in the case of Bouchereau, Magnan, and Lunier, and to others' credit, in the case of Brierre de Boismont. The psychiatric community had spent the first seven decades of the nineteenth century demarcating their professional role, and all alienists were keenly aware of their duties, both as doctors and as men. Many confronted situations during the invasion that made it difficult for them to live up to their own expectations. Still, when they narrated their experiences, they sought to present weakness as a source of strength.

The Doctor as National Hero

It is much easier to identify the strategies used by medical men to promote their professional reputations than it is to assess the extent to which those efforts succeeded or failed. Fortunately, one doctor who published his recollections of the events of 1870–1871 received official accolades from the government of the Third Republic, thereby affirming that his actions reflected well on the state. Arguably the most adept example of professional self-promotion performed by an asylum doctor in the aftermath of the Franco-Prussian War was that of Eugène Billod, an alienist and administrator of the public institution Vaucluse. In addition to presenting himself as a member of a worthy profession, as was the case for our doctors in the previous section, Billod's account of his actions served to enhance the honor of the French nation itself—a welcome addition in a country reeling from military defeat and the recent loss of its eastern territories, Alsace and Lorraine.

In *Les aliénés de Vaucluse et Ville-Evrard pendant le siège de Paris*, Billod describes the day-to-day operations of his institution, offering invaluable insights into one doctor's behavior during the invasion and how he subsequently chose to narrate his experiences. Unlike mental institutions within Paris itself, Billod's facility was never under siege. However, the Prussian army occupied the territory surrounding Vaucluse because of its location just outside the city. Prussian soldiers cut the asylum off from both the capital and the hinterland, and it was under constant threat of physical occupation. Billod and his patients were alone in a way other asylum administrators could not truly comprehend. Despite the extreme nature of his position, Billod's preoccupation with the reputation of French psychiatry had much in common with the views of his Parisian contemporaries. He consistently implied that maintaining both personal and professional honor would affect Vaucluse's very survival. All Billod had was his image: he could not rely on anything or anyone else.

The isolation the alienist found himself in was unexpected, for the administrators of the Assistance Publique had considered the fate of the department's asylums and attempted to plan for the worst. Vaucluse served the city of Paris along with the asylums Sainte-Anne, Bicêtre, the Salpêtrière, Charenton, and Ville-Evrard. Both Ville-Evrard and Vaucluse were located outside Paris on large tracts of land the patients cultivated as a form of treatment and a source of revenue. As news of French defeats in the East reached Paris, the administrators of the Assistance Publique decided to combine the populations of the suburban asylums, transporting the patients residing at Ville-Evrard to Vaucluse because they believed Ville-Evrard was in greater danger. This proved not to be the case. However, by the time people realized the more precarious situation of Vaucluse, the patients had already been transferred and there was nothing to do but wait out the occupation.[34]

The vast, village-like institution is located approximately twenty-seven kilometers from Paris, near the village Épinay-sur-Orge. Under normal circumstances one could reach the suburban asylum easily by train from Paris because a railroad station had been built for this purpose. The Prussians blocked access to the tracks in both directions once the occupation began, however, at which point communication and transport between Vaucluse and the capital ceased. Neither goods nor information traveled in or out between October 1870 and the end of the siege in February of 1871. Whatever food and supplies the asylum possessed were either gathered locally, procured before the occupation, or furnished on-site.

Billod comes across in his account as a man profoundly aware of the power of appearances. He consistently avoided the semblance of desperation and aimed to display the dignity he considered befitting his gender, class, profession, and nation. His behavior likely represented both a practical and an emotional response to living and working in a territory occupied by the enemy, but it was also a personal and professional imperative. In a situation in which he held so little "real" power, Billod's ability to project an image of authority was a matter of life and death. He needed to convince various people—from members of the surrounding community to Prussian army officers—that he deserved to be treated with respect and that the needs of his patients truly mattered. This was no small feat at a time when the threat of starvation afflicted nearly everyone. The asylum director drew on rich reserves of cultural capital when other resources were severely lacking. In the process he elevated his personal reputation and that of the psychiatric profession. Narrating his experiences for a broad audience after the fact was itself an exercise in self-fashioning that cemented his reputation as a man of distinction.

Billod published his account in late 1872, nearly two years after the Prussian occupation. Reprints of letters lauding Billod's behavior during the siege precede the text itself. These include a note from his superiors at the Assistance Publique highlighting his "praiseworthy" conduct, his "courage," and his "devotion," without which neither his patients nor the asylum could have survived the war. This letter is followed by an attestation from Jules Ferry—prefect of the Department of the Seine during the siege and future prime minister of the Republic—authorizing a public monument to be erected at the asylum in honor of Billod and his personnel, as well as a letter from Billod's male employees expressing gratitude for his wise actions. The mayor of the nearest village, Épinay-sur-Orge, added his voice to the chorus in a note thanking the alienist for services rendered to "the community." The final document is a notice of Billod's induction into the Legion of Honor in September 1872, just before the memoir's publication.

This outpouring of official praise attests to Billod's success in keeping Vaucluse operational during the war, but it also indicates his expertise in crafting his public image. Like asylum doctors in less trying times, Billod aimed to present himself as both authoritative and benevolent, as can be seen in his explanation of his major goals during the siege. First, Billod wanted to preserve the establishment and keep his personnel out of harm's way. Second, he hoped to sustain patient services. Third, he needed to maintain a rigorous sense of order. In other words, he sought to simultaneously control and protect the establishment and those who lived there. Billod's fourth and final goal was to "secure this triple result all while safeguarding, in the most scrupulous manner possible, the honor and dignity of the administration."[35] He left it up to the reader to determine whether he accomplished these tasks, but it can be assumed his success was self-evident. After all, he would not have been asked to publish his account nor been inducted into the Legion of Honor if state officials did not think his story reflected well on the bureaucracy in charge of asylum administration, not to mention the nation. We can therefore read Billod's account of the siege as a lesson in professional behavior, one that shows how an alienist could effectively present himself as a man of authority, dignity, and self-respect under the most difficult of circumstances.

Interactions with the Prussians proved especially consequential, both for the survival of the institution and as proof of Billod's status as a man of honor. These moments were invariably tense because they held high stakes for the asylum and its inhabitants. Vaucluse constantly faced the threat of requisitions of already limited supplies of food and fuel. As early as September 15, the lines of transportation between the institution and Paris had been cut, and shortly thereafter the Prussians ordered the local baker to stop selling bread to the asylum. The threat of occupation was even more troubling, for the Germans hoped to station troops at Vaucluse and take the food produced on the asylum farm for themselves. Having anticipated this possibility, Billod tried to secure Vaucluse's status as a Red Cross outpost before the arrival of the Prussian army. While he had received permission to house twelve wounded for the Red Cross, the Prussians refused to recognize the international flag because the wounded never arrived, leaving the asylum open to forced requisitions and the billeting of soldiers. Prussian officers met Billod's attempts to resist their incursions with indifference. The Prussian commander stationed at the nearby town of Breuil even remarked that "the lives of Prussians were more precious than those of the mad."[36]

Under the threat of requisitions, Billod decided to appeal to Prussian leadership. The doctor initiated this interaction with a letter addressed to the Prince Royal, commander of the Prussian Third Army, who had stationed one of his battalions near the asylum. Billod assured his readers that he decided to take this step only when it became clear it was a "question of life and death for my unfortunate patients."[37] He explained in dramatic terms, "I did not hesitate further, although I knew it would cost me greatly to say it, to do what was the greatest hardship of my life in the interest of what was proper, that is to say, to call upon the human sentiments of the Prince Royal."[38] Despite Billod's reticence to supplicate the invader of his homeland, he framed his decision as a worthy act of self-sacrifice. As a representative of the French state and as a professional man, he could not risk prostrating himself at the feet of the German prince. "Aware of the importance of the path I was about to attempt," wrote Billod, "I committed myself to weighing the terms of my letter in a manner in which not one word of that document impinged to any degree the dignity of the administration or myself."[39] The doctor chose his words carefully, attempting to achieve a balanced tone that conveyed neither obeisance nor disrespect.

His letter apparently struck the right chord. The day after receiving Billod's note the Prussian Prince of Gottberg declared that Vaucluse would not be required to house soldiers and was officially freed from any future requisitions. He also granted the doctor liberty to travel within the occupied territories in order to secure necessities for the institution. While Billod's conception of personal, professional, and national esteem made him reticent to contact the prince, his ability to express himself with dignity ultimately served him well. A shared understanding of what constituted correct behavior seems to have helped persuade the Prussian general to grant Billod's request. The desire of both men to act honorably provided them a mechanism to manage conflicts while maintaining a sense of independence and self-respect. If masculine honor could be a source of contention, it was also a source of connection, even among enemies.

The asylum doctor again made use of his interpersonal skills toward the end of the occupation. Several Prussian officers arrived at Vaucluse in February 1871, having received orders to billet ninety horses and soldiers on the asylum grounds in spite of the prince's earlier promises. A very tense series of interactions followed their arrival and, despite his vulnerable position, Billod managed to secure the safety of the institution. He refused to allow the occupation of Vaucluse until he saw an order from the prince contradicting his original promise. One of the German officers replied, "You ask for an order. Well, here it is," as he tapped on his sword threateningly. The alienist responded, "I regret to have to tell you . . . that what you have just shown me is not an order, it's an expression of brutal force, and in my showing you an order from the head of your army [the original letter from the prince], I prove to you that I know no force aside from moral force."[40] The major reacted angrily, motioning as if he were going to slap the doctor in the face. To this insult Billod declared, "No more of these movements, I don't like them, and don't forget you're in my house."[41]

The officer then changed his tone, at least according to Billod's recollection of events, now acting as one gentleman would toward another, touring the asylum with Billod and impressing him with his "perfect urbanity."[42] The doctor had successfully mobilized his personal self-presentation as his best defense against Prussian encroachment, calling attention to an apparently shared sense of decorum to convince the soldiers to treat him with respect. Furthermore, it was by drawing on the domestic metaphor (and the paternal authority it implied) that Billod was able to shame the officer into recognizing the incivility of his attitude. The asylum was not a neutral space, but "chez moi"—and to insult Billod in his own home was a step too far. The end of hostilities came in time for Vaucluse to avoid more requisitions, and it is unclear whether Billod's stalling tactics would have worked indefinitely, but they were surprisingly successful in the short term.

The conceptions of ideal masculinity whose spread this book has traced continued to hold relevance during and after the Franco-Prussian War, as evidenced by Billod's account of the siege and the accolades he received for his efforts. The bourgeois Billod embodied rational savoir-faire, making use of his skills as a negotiator when exerting physical strength to counter his opponents was out of the question. His courage was expressed not via brute force but through persistence and know-how, his decisions the products of deliberate consideration rather than emotion. Furthermore, like other members of his class and profession, Billod embraced the honor code as a way to navigate disputes with other men—men who physically had the upper hand and whose very presence signified the humiliating defeat of France. More important, Billod's actions, his narration of those actions, and the reactions of other French men all point to an essential link between the expression of masculine honor and the preservation of national esteem. As Venita Datta has shown with respect to press accounts of men's cowardice later in the century, "the valor of elite males also reflected on that of the French nation itself."[43] France could use all the valor it could get in the immediate aftermath of the Franco-Prussian War, as those who lauded Billod must have sensed.

The experience of the Franco-Prussian War also suggested to many men that the inculcation of bourgeois habits had perhaps left them unprepared for combat. Had French society spent the first part of the century elevating martial attributes of masculinity instead, there might have been no need to celebrate the victories of someone like Billod in the first place. The cultural promotion of masculine self-control did much to prop up the social and political authority of bourgeois men whose lifestyles were considerably more sedentary than those of their aristocratic predecessors or their lower-class contemporaries. We must remember, however, that older expectations of masculine comportment never disappeared and that anxiety over men's apparent "domestication" has represented a central feature of Western civilization since the early modern period.[44] Billod attempted to present himself as both the ideal male professional and a manly defender of the innocent.[45] It was in the best interests of the nascent republic to reward him for his efforts, but the cultivation of Billod's self-presentation still required an uneasy balancing act. Overt expressions of virility and strength among bourgeois and middle-class men would become more prominent in the period between the Franco-Prussian War and the start of World War 1, at least in part owing to rising concerns over the physical debility of potential French soldiers.

Nonetheless, because Billod was a bourgeois professional who saved the inhabitants of a state-run institution during a period of national calamity, it still made sense for officials to frame his story of the siege as a point of pride. The doctor had set out to preserve the "dignity" of the administration while securing the safety of his establishment. The publication of his story is proof of his success. And while Billod's experiences were more exceptional than most, the Prussian invasion confronted all French alienists with unprecedented circumstances. Violence, isolation, and hunger threatened the lives of doctors and patients alike. Yet psychiatric professionals consistently took the catastrophes of 1870–1871 as opportunities to shape their professional identities and present themselves and their colleagues as resilient, honorable, and even heroic men. Their interpretations of the Paris Commune would further solidify the alliance between medicine and the state, this time through the vilification of common enemies.

Prescient Doctors and Furious Revolutionaries

The image of the psychiatric profession presented by Billod and others who wrote about the Prussian siege depended on a very particular conception of the doctor-patient relationship. Doctors styled their patients as children in need of care and protection whose apparent vulnerability justified medical intervention. They fashioned themselves as father figures, strong but benevolent, the only people capable of saving their patients from the dangerous influences of the outside world (their own families included). Yet doctors also had a stake in spreading the belief that those considered insane were threats to the communities in which they lived, a fear that justified the expansion of doctors' social roles.[46] In other words, mad people were at once dangerous and in need of protection. The spread of such assumptions helped psychiatric professionals establish their authority within the asylum and beyond.

Doctors' depictions of 1870–1871 perpetuated both of these tropes. Mentally unstable individuals already living inside psychiatric institutions appear in doctors' writings as vulnerable and childlike, whereas doctors depicted the Communards of Paris as "mad" and even contagious. All the world could agree, wrote the doctor Jean-Baptiste Vincent Laborde, that "a wind of madness" had passed through the French capital when its citizens rejected the Third Republic and formed a new municipal government in its stead.[47] According to Laure Murat, French alienists had long noted how revolutionary upheavals colored their patients' delusions. This, however, did not necessarily imply that doctors were politically opposed to the idea of revolution nor that they pathologized revolutionary activity in and of itself. As we have seen, Pinel secured his position as the head of Bicêtre in the 1790s, and those who followed in his footsteps often played lip service to *liberté* even when contradicting this revolutionary value in practice. Furthermore, Murat has identified only two alienists after the revolution of 1848 who claimed revolution was a product of madness rather than one of its potential inspirations.[48] The most prominent advocate of this position was the politically conservative and devoutly Catholic Brierre de Boismont, who also maintained that the revolutionaries of the Paris Commune were clinically insane. This time, however, he was joined by his colleagues in far greater numbers. The differences between doctors' interpretations of 1848 and 1871 were profound, with most psychiatric commentators taking the madness of the Communards for granted even when disagreeing on other medical matters.

To those at odds with the national government the decision to revolt during the spring of 1871 was hardly unreasonable. Many Parisians felt betrayed by the

Third Republic in the aftermath of the Franco-Prussian War, especially because they had borne the brunt of the siege. Two economic policies announced by the National Assembly in March 1871 were especially unpopular: the requirement that the city's inhabitants immediately pay back rent to their landlords and the establishment of a short deadline to repurchase items they had been forced to pawn. Citizens were already frustrated by the new government's decision to capitulate to the Prussians and allow them to march through Paris victorious, and such policies posed an almost inconceivably cruel predicament for anyone of limited means who lived in the capital. A citywide revolt, led mainly by members of the popular classes, broke out when the conservative first president of the Third Republic, Adolphe Thiers, sent troops to Montmartre to preemptively seize cannons from the city's armory.

While Marxist historians have perhaps overstated the protosocialist elements of the Paris Commune, which constituted an expression of neighborhood solidarity as much as class consciousness, contemporary discussions of the revolutionary government and its ultimate destruction almost universally reflected class prejudices.[49] This was certainly the case among doctors attempting to diagnose Communards after the fact. Medical men writing about the Commune made no secret of their political commitment to the Third Republic and their disgust for the working-class Communards. J. V. Laborde, the neurologist and founder of the journal *La Tribune médicale*, was among the most outspoken medical critics of the Commune.[50] A self-described republican and friend of Leon Gambetta, Laborde's antirevolutionary conclusions were reflective of the relative conservatism of mainstream republicanism by this time. In 1872 Laborde published a widely reviewed book about the Commune, *Les hommes et les actes de l'insurrection de Paris devant la psychologie morbide*, in which he medicalized revolutionary sentiment to an extreme degree. Murat has analyzed numerous other psychiatric treatises published around the same time that made similar arguments. Those who condemned the Commune consistently implied that the interests of the psychiatric community aligned precisely with those of the state.

While Laborde suggested that some revolutionaries had been driven to revolt by harsh circumstances and the effects of drink, he also provided numerous examples of what he considered clinical insanity among the Communards. The disordered political climate supposedly gave madness a chance to reveal itself and even flourish. Mental disturbances that had lain dormant in more peaceful times eerily rose to the surface in the face of war, siege, and famine, and the insane of Paris supposedly flocked to revolutionary organizations across the city. Even those hereditarily predisposed to madness who had never before been politically inclined found the disorderly atmosphere appealing. For Laborde, the adage "Qui se ressemble, s'assemble" was never truer than during the three months of urban revolt.[51] He claimed those who might have been committed to asylums in other times were celebrated during the Commune for the originality or their ideas and their passionate forms of self-expression.

Laborde argued that politics was a milieu well-suited to the unleashing of passions and impulses, all the more so during moments ripe with possibility and rebellion. In this respect he echoed the theories of early alienists who believed madness was the result of passions run amuck. His descriptions of male revolutionaries likewise mirrored earlier psychiatric discussions, with some novel additions. Men suffering from delusions of grandeur, whose messianic ramblings might once have been ignored, supposedly embraced the opportunity to become revolutionary leaders: those who had once been objects of pity or disgust "were taken in triumph [during the insurrection], the martyr's wreath upon their heads."[52] Men who exhibited signs of *délire de persécution* also fit right in because this particular condition manifested when ambitions had not been realized. Laborde claimed that failed intellectuals, journalists, and artists lashed out wildly during the Commune, finding large audiences for their vengeful diatribes against a society they perceived as having wronged them. Asylum doctors after the French Revolution had also tied professional frustration to mental illness in men, implying that new possibilities for financial success caused so much anxiety that some men went mad. Such diagnoses served to police the behavior of men by defining insanity as a failure to conform to bourgeois expectations. But the gender-based treatment scenarios concocted in the course of the moral treatment also suggested that doctors believed these patients could become productive citizens once again. By 1871, this was not the case.

Laborde presented a vision of society in which the consequences of madness had reached apparently unprecedented depths: revolutionary Paris was a space in which "perversions, ambitions, and madness swarmed and agitated," an upside-down world where the irrational momentarily ruled the sane. The inclusion of "ambitions" between "perversions" and "madness" is noteworthy. For Laborde, mental illness inspired by professional disappointment reflected a mismatch between a man's expectations for social success and what he truly deserved—which, in the case of those who sought to rise above their station, was apparently very little. To put it another way, Laborde's prototypical mad Communards were precisely those individuals who understood meritocracy to be an illusion and who dared to envision a world in which this was no longer the case. "Unrealistic" aspiration therefore constituted not only a dangerous sign of insanity, but a source of social chaos. If the minds of individual revolutionaries evinced the disease of unwarranted expectations, the Commune itself seemed to confirm elite fears that such hopes had spread throughout the body politic.

Shifting conceptions of the political and social consequences of madness served to reinforce its stigma. So too did changing psychiatric attitudes toward alienation's source. Although Laborde linked insanity to the overexcitement of the passions—especially ambition—he did not argue, à la Pinel, that all people were susceptible to mental illness, claiming instead that madness was primarily the result of hereditary degeneration. First elaborated by the asylum doctor Benedict Morel in 1857, degeneration theory pinpointed insanity as one of many seemingly distinct afflictions whose appearance in a family's medical history supposedly signaled the inevitable physical decline of future generations. Laborde similarly found that "transmitted predisposition can ... proceed from very different pathological states of departure,"[53] including but not limited to the insanity of a parent or other relative. Everything from epilepsy to headaches to slight physical deformities, in relatives living or dead, constituted evidence of a family's pathological nature for degeneration theorists: for this reason, it was never hard for a doctor to "confirm" a diagnosis of hereditary insanity. Laborde connected individuals' participation in the Commune to this sort of family history time and again, suggesting not only that madness and revolutionary politics were one and the same, but that a person's eventual psychological state was practically predetermined at birth.

As a neurologist and physical anthropologist, Laborde's conviction of the hereditary basis of mental illness was more pronounced than that of most alienists who actually operated asylums, many of whom still interpreted insanity as a "moral" condition to some extent. Even Morel, the originator of degeneration theory, rejected hereditary insanity as an explanation for revolutionary activity because he believed this would unjustly pardon the Communards for their rebellion.[54] As one of Laborde's reviewers noted, "monsters" should not be absolved of their actions just because "their father was sorrowful and depressed."[55] Nonetheless, even those who disagreed with Laborde on the question of heredity readily accepted his equation of madness with participation in revolutionary politics, thereby providing a ready-made rationale for dismissing Communard demands and supporting any actions taken by the state to curtail revolutionary activity, no matter how violent.[56]

Expressions of fear and condescension toward popular politics were not unusual. Most bourgeois commentators were horrified by the Commune's endorsement of egalitarian initiatives—such as universal secular education, nurseries for working parents, and the elimination of night baking—and physicians were not alone in explaining away social radicalism in terms of insanity. Drawing particular ire were women revolutionaries, whose actions came to symbolize for bourgeois critics all that was wrong with working-class politics more broadly. Depicted as wild-eyed furies, the women of the Commune were supposedly out of control, sexually licentious, and gleefully destructive. Gay Gullickson has extensively chronicled contemporary depictions of the "unruly women of Paris," and her evidence indicates that already prevalent assumptions about women's irrationality shaped people's impressions of Communardes. The conservative columnist Francisque Sarcey, for example, claimed the *pétroleuses* were "under the epidemic influence of incendiary mania" when they supposedly burned down parts of Paris in the traumatic final days of the Commune.[57] The writers Edmond and Jules de Goncourt noted that many captured women revolutionaries "had the eyes of madwomen."[58] These sorts of commentaries fueled sexist assumptions about politically engaged women, implying that the Communardes represented horrific deviations from the domestic ideal and, at the same time, were precisely what all women would become if granted political rights. Members of the medical community unsurprisingly reproduced these stereotypes in their discussion of women who participated in or even sympathized with the Commune, conceptually linking "unwomanly" behavior to madness and legitimating the opinions of lay observers.

The writings of the Brierre de Boismont family offer a case in point. Alexandre Brierre de Boismont worried "this frightful social and political convulsion" would eventually have "sad effects on mental health," while his daughter Marie Rivet described her impressions of Communardes in particular.[59] She made special note of a tense interaction with a woman preaching atheism at the Place du Trône who responded to Rivet's questions about the possibility of rejoining her husband in the afterlife with the assertion that she had "never been married, thank God."[60] The *directrice* also recounted meeting a widow, Madame A., whose children sought to intern her for profligate spending; they realized their goal following the Commune's defeat, when military doctors took the woman's fraternization with revolutionaries as evidence of her insanity. Having been captured on the barricades dressed as a *fédéré*, "her rifle still hot," it was almost certainly Madame A.'s elite background that kept her from being executed or sent to a colonial prison along with her compatriots.[61] She reportedly told Rivet that the insurgents had impressed her with their "energy and their assurance that they would die for a great humanitarian principle; that one could kill their bodies, but the idea would remain."[62] The woman's support for the

Commune—particularly because she was wealthy—represented clear evidence of insanity for Rivet, an opinion her male colleagues would almost certainly have shared.

Laborde's descriptions of the Commune were therefore lurid, but not especially original. Nonetheless, as a medical doctor, he was in a singular position to act as both witness and expert. He even claimed it was possible to anticipate who might succumb to madness during times of political agitation by looking for signs of inherited predisposition and clues in past behavior.[63] Doctors represented France's best chance for redemption because they could pinpoint future revolutionaries with scientific precision before they caused unrest. The post hoc "diagnosis" of Communards therefore represented an important public relations strategy for the psychiatric profession, in that decrying the Commune allowed medical practitioners to establish their political commitment to the Third Republic and link its survival to their own. Furthermore, if doctors' condemnation of the Commune was a form of self-promotion, it was also a method of self-defense. It is entirely possible that French alienists feared the Commune because the municipal government, given time, might have turned its attention to questions of asylum reform. There was at least one incident of a crowd attempting to free a patient from Saint-Anne against doctors' orders, and Bouchereau and Magnan reported that a political club had actually made plans to debate revising the law on asylum sequestration.[64]

When doctors presented revolutionary Paris as disorderly and irrational, they conveniently upheld the political claims of the bourgeoisie, as well as their own professional and masculine prerogatives. Doctors drew upon and helped cultivate widespread prejudices against those considered insane to justify dismissing revolutionary demands. In the process, they further stigmatized mental illness, thereby creating an even more powerful justification to continue to deny rights to anyone who dared question the political or economic status quo (especially workers and women). In this sense, medical discussions of madness and the Commune are poignant examples of the ways psychological disability has operated historically as an essential marker of difference used to legitimate hierarchies of all kinds.

These cultural outcomes meshed with the material interests of individual alienists and elevated the status of the French psychiatry as a whole. Laborde positioned men like himself as society's best defense against the dangers of social revolution. He also implicitly provided a strong argument for increased asylum incarceration by linking psychological and family history to revolutionary sentiment. Alienists who found Laborde's claims about hereditary madness overstated did so as well. They might not have believed doctors capable of discovering future revolutionaries before they wreaked havoc, but they nonetheless agreed that such individuals should be incarcerated at the first signs of "trouble." Eugène Billod, the embattled director of Vaucluse, likewise presented asylum sequestration as a social good. He depicted his patients as basically harmless, choosing to relate charming stories of patriotism during the siege rather than examples of conflict or disruption (at one point the inhabitants of the women's quarter met Prussian soldiers with shouts of "Vive la France!" and "Vive la paix!" although Billod suspected few patients understood the larger implications of the war).[65] Compared with Laborde's descriptions of the supposedly mad men and women of Paris, the inhabitants of Vaucluse remained remarkably placid during the wartime period. Living through desperate times had not encouraged violent or disruptive behavior: the asylum setting had effectively pacified its inhabitants. This was, of course, the point.

MEDICAL COMMENTARIES CONCERNING the events of 1870–1871 did not exhibit the same defensive tone as psychiatric discussions of unjust internment from around the same period, but they still promoted a view of the profession that implied the aggrandizement of psychiatric power was in the best interests of French society. Some writers were content to highlight the efforts taken by asylum doctors to safeguard their institutions during the siege. Such narratives implied that these men were well-suited to their authoritative roles, perhaps especially in times of stress and anxiety. These write-ups gave doctors credit for maintaining patient services and advertised the heroic efforts of individual alienists in France and abroad, often in a fashion that drew upon well-established features of psychiatric masculinity (including benevolent paternalism and professional honor). They therefore made a subtle case for the asylum system's continued utility in the fledgling republic, despite the near constant drumbeat of criticism coming from anti-alienist corners. Medical discussions of the Commune went even further in defense of the profession, implying that the fate of France depended on the diagnostic capabilities of medical men and their elevation to positions of power.

This era was similar to the first French Revolution in that it gave doctors the chance to align themselves with the state in a fashion that proved mutually beneficial. But there was a major difference: the bourgeoisie was no longer a revolutionary force, and neither was French psychiatry. Where the association of psychiatric and state power during and after the French Revolution inspired medical efforts to incorporate diverse segments of the population into the emergent social and political order, asylum doctors' triumphs in the immediate aftermath of the Franco-Prussian War and the Paris Commune had the opposite effect on medical understandings of treatment and cure. For one, psychiatric commentators like Laborde began to emphasize in ever more strident terms the hereditability of mental illness. Unlike their counterparts at the high point of the moral treatment era, degeneration theorists emphasized seemingly immutable differences between healthy bodies and pathological ones. Eventually the push toward hereditarianism would undermine doctors' faith in the gender-based treatment regimens developed earlier in the century and contribute to an even greater marginalization of those deemed mentally ill. Furthermore, the war and the Commune would come to play oversize roles in what we might call the French medical imagination. While Laborde somewhat dramatically positioned psychiatry as France's best defense against chaos, his descriptions of the revolutionary city implied that the resuscitation of French society could prove a lost cause, no matter what doctors like him had to say about it.

One final description from Laborde should make this clear. A particularly vivid episode in his narrative took place during the republican invasion of western Paris, just before the notorious "Bloody Week" that ended the experiment of the Paris Commune. He tells the tale of a friend and "fellow doctor" traveling through the city who supposedly witnessed a number of disturbing street scenes. Amid explosions and gunfire, a man danced in the middle of the road.[66] Injured revolutionaries sang raucously as their comrades were blown to pieces.[67] The streets ran "red with wine and blood" as men consorted with women of ill repute.[68] Again, the revolutionaries were not simply misguided, but out of control to the point of insanity.

Descriptions of this sort provided powerful "proof" of civilizational decline in the years to come. Those who emerged socially and politically victorious in the aftermath of the Commune—people like Laborde himself—recalled the period in terms of frenzied delirium rather than considered struggle. This image of the Commune contributed to a growing conviction that French society was as degenerate as the supposedly ravaged minds of the Communards. The dramatic loss of the Franco-Prussian War and the subsequent civil conflict indicated to many that France was a nation in free fall, a society whose diseased nature could be read in the very biology of its citizens. Specialists in mental medicine would soon come to see that this sort of thinking was incompatible with the basic tenets of the moral treatment, including its emphasis on gender as cure, which would lead some to rethink the asylum system in its entirety.

CHAPTER 6

Reforming the Asylum and Reimagining the Family

D OCTORS SUSTAINED AND EVEN INCREASED their legal and cultural authority throughout the early Third Republic, but this did not mean their critics were silenced. The French anti-alienist reformer and former city councilman J. Manier, for example, published a lengthy diatribe in 1886 in which he described a number of incidents typifying the abusive nature of psychiatric power.[1] Many of these cases were well-known at the time, such as the commitment of the talented woman musician Hersilie Rouy by her estranged brother in the 1840s, and a more recent case of unjust internment involving a young heiress, Antonia Monasterio. Other examples were less familiar, but all featured family members cruelly acting in their own self-interests—be it a husband committing his wife as to more easily carry on an affair or a wife seducing an asylum doctor to get rid of her husband—with the complicity and encouragement of the psychiatric community. Doctors had recently taken the events of the Franco-Prussian War and the Paris Commune as opportunities to strengthen their relationship to the state and reaffirm their commitment to bourgeois class interests, but they had clearly done very little to appease critics calling for the reform and even the abolition of the asylum system.

While asylum doctors and their most vocal critics saw one another as enemies, their proposed reforms were sometimes quite similar. The introduction of care in the community was the most serious reconsideration of the asylum system in the late nineteenth century, and its advocates came from within and outside the psychiatric profession. Manier, who considered himself an ally of the unjustly interned, believed the French asylum system was beyond repair. He did not dwell so much on the particulars of care in the community but used it instead as a rhetorical weapon against those who championed institutionalization despite the growing list of injustices committed inside asylums. French alienists focused more sustained attention on the question of community care than did any of their critics. Some advocated a form of "family colonization" in which particular villages would accept large numbers of mental patients into the local community, housing each patient with a host family. Others saw advantages in spreading mental patients throughout a given region or even the country as a whole. Still others envisioned opening up the asylum itself, allowing patients freedom of movement while still keeping them under medical supervision.

The key to the wide-ranging appeal of community care rested in its ability to simultaneously challenge and sustain the central tenets of asylum psychiatry, including those related to gender, class, and the family. Those who hoped to shutter asylums viewed care in the community as a form of liberation from medical authority. Reformers within the psychiatric community did not. Rather, their discussions of community care showed that some doctors were willing to surrender the physical space of the asylum as long as they could maintain its hierarchies, which they viewed as compatible with community care in ways someone such as Manier failed to recognize. Care in the community posed an undeniable threat to the moral treatment regime—notably its emphasis on patient cure through continuous interactions between the patient and a trained alienist—but it supported enough of the moral treatment's component parts that few doctors recognized (or cared to recognize) their own role in the destruction of Pinel and Esquirol's mission. Almost all reformist asylum doctors took great pains to show the ways in which community care maintained the relationship between the family, the patient, and the doctor elaborated during the performance of the moral treatment: familial isolation, patient surveillance, and the assertion of masculine scientific authority were just as readily accomplished outside asylum walls as within, perhaps even more so.

Debates over care in the community thus constitute a natural endpoint for a book examining the contradictory effects of doctors' efforts to "institutionalize gender" in the hundred or so years following the French Revolution, as they allow us to see what had changed, what had not, and why it mattered. This chapter explores three distinct approaches to late nineteenth-century asylum reform, all tied in one way or another to the concept of community care, moving chronologically from the earliest initiatives spearheaded by doctors in the 1860s to more urgent calls for change reflecting the supposed threat of hereditary degeneration in the 1880s and 1890s. Like the earliest practitioners of the moral treatment, doctors active in these debates reified bourgeois class and gender values while simultaneously expressing suspicion toward families of all backgrounds. For many of these medical reformers, however, community care also signified a loss of faith in curability and, as such, the abandonment of the gender-based treatment scenarios of the early- and mid-nineteenth century. Yet this shift in medical thinking was neither inevitable nor universal. It took time for theories of hereditary degeneration to solidify their ascendancy within psychiatric circles, and even then there were outliers. I therefore conclude by discussing the most groundbreaking medical reconsideration of the asylum—Évariste Marandon de Montyel's "open door" method at Ville-Évrard—to show that only through liberalizing their attitudes toward the family could doctors reform the hierarchical relations embedded in the psychiatric enterprise.

"From Paris to Gheel"

The first wave of psychiatric reformers focused their investigations on the Belgian "family colony" Gheel, as did the critic Manier, who laid out his case for the reorganization of the French national asylum system in a tract aptly titled *From Paris to Gheel*. In Gheel, located in what is now the Belgian province of Antwerp, patients lived in the homes of host families rather than under the lock and key of an asylum administrator. While Manier portrayed asylums as prison-like "Modern Bastilles," he spoke of Gheel in glowing, quasi-spiritual terms:

> Our mad are imprisoned and they are not criminals: let us give them air and liberty! Humanity, justice, and our finances demand it.... Gheel will see a day when it is held up as the most glorious monument of the entire world: To individual liberty! To social charity! To the universal redemption of the mad![2]

The seemingly more relaxed atmosphere of the family colony made it a useful comparison for those seeking to draw attention to the many deficiencies of the French asylum system. This certainly included those who hoped to destroy that system entirely, but the example of Gheel also intrigued doctors, many of whom were no longer convinced that the moral treatment was necessary for every patient. The asylum critic and medical doctor Léopold Turck urged French legislators to consider implementing a Gheel-like system in France as early as 1865, and the notable alienist Moreau de Tours celebrated the singular atmosphere of the colony after visiting in the 1840s.[3]

According to legend, Gheel's association with mad people began in the seventh century.[4] After fleeing from Ireland, a princess arrived in the village only to be tracked down by her angry and lustful father, a pagan king who intended to force his young Christian daughter to marry him. When she resisted his advances he murdered her: the martyred princess, Dymphne, came to be known as the patron saint of mental illness. The wandering mad arrived in Gheel on redemptive quests of pilgrimage, at which point locals brought them into their homes in Dymphe's honor. For many centuries, those hosted by the villagers of Gheel could hardly be considered patients at all, as the peasants made no attempts to heal their visitors. Instead, they simply lived within the community, apparently free of the stigma experienced in other parts of Europe. Intervention by medical professionals in day-to-day care became standardized during the nineteenth century when the town constructed an infirmary and the state involved itself in the commitment process. Patients still lived in local homes, shared meals with their caregivers, and worked either on farms or in town doing manual labor. Although a trained physician oversaw the placement of individual patients and kept track of their physical and mental states, these were limited forms of oversight compared with the levels of control exercised in more traditional asylums. The state provided host families a modest payment for their efforts.

Manier's appeals to individual liberty, in addition to his emphasis on treating patients as "free men," aligned with the stated goals of French alienists, if not their actions.[5] Following Pinel, whose decision to treat those labeled insane as patients rather than prisoners represented the fulfillment of some of the most progressive impulses of the French Revolution, nineteenth-century asylum doctors aimed to rehabilitate patients and eventually reintegrate them into their communities. Not surprisingly, proponents and critics of the asylum disagreed on how to best accomplish these ends. Manier believed doctor-patient relations were inherently authoritarian and abusive, and he found the living conditions inside both public and private asylums deplorable. He also thought alienists had a financial interest in admitting new patients and sequestering them as long as possible, giving lie to doctors' claims of scientific objectivity. The best path to reform would therefore involve introducing something entirely different, and Gheel functioned as an ideal model asylum because it was not truly an asylum at all. Manier claimed patients in Gheel were valued members of local households rather than perpetual objects of surveillance and scrutiny.

Envisioned by psychiatry's critics as the anti-asylum, the system of treatment in place at the Gheel colony elicited the skepticism of many French alienists. Yet they also expressed genuine concern about the underfunded and overcrowded conditions that reigned in their own institutions, leading doctors to explore alternatives. Representatives of the editorial board of the *Annales médico-psychologiques* undertook the most serious medical investigation into the Belgian system when they visited in 1860. The psychiatric community's interest in Gheel heightened over the course of the decade, as criticism of the asylum system reached a fever pitch and governmental reform initiatives allowed for the construction of new mental health facilities. French alienists considered a number of reform schemes, especially during the era of Haussmannization, because the Baron's intentions for Paris included plans to modernize asylum care throughout the Department of the Seine. Doctors used their discussions of Gheel to determine whether psychiatric treatment always necessitated sequestration in an institution, or if it might be possible to maintain both patient oversight and medical authority in a less restrictive environment.

Where someone like Manier celebrated the apparent freedom enjoyed by the patients in Gheel, some doctors worried that the situation encouraged a frightening lack of medical surveillance: patients "at liberty" could prove dangerous to the community, and unsupervised caregivers without medical training might do more harm than good. Certain doctors, notably the director of the Sainte-Anne asylum, Guillaume Ferrus, believed that insufficient administrative control in Gheel allowed villagers to treat their boarders abusively. Ferrus had been one of Esquirol's most promising students and he famously developed a method of treatment requiring patients to spend time out-of-doors doing agricultural labor. He described his visit to the Belgian colony in the 1840s as a step back in time, before the advent of the moral treatment. Some patients filled their days wandering the village without companionship or supervision, then spent their nights in irons.

Ferrus faulted the host families for behaving in a draconian fashion, arguing that the harsh living conditions within the family homes contributed to boarders' mental and physical deterioration. He witnessed a number of people chained inside filthy rooms in peasant dwellings where they were poorly fed and insufficiently clothed. "I believe," he wrote, after visiting Gheel in 1849 ". . . that treatment and liberty cannot go together."[6] Doctors rarely visited the boarders, and those who walked freely supposedly committed "immoral acts," as evidenced by the births of illegitimate children. He did not dwell on this observation, but it likely refers to the sexual abuse of women patients by members of the community. Additionally, according to Ferrus, the host families had no interest in caring for their charges and merely sought to collect compensation, as did the unscrupulous "intermediaries" who delivered mad people from surrounding territories for "treatment" in Gheel.[7] Alexander Brierre de Boismont, the private asylum director and longtime contributor to the *Annales médico-psychologiques*, also visited the Belgian colony in the 1840s and spoke out against what he considered the substandard treatment of the patients who resided there (which should come as little surprise considering his belief in the curative properties of bourgeois family values).[8]

By the 1860s, Brierre de Boismont admitted that a number of improvements had been made: the town constructed an infirmary and a Belgian alienist, Dr.

Bulkens, now controlled the colony's operations. Increased medical oversight seemed to satisfy the French medical community. Ferrus himself planned to revisit the site along with other French asylum doctors in 1860, but he died shortly before the expedition took place. Had he made the trip, he might have changed his dire opinion of the family colony. The doctors Trélat and Baillarger took his place on the exploratory mission, accompanied by fellow alienists Moreau de Tours, Michéa, Mesnet, and Falret. Those who visited in 1860 did not dwell on the frightful conditions previously highlighted by Ferrus. Instead, these medically trained visitors tended to consider both the strengths and weaknesses of family colonization, while also insisting that a Gheel-like system would never be possible in France.

Reporting on the commission's trip to Gheel at a meeting of the Société Médico-Psychologique in late 1861, Jules Falret that noted the colony often inspired extreme reactions. Most writing on the subject served to either "glorify Gheel, or fight against it."[9] His report took a descriptive tone, and he began by explaining that the town and its surrounding villages had approximately ten thousand inhabitants and eight hundred patients in total. Until 1851, the colony had largely gone unsupervised by regulatory authorities, and the "absolute abandonment of the mad to the hands of ignorant and greedy peasants" resulted in abuses like those described by the physicians Ferrus, Brierre de Boismont, and others.[10] By midcentury, however, the reforming zeal that had long since taken hold of the French psychiatric enterprise made its way to Belgium. Along with heightened state involvement came new regulators who paid scrupulous attention to deciding which families were allowed to take patients, and closely supervised those deemed worthy of the responsibility.[11] According to Falret, the active involvement of governmental and medical authorities created better living conditions for patients and increased the likelihood of cure.

Furthermore, when Falret spoke with the patients of Gheel, he noted with satisfaction that despite their "confusions of ideas, one habitually discerned a sentiment of satisfaction and interior tranquility."[12] He also expressed amazement that there was no noticeable increase in crime, accidental fires, or violence of any sort in a community inhabited by eight hundred mental patients. For Falret and his traveling companions this represented quite a mystery—the solution to which revealed precisely why Gheel could not be replicated in France. He wondered "how it was possible to give the mad the same degree of liberty that one gives men of healthy intelligence, and how, in these conditions, are accidents not more frequent, since the patients are left to themselves, without any surveillance."[13] He replied to his own question, noting that while it might appear there was little patient supervision, the legally appointed guardian and the other sane members of the household closely observed the patients living among them. Moreover, all ten thousand regional inhabitants oversaw the patients who moved freely throughout the town and countryside without attendants by their sides. This sense of communal responsibility supposedly stemmed from Gheel's unique history, particularly the religious origins of the town's relationship to the insane.

While recreating Gheel in France might have been desirable solution to the overcrowding of public asylums, the commission from the Société Médico-Psychologique did not think this was possible in the 1860s. A number of factors apparently worked against the development of such a system. In addition to Gheel residents' accepting attitudes towards the mentally ill, the region's geography and relative socioeconomic underdevelopment also contributed to the colony's success. Aside from a particular river bend, the region's terrain was safe for patients to meander unsupervised, and a thick belt of heather encircled the town and its environs. This made it difficult for patients to escape, with the added benefit of discouraging outsiders from passing through. Lastly, the town was large enough that it possessed a number of modest amenities, but it did not support any modern industries. This created an atmosphere in which "patriarchal morals" supposedly dominated.[14] In other words, the peasants treated the local bourgeoisie with an appropriate level of deference, and there were few members of the working class whose influence might provoke the already mad to greater levels of insanity.[15] Suffice it to say, there were few locales in France with a similar combination of environmental, social, and cultural attributes.

The eventual director of the suburban Parisian asylum Vaucluse, Eugène Billod, also expressed doubts over the applicability of the Gheel system to France. Like the members of the Société Médico-Psychologique, Billod paid a visit to the Gheel colony around 1860. He was less than impressed by the atmosphere cultivated by Dr. Bulkens, and soon published a rebuttal to the commission's findings. While he admired Falret's descriptions of the family colony's operations, he disagreed with some of the group's overall impressions. Falret spoke of the tranquility exhibited by patients living in Gheel, whereas Billod found the town's atmosphere rather depressing. He wrote, "If I had traversed Gheel in a fortuitous manner and without forewarning of the particularity that characterized it, nothing would have revealed itself positively to me. I even regret to add that I was taken aback by the absence of movement, of a mournful and silent aspect, that must make the patient's stay [in Gheel] no more attractive than [a stay] in a closed asylum."[16] This first impression was not one that he had expected, having read Falret's report, and he immediately sought an explanation.

Billod concluded that the sense of liberty that purportedly distinguished Gheel from other sorts of institutions did not truly exist. He blamed this state of affairs on the families who served as patient guardians. Despite the recent uptick in medical supervision, they focused their energies on controlling patients' actions rather than truly integrating them into the community. Falret suggested that Dr. Bulkens's innovations had introduced a more standardized form of treatment throughout the colony and that patient abuse was relatively uncommon, yet Billod suspected guardians resisted the efforts of medical men and sought only to maintain order within their households. This might not have led to physical abuse, but neither did it encourage liberty in any real sense. In essence, Billod argued that the atmosphere cultivated in Gheel was more authoritarian, more tightly controlled, and patently less free than that of French public asylums. "The guardians," he said, "are particularly interested in maintaining order, to prevent accidents" that might reflect badly on themselves and the colony as a whole.[17] They rarely accompanied their boarders on walks and the patients "gave in soon enough to apathy and did not delay . . . in taking up sedentary habits." At the time of his visit, "order reigned" at Gheel, thanks in part to "its new organization," which, he wrote, "was more or less restrictive of liberty."[18]

Billod supported the psychiatric enterprise. He was the first director of the newly built Vaucluse asylum, where he successfully maintained operations during the Prussian siege of 1870 and earned entrance into the Legion of Honor for his efforts. But in his criticisms of Gheel, he undermined some central assumptions held by major figures in the French psychiatric community. Namely, he questioned whether a correlation always existed between order, surveillance, and successful treatment. As an outspoken partisan of the French national asylum system, Billod failed to take his observations to their logical conclusion: he did not extend his point regarding order and the destruction of the patient's spirit in Gheel to the asylum itself. Instead, Billod noted that the Belgian case served as an example of why colonization would have to emerge from existing institutions in France rather than through replication of the Gheel model. A deep suspicion of families willing to house mental patients lay at the heart of his critique, as it had in the work of Ferrus twenty years prior. The people of Gheel felt overly responsible for the behaviors of their charges, so they repressed liberty in the name of safety, security, and their own reputations. Billod was far more comfortable placing this responsibility in the hands of asylum doctors like himself, whose authoritative but still benevolent relationship to their patients stemmed from a scientific and supposedly disinterested rationale.

Neither Billod nor his better-known contemporaries found the creation of a "French Gheel" particularly wise or realistic, yet the stage had been set for more radical reform initiatives. The commission from the Société Médico-Psychologique concluded that the asylum and the family colony would each benefit from adopting certain elements of the other. As Falret explained, "for each of them progress consists of this double movement. . . . Gheel can only perfect itself by approaching the closed asylum. [Asylums], for their part, can only ameliorate themselves while walking with a prudent slowness, but with perseverance, on the path of liberty."[19] Aside from two obvious differences between Gheel and the asylum ("liberty of circulation and living in the milieu of non-insane families"), the two methods aimed to implement, albeit in different forms, "the same principles."[20]

The moral treatment had been established in the late eighteenth century in order to rid institutions of "everything that recalls the prison." According to Falret, Pinel and his intellectual descendants sought to create an atmosphere that recalled "ordinary habitations more and more, and the life of man in general" by furnishing patients with diversions in and out of doors, allowing them to socialize and dine with one another, and eliminating all unnecessary forms of physical restraint.[21] These goals could just as easily describe those of the family colony's overseers. The medical sojourners of the Société Médico-Psychologique therefore insisted the two systems displayed "secondary" rather than "fundamental" differences.[22] As time wore on, however, the discussion over asylum reform focused less on how to best implement the original goals of the moral treatment and more on whether those goals remained compatible with the priorities of French society at all.

Asylum Reform and Degeneration

In 1877, Emile Zola published *L'Assomoir,* the seventh volume of his series of twenty novels chronicling late-nineteenth-century France through the stories of various members of the sprawling Rougon-Macquart family. *L'Assomoir* relates the relentlessly bleak fate of Gervaise, a hardworking laundress who succumbs to the ravages of alcoholism. Following a long period of social, psychological, and physical decline, Gervaise eventually dies alone under a stairwell, all but forgotten by her friends and neighbors. Her fall from respectability is precipitated by her husband Coupeau's literal fall from a roof. The resultant injury keeps Coupeau from working—a fate he ultimately seems to embrace because it allows him time to drink. As in the case of Gervaise, alcoholism kills her husband. Yet his end lacks even the dignity of privacy, for he spends his last days institutionalized in the Parisian asylum Saint-Anne, having lost control of his bodily functions along with his grasp on reality.

Coming near the end of the novel, the scenes at Saint-Anne portray French asylum psychiatry as authoritative and self-assured. The indifference of expertise melds with a sense of bourgeois disdain as the doctor, modeled after the alienist Valentin Magnan, casually announces to Gervaise her husband's incurability.[23] The portrayal of medical men as unfeeling and disinterested was not unique to Zola, particularly with the rise of scientific positivism and its emphasis on observation and objectivity. Psychiatric treatises themselves had largely lost the relative sentimentality apparent in the writings of the discipline's founders, which was replaced with a studied clinical remove. At the same time, many asylum doctors in the 1870s still proclaimed the value of their profession in terms of patient welfare and, crucially, patient cure. It is therefore noteworthy that Zola, the writer of realist fiction, understood something that alienists were as yet unwilling to admit: their own evolving theories of the mind were moving in a profoundly cynical direction, and some had all but given up on the moral treatment's mission even if they continued to claim Pinel and Esquirol as their masters. Asylum psychiatry faced multiple threats at century's end, and members of the profession dwelt extensively on the chronic underfunding of public institutions, as well as the various unjust commitment scandals that seemed to draw constant attention from the press. Yet few practitioners acknowledged that one of the most profound dangers to the implementation of the moral treatment—the rise of biological, hereditary explanations for mental illness—emerged from within the profession itself.

Zola suggests as much in his *L'Assomoir* asylum scenes. He famously conceived of the Rougon-Macquart cycle as an exploration of the relationship between social decline and heredity, showing the ways in which members of the family failed to escape the stain of their degenerate origins (including Gervaise and her daughter, the eponymous prostitute of *Nana*). Coupeau's doctor at Saint-Anne thus inquires into his patient's pathological family history as his patient's body thrashes in a cell like a marionette. A hereditary explanation for Coupeau's condition simultaneously confirms the doctor's theories on the origins of the patient's addiction-fueled mania and provides a ready-made excuse to give up on treatment. "Magnan" soon determines that Coupeau is a hopeless case, as were presumably thousands of others in fin-de-siècle France whose lineage predisposed them to all manner of mental and physical impairments.

Like the various characters of *L'Assomoir*, real mental patients in the late 1800s were increasingly viewed as incurable victims of their own family trees. Hereditary explanations for madness gained steam at the precise moment when the inadequacies of asylum psychiatry became evident to anyone paying attention. In fact, the increasing prevalence of such attitudes might best be understood as reactions to the apparent failures of the moral treatment regime since its implementation in 1838 (reactions that, in turn, hastened that system's decline). Somatic interpretations of insanity had always existed alongside psychological ones, and even Pinel acknowledged the impact of nonenvironmental, physical factors on the emergence and progression of mental illness. Hereditarianism tilted this balance sharply toward the somatic over the psychological by combining the already widespread belief in the physical origins of insanity with the recent vogue for evolutionary theory.

The asylum doctor Benedict Morel published his *Traité des dégénérescences physiques, intellectuelles et morales de l'espèce humaine et des causes qui produisent ces variétés maladives* in 1857, and his ideas regarding madness as a sign of evolutionary decline influenced the profession immediately, if unevenly. As Robert Nye has expertly shown, hereditary degeneration was a theory well suited for its time.[24] In an era of intense instability and national soul-searching, especially after the loss of the Franco-Prussian War, the relative optimism of the postrevolutionary psychiatric community seemed profoundly out of place. Magnan, the Saint-Anne doctor who inspired Zola's character and was known for his studies on hereditary alcoholism, was one of Morel's many students and followers, the numbers of whom would multiply both within and outside the psychiatric profession in the decades leading up to the First World War.

The rise of degeneration theory led psychiatric professionals to reconsider their long-held assertion that every mental patient required isolation from their family in an asylum. The sad irony was that this had little to do with the charges leveled at the profession by its critics, but instead reflected doctors' loss of confidence in their own ability to truly reintegrate patients into French society. Pinel understood the asylum as a sort of way station where patients could relearn proper behavior before returning to their homes as fathers, mothers, and citizens. Few of the men running psychiatric institutions sixty years after his death held such hopes. When doctors started to equate heredity with destiny, the moral treatment itself suffered a fate much like that of *L'Assomoir*'s Coupeau and Gervaise. It wasted away, another French casualty of "degeneration."

Debates during the mid-nineteenth century about the applicability of Gheel's example to France did not refer to contemporary theories of hereditary degeneration, although Morel first published on the subject in the late 1850s. One of the complaints of alienists regarding Gheel actually involved the comparatively low rates of cure among family colony patients, indicating that doctors in the 1860s still considered most forms of mental illness curable when treated in an asylum. This perspective would begin to change following France's defeat in the Franco-Prussian War of 1870 and the subsequent civil conflict of the Paris Commune, as intellectuals of various stripes began to obsess over the widespread perception of national decline.

Most of these social and cultural commentators had little practical interest in asylum reform and instead dwelled on the myriad signs of degeneration apparently afflicting France on the national, familial, and individual levels. Charles Féré, a physician and one-time assistant to Jean-Martin Charcot, was a notable exception. He published widely in the late decades of the nineteenth century on topics ranging from animal magnetism to criminality to the "neuropathic family"—a term he coined for an astonishing array of symptoms he insisted were linked to one another despite their differences in character and severity, any one of which constituted evidence of hereditary degeneration.[25] Féré served as a the chief physician of Bicêtre from 1887 until his death in 1907. In 1889, he published the most detailed discussion of family care written in France before the First World War, and a second edition came out several years later. Féré's *Traitement des aliénés dans les familles* addressed a number of practicalities related to family colonization that other doctors alluded to only in passing. In the process, he made manifest certain assumptions regarding the class and gender dimensions of this form of treatment that had remained latent in earlier discussions, while adding a fresh focus on heredity. His writings show the ways degeneration theory complemented the moral treatment in fundamental respects, in particular its insistence on the patient's isolation from the family, while ultimately undermining that method's commitment to patient cure.

In his work on the neuropathic family, Féré's most fully developed contribution to degenerationist thought, he presents a rather desperate picture of French society. Echoing Charles Beard, Féré believed nervous conditions stemmed from life in modern, urban environments, noting "the best cure for civilized life is a return to barbarism."[26] The conditions of modern life intensified the threat of mental and physical breakdown for those born with hereditary predispositions, whose numbers appeared to be on the rise. Féré also thought, like Morel, that hereditary degeneration ultimately resulted in sterility, putting him in the seemingly contradictory position of seeing potential degenerates everywhere while also claiming that their own pathological natures would cause their family lines—insufficiently prepared for the evolutionary battle of all against all—to eventually die out.[27] Thus, unlike some of his contemporaries, Féré opposed forced sterilization or even some of the more "positive" eugenicist interventions promoted by the likes of Francis Galton, such as the issuance of eugenic certificates or the required revelation of family health histories before marriage. Instead, he believed the best way to reduce the number of French "degenerates" was to keep them as healthy as possible for as long as possible (he emphasized nutrition and sleep habits), and away from potentially triggering situations.[28] That said, he expressed little hope that an individual might fully recover once having exhibited symptoms of degeneracy.

For people showing signs of mental illness—which constituted a major branch of Féré's neuropathic family—treatment entailed separating them from their relatives, who, naturally, were also predisposed to hereditary afflictions. Féré believed the family home represented a dangerous combination of environmental and biological inspirations for nervous ailments like hysteria and neurasthenia, explaining "the neuropath often lives in an atmosphere of nervousness."[29] He therefore concluded that living in a stranger's home might represent an effective form of treatment. Hysterical women who refused to eat, overly emotional and indecisive men, children with infantile neurosis—all these types would supposedly benefit from fresh air, discipline, and a safe distance from their overly permissive relatives.

Furthermore, the care of an insane family member could be overly taxing for someone with an emotional involvement in the case. Citing the American physician Silas Weir Mitchell, Féré likened the ill patient to "a vampire sucking the blood of the healthy people of the house," and he suggested that children in particular could be harmed if they lived with and tried to care for their unwell parents.[30] The danger of mental contagion between family members was dire, and not just for women. Féré warned his readers "the strong sex" was susceptible as well and even brought up the example of sympathetic pregnancy.[31] Familial isolation would keep each member of the family safe from the pathological influence of the others, while removing the mental patient from the environment in which their illness initially took root.

On the surface, Féré maintained that family colonization could lead to cure, at one point noting that "the happy termination of the illness depends in large part on the influence that the nurse [i.e., the in-home caregiver] can acquire over the patient."[32] He consistently belied this statement, however, with his insistence that the most appropriate patients for family colonization were "incurables." Public asylums in France—Féré himself worked in one the largest and best-known—remained overcrowded and chronically underfunded. His experience as the lead physician at Bicêtre convinced him that most patients in public institutions were hopeless cases draining limited resources from those who could still be rehabilitated. He wanted asylums to function more like hospitals, where he and his fellow doctors and interns could experiment with new methods on people they deemed more medically interesting than those experiencing symptoms of dementia, mania brought on by alcoholism, or the ravages of syphilis (which he did not consider a hereditary affliction, although he argued that a predilection toward sexual promiscuity and other risky behaviors was passed down through generations). Removing such patients from asylums would do them no harm because their conditions would never improve in any case.

Féré championed family colonization more stridently than any of his predecessors, always under the condition that patients would be placed in the households of strangers. The physical and emotional isolation from people associated with the patient's former life could be accomplished just as well inside the home of a host family as it could within a closed institution. Like previous medical commentators, he saw a great deal of potential in the example of Gheel. Yet, again like other French observers, he thought the Belgian case was too unique to be replicated in France. He argued that the example of the Scottish "cottage system" held greater promise because it isolated the mad from their families, but had the added benefit of stricter medical oversight. Patients in Scotland were also spread throughout the country instead of clustered in one particular village, making it a more easily replicable system. For Féré this practice entailed a number of important benefits, including ease and cost of treatment. It allowed more patients to be cared for without constructing new psychiatric facilities, and it let asylums serve as hospitals rather than permanent rest homes for incurable patients. It also supposedly ensured patients' "comfort, satisfaction, happiness, and good health" without compromising public security.[33]

While psychiatric observers like Falret, Billod, and the head physician of the asylum of Antiquaille, Joseph Arthaud, had previously endorsed family care when under the strict supervision of medical professionals, Féré elucidated what this should look like in practice.[34] He aimed to enforce a very specific vision of order, authority, and discipline within the host homes by training guardians to oversee the patients when the doctor was not present. Families were to house patients and provide them with sustenance, but Féré also expected them to observe patients closely and act as exemplars of normative mental health. The families, in turn, were to operate under the watchful eyes of the local asylum doctor. In this fashion the hierarchies of the asylum could be maintained without the associated costs and inconveniences.

The most important aspect of family care was the choice of "nurse" or guardian. This companion performed a diverse number of activities vis-à-vis the patient living in their home, from providing them with intellectual and physical stimulation to feeding them and delivering medications.[35] Yet Féré did not imagine the guardian's duties as merely a list of tasks. He or she also needed to craft a thoughtful self-presentation. Similar to the psychiatric persona developed by Pinel and later elaborated by Leuret and others, Féré's ideal attendant should sustain an authoritative demeanor that would encourage the patient's acceptance and obedience.

While taking responsibility for a mental patient was an "arduous and tiresome task" that depended on "the strength of a sole individual," there were often multiple guardians in the home.[36] One person should be designated as the primary caregiver and, again like an asylum doctor, he or she should approach all interactions with the patient on an even keel, acting "firmly and without indecision."[37] Maintaining this sense of comportment was especially vital considering the consequences that might ensue if the patient lost respect for the guardian. The guardian's slightest "weakness" could have a long-term effect on their ability to control the patient inside their home. Féré noted that it "often becomes necessary to change the caregiver who bends under the heavy weight that is imposed on him."[38] All these warnings could be directed equally toward alienists themselves as to family care guardians. However, as Féré made clear, the guardian should never act as a counterpoint to the doctor, whose authority was to remain supreme at all times. Furthermore, unlike the doctor-patient interactions carried out in the course of the moral treatment, Féré gave no indication that family care guardians should engage in carefully plotted treatment scenarios to convince patients to return to rationality.

Who, then, was the perfect guardian? According to Féré, the position required above all "a vigorous person, of good will, and ready to accept the direction of the doctor who is in charge of the treatment."[39] He argued that it was convenient for the patient and the guardian to share a similar class background, considering the amount of time the two would spend together and the importance of maintaining the patient's respect for their caregiver. Féré found that women often proved more suitable than men, particularly those "women who have had a reverse in fortunes in which they played a purely passive role, and have accepted definitively their situation."[40] Women who had fallen from their station presumably had a number of attributes Féré found agreeable. First, they came from respectable class backgrounds, but were nonetheless eager to augment their finances. They also played no role in their declining fortunes and were therefore likely to serve as examples of respectability. In accepting their new station, they proved themselves likely to commit to guardianship in the long term and be willing to follow the directives of a medically trained man. Male guardians with a similar life history were generally unappealing precisely because they "accept with less resignation their new position."[41] The gender dynamics ensuring a downtrodden bourgeoise would cede authority to the male doctor did not imply she would be subservient to her male wards, suggesting that Féré considered male patients already emasculated by virtue of their illnesses. Like the female directors of private asylums discussed in a previous chapter, rational women who served as family care guardians could conceivably act as authority figures over the men in their care without subverting nineteenth-century gender values.

An entire chapter of Féré's *Du Traitement des aliénés dans les familles* was devoted to "indispensable notions for persons charged with the care of the mad." Guardians had accepted a heavy responsibility, especially from the perspective of their patients' families. They therefore owed it to them to become as knowledgeable as possible about the manifestation of mental illness; they were not to diagnose or come up with treatment regimens on their own, but they "could not give useful information to the doctors if they do not have some general knowledge of the most common symptoms of psychosis."[42] Guardians thus served as the doctor's eyes and ears when he was not present.

Even more important than knowing what to look out for was knowing how best to behave while in the patient's presence. It was vital that the alienated "have always under their eyes the example of order and the most scrupulous cleanliness" because they often failed to practice good hygiene or dress themselves with care.[43] While patients might have lost their own sense of propriety, they could apparently still judge it in others. A shabbily dressed guardian risked earning the approbation of the patient and might then lose respect and control. Caring overly much about one's appearance was also a dangerous trait because the patient might find vanity a source of irritation. In the realms of "moral and intellectual discipline"[44] the guardian must likewise serve as an upright example. He or she should react calmly to all insults and eschew excessive language. In fact, the caregiver ought to refrain from speaking too much at all in order to avoid saying something potentially disruptive. It was especially important for Féré that the guardian never talk about the patient while he or she was present and that they should present themselves as deserving of respect without seeming arrogant. The doctor ends the chapter with a brief aside: guardians should "particularly avoid familiarity with servants from whom they must always distinguish themselves."[45]

Féré's treatise showed it was possible to reimagine the asylum without truly questioning the power relations embedded in its architecture, legal mechanisms, or personnel hierarchies. For a proponent of the family care system, he proved consistently suspicious of those on whom the treatment depended the most: he did not trust caregivers to develop relationships with their charges without the intervention of a medical expert like himself. The close supervision of guardians maintained the family, class, and gender dynamics asylum doctors had elaborated earlier in the century, and his statements regarding the ideal family care guardian clearly upheld dominant notions of bourgeois domestic femininity. Furthermore, like the practitioners of the moral treatment who preceded him, his understanding of the symptoms of degeneration often pathologized gender and sexual nonconformity: nymphomania, homosexuality, and impotence all constituted evidence of degeneracy for Féré.

Yet, in contrast to his predecessors, Féré never envisioned the family care system as a means of cure. He might have turned the structure of institutionalization on its head, but many of the fundamentals remained the same, for he questioned neither the paternalistic authority of the asylum doctor nor the concept of familial isolation. Owing to his concern over degeneration and the threat of hereditary madness, Féré insisted even more stridently than the first French alienists that patients must remain isolated from their own families, now in the name of containment rather than cure. The nineteenth century began with doctors modeling asylums on the interpersonal dynamics of the family home to aid them in their efforts at patient rehabilitation. It came to a close with at least one influential doctor hoping to turn family homes into miniature asylums, now with a different mission.

An Alternate Path

Much of the French psychiatric community began to support the use of family colonization for "chronic, inoffensive" patients by the end of the century, mainly owing to the expense and overcrowding endemic to more traditional institutions.[46] As an asylum doctor in the Rhône noted in 1901, his institution was so overcrowded that the department was considering plans to build a new asylum, but he thought creating a family colony would be "equally practical and less expensive."[47] Two such colonies opened in France in the 1890s: a women's facility at Dun-sur-Auron followed by a colony for men at Ainay-le-Château. By 1900, the women's colony housed upward of one thousand patients in the homes of thoroughly vetted villagers. Family care guardians at Dun were allowed to host up to six patients at a time, and two staff doctors made rounds throughout the colony to observe the patients and prescribe medications. Significantly, the majority of patients were considered incurable—43 percent of the women exhibited signs of senility and dementia and, at least initially, all women patients were required to be post-menopausal. There was little indication that patients who lived in French family colonies were expected to recover and eventually leave, although it is likely that the experience of residing in a family colony was more comfortable than remaining in an overcrowded asylum.[48]

The asylum director Évariste Marandon de Montyel was arguably more innovative in his attempts to reform the nature of asylum care because he purposely sought to overturn what he considered outdated attitudes towards the patient's own family. Appointed director of the Parisian suburban asylum Ville-Évrard in 1888, Marandon de Montyel immediately began experimenting with new forms of institutional administration. His major innovation in patient care was the inauguration of the "Open Door" method.[49] Like family colonization, the origins of the Open Door were Scottish, but the practice had also been implemented in continental and North American contexts.[50] While the original practitioners of asylum psychiatry sought to isolate and sequester patients from the potentially harmful influence of their families, Marandon de Montyel believed maintaining contact between mental patients and the rest of society would have a positive effect.

He thus tried to create what many at the time considered a contradiction in terms—an asylum without walls. Rather than keeping patients in individual cells with only limited access to one another and the outside world, Marandon de Montyel opened the doors inside the asylum as well its front gate, creating a situation where patients could move about with relative freedom while still under the surveillance of asylum employees. Despite generating serious interest from alienists throughout Western and Central Europe and the United States, Marandon de Montyel noted with disappointment that French doctors generally ignored the Open Door as a treatment option.[51] He attempted to bring attention to his cause with some success during the 1890s, but died in 1908 after a prolonged illness (making his time at Ville-Évrard exactly contemporary with Féré's tenure at Bicêtre). The French national asylum system never implemented the Open Door in a concerted fashion.[52] Nonetheless, as the reformer himself noted, certain aspects of the Open Door had become mainstream by the turn of the century.[53]

It was fitting that Marandon de Montyel articulated the "Open Door" policy at Ville-Évrard. The institution was founded in the 1860s in the midst of psychiatric debates over asylum overcrowding and the merits of the Gheel colony. Most asylum doctors determined that full-fledged family colonization was not a realistic option for France at that time, but those of the Seine Department concluded that some reformation of the asylum system should indeed take place. Not only was Paris the center of psychiatry's intellectual community, as an educational center and meeting place for the discipline's major professional organizations, but the region experienced asylum overcrowding to a greater degree than other parts of France because of the influx of emigrants from the provinces. For these reasons, along with the general reformist zeal that marked Haussmann's Paris, asylums built in the 1860s were distinct from those that came before. Ville-Évrard and its sister institution, Vaucluse, were designed as agricultural colonies where patients were expected to internalize both discipline and a limited sense of liberty by working in the fields.

Ville-Évrard constituted an innovative institutional space from the start. It was not until Marandon de Montyel took over, however, that the asylum's operating procedures began to undermine foundational assumptions of psychiatric medicine. In many respects, the Open Door was simply the logical conclusion of psychiatry's goal to increase patient freedom. Just as Pinel had released the mad from their chains, so too did Marandon de Montyel free them from the walls of the asylum—or so he claimed. Like most alienists, whether or not they considered themselves partisans of asylum reform, the head of Ville-Évrard explained his innovations in the language of psychiatry's founders, praising Pinel and Esquirol for treating patients like potentially useful members of society instead of prisoners or animals. Marandon de Montyel argued that despite the changes implemented by "our fathers" early in the century,

> ... the mad person is still locked up in his special environment. This special environment, sirs, is dangerous and painful; dangerous and painful as were the chains, dangerous and painful as was idleness. Let us march upon the glorious paths of our illustrious predecessors, and, for our part, deliver the patient who is dear to all of us from his hospital prison.[54]

This was a variation of the same idea celebrated by the proponents of Gheel, who insisted the arc of the asylum should always bend toward liberty. Yet Marandon de Montyel criticized the failures of the psychiatric enterprise far more boldly than previous commentators, who typically justified their experimentation with care in the community on the basis of cost rather than the outright failure of the asylum system. Indeed, Marandon de Montyel's comparison between the asylum and the prison mirrored the language of writers affiliated with the anti-alienist movement, who often referred to asylums as "Modern Bastilles."

Marandon de Montyel was not prepared to abandon the asylum altogether. Instead, he hoped to redesign mental institutions in such a way as to promote feelings of connection and inclusion rather than loneliness and isolation. A major aspect of the Open Door revolved around asylum architecture, again in a fashion that served to link his heterodox ideas to those of psychiatry's founding fathers, in this case Esquirol. In a response to his harshest critic, Dr. Christian of the Parisian asylum Charenton, Marandon argued "Esquirol was absolutely right to say that the asylum must be the principal instrument of cure."[55] The reformer even claimed that if Esquirol were alive in the late nineteenth century, he would be a proponent of the Open Door. (Esquirol, the doctor who most forcefully elaborated the principal of isolation to begin with!) Marandon de Montyel was horrified by the cloistered nature of midcentury asylums, especially the various closed off symmetrical "covered galleries," which, he argued, created asylums within asylums where patients were not only isolated from the outside world, but from one another as well.[56] He thought patients should instead be housed in villas spread out in a park-like atmosphere and watched over by asylum employees. The doors and windows would remain open at all times, and all but the most dangerous of patients would enjoy freedom of movement.

Patients earned the privilege of liberty through labor. Ville-Évrard consisted of numerous buildings and studios in addition to a functioning farm. There were multiple pavilions, workshops, and other buildings scattered over 285 hectares. The asylum farm took up some of this space, and patients spent much of their time there. As was the case inside the asylum's buildings, patients did not experience physical restraint in the fields, although guardians provided oversight. If a patient failed to work assiduously, they would be transferred to a more secure part of the facility, having proven themselves undeserving of the limited freedoms possessed by others. According to Marandon de Montyel, labor was essential to successful treatment because if a patient could not work, he would never succeed in "the struggle for life" upon release.[57] This attitude was not particularly original, and most doctors shared Marandon de Montyel's patently bourgeois perspective on the link between rational self-control and productive, disciplined labor.[58]

With respect to patients' families Marandon de Montyel proved more radical. The isolation of patients from their relatives had long been a central principle of psychiatric care, and most doctors were unwilling to consider the benefits of family life for rehabilitation (that is, when the family in question was the patient's actual family, rather than a stand-in family of paid strangers). Some doctors had nonetheless insinuated that isolation from the family might be ignored in certain cases, most often as a cost-saving measure. Billod, in his 1861 critique of Gheel, made the surprising suggestion that patients might be returned to their own families for treatment. Like Falret and the other commissioners from the Société Médico-Psychologique, Billod believed Gheel's methods were most useful when it came to "chronic, incurable, and inoffensive" patients, but he also noted that "for the same patients, I would know a much more preferable system": entrusting to their own families those individuals whom, at Gheel, "we charge to the families of strangers."[59] Few doctors in the 1860s actively questioned the central precept of familial isolation, and Billod did so mainly for financial considerations, explaining that families who took care of their relatives at home could receive a monetary allowance from the state for their efforts. This subsidy would "always be inferior to the pension paid in the asylum, [which] will result, for the department, in a certain reduction of their burdens."[60] He also noted, much like the proponents of the Gheel colony and the degenerationist Féré, that urban workers should never be tasked with the responsibilities of guardianship.

Psychiatric suspicion of families infused all discussions of possible reforms, and Billod was not typical in his belief that returning patients to their own families prior to recovery could constitute anything but a last resort. Of course, many families chose not to commit their relatives to begin with, whether because they could not afford the fees involved in private asylum internment or even the less expensive option of "voluntary" commitment to a public asylum, or because they did not want to subject their loved ones to the conditions of institutionalization. Private asylum doctor Brierre de Boismont claimed there were 84,214 mad people living in France in 1861. Among them, 31,154 inhabited asylums, whereas a full 53,260 still lived with their families at home.[61] As shown in the previous chapter, doctors in Paris returned patients to their relatives during the Prussian siege in 1870 as a preventative measure against the possibility of mass starvation.[62] Many doctors nonetheless believed keeping patients with their own families was a stopgap measure at best.

Marandon de Montyel went much further by suggesting isolation from the family almost always caused more harm than good. Those like Féré still insisted patients should reside with strangers because their pathological home lives contributed to insanity. It was essential to remove patients from the environment in which their illness had first manifested, and this meant keeping patients away from the negative influence of their families above all else. Conversely, the director of Ville-Évrard believed that continued interaction between patients and their relatives would encourage a more speedy recovery, even when the patient lived in an asylum. This controversial aspect of the Open Door would face considerable resistance from the psychiatric community, but Marandon de Montyel insisted that doctors who cut ties between patients and their families confused two interrelated principles: "change of milieu" and "isolation."[63] Altering a patient's environment remained fundamental to the treatment process, whereas isolation from their loved ones imperiled attempts to heal them and later reintegrate them into their communities. Marandon de Montyel wondered whether if a patient "still loves his family, how can isolation from them be a good thing?"[64] In such a case, isolation would only make the patient feel abandoned, while one who already distrusts his relatives would have all his worst suspicions confirmed.

Furthermore, regular family visits could prove curative. They showed the patient in a concrete fashion that he was not a source of shame. Visits also underscored the fact that patients were not prisoners, especially when relatives spent time together outside the asylum. Marandon de Montyel took practical steps to encourage visitation, the most effective of which was the elimination of strict visiting hours. He recognized that organizing a trip to the suburbs took quite a bit of time and effort, especially for working people. He allowed those who made the trip to bring meals and special treats. Again, this made patients feel less like inmates forced to do without the conveniences of everyday life. So too did brief sojourns in the countryside, where relatives often accompanied patients on Sundays. These sorts of interactions had positive mental and physical effects and also served to decrease tensions between families and doctors, according to Marandon de Montyel. All of this represented a great divergence from the suspicion of families long expressed by alienists. Marandon de Montyel considered his patients' families partners. This new attitude had the potential to undermine the power relations that had structured the asylum system for decades. Someone like Féré hoped to avoid this at all costs, going so far as to reproduce traditional asylum hierarchies within the seemingly distinct setting of the home, whereas Marandon de Montyel seemed to embrace this result.

He was not alone in his ambitions. The innovative asylum doctor had at least one ally in Dr. Bourneville, the socialist asylum director of another suburban asylum, Villejuif.[65] The doctors Colin and Toulouse also came to Marandon de Montyel's defense in the pages of the *Annales médico-psychologiques*.[66]

Nonetheless, he faced severe backlash for having dared to so openly critique the status quo. Numerous colleagues were offended by Marandon de Montyel's suggestion that asylums—and by extension, asylum doctors—transformed patients into incurables through sequestration and isolation. They even attacked the Open Door at a special session of the Société Médico-Psychologique in 1897, bringing up the old argument that "the families of the mad are often their worst enemies."[67] Most asylum doctors still aimed to maintain a safe distance between relatives and institutionalized patients at the turn of the century, perhaps more than ever owing to the constant drumbeat of degeneration-fueled anxieties preoccupying French society more broadly.

Marandon de Montyel and other advocates for the Open Door represented a new type of alienist, one who envisioned the ideal doctor-patient relationship less hierarchically than the founders of the moral treatment, the degeneration theorists, or the proponents of the Gheel colony. The family occupied a central position in this novel conception of psychiatric power, for Marandon de Montyel viewed relatives as potential allies rather than sources of madness. This simple alteration encouraged him to reimagine the asylum system in its entirety. It was not practical to demolish the nation's asylums and rebuild new ones without doors, but the attitudes expressed by Marandon de Montyel and his supporters became more widespread over time. And while he did not succeed in reorganizing the nation's asylums beyond individual institutions in the Department of the Seine, France implemented a version of community care in which patients remained in their own homes at the end of World War I.[68]

The timing was not coincidental. For if numerous doctors in the late nineteenth century felt comfortable labeling those experiencing the symptoms of insanity as degenerates or incurables, the traumas of the First World War contradicted these assumptions in dramatic fashion. When the minds of all men—indeed, the "best" of men—showed vulnerability to mental breakdown under the stress of trench warfare, doctors sought to reincorporate them back into French society when they finally came home. Considering the staggering numbers of French soldiers who never returned from the field of battle at all, what other choice did they have?

BY THE END OF THE 1800s, psychiatric professionals faced circumstances resulting in the widespread abandonment of the moral treatment. These threats were threefold. First, asylums after 1838 never received the monetary support needed from the state to enact the moral treatment on a large scale. Where

Pinel, Esquirol, and their immediate intellectual descendants had been able to carry out the moral treatment in a piecemeal fashion over the first decades of the nineteenth century, legislators did not give public asylum doctors the tools with which to put their theories into action nationally. This lack of resources resulted in overcrowded and unsanitary conditions in asylums, in addition to abuse and insufficient oversight. Instances of unwilling asylum commitment represent a second and related challenge to the profession, and to the moral treatment regime in particular, because cases of unjust internment so clearly contradicted the method's stated aims. The third threat emerged from within the profession itself, as more and more practitioners became convinced that Pinel's methods were incapable of curing the ever-growing population of asylum patients, even if they still gave lip service to his aims. In the face of failure, doctors homed in on physical explanations for the onset and treatment of mental illness, particularly those that incorporated new conceptions of heredity and degeneration. As we have seen, the events of the Franco-Prussian War and the Paris Commune gave inspiration and credence to these theories.

This state of affairs realigned psychiatric understandings of family life in ways that undermined doctors' faith in the connection between bourgeois values and cure, creating a situation in which alienists continued to naturalize gender and class difference without even pretending to use these ideas in the name of rehabilitation. This tendency can already be seen in the investigations of the Gheel colony, which French doctors celebrated for maintaining class divisions between patients and community members and for shielding patients from the supposedly dangerous influence of workers despite the low rates of cure. The degeneration theorist and outspoken proponent of family colonization, Féré, took these notions even further. He consistently linked gender nonconformity to mental illness and also promoted family colonization as a way to isolate the mad from their own families—not to free them from their supposed maladies or the inhumane conditions of the asylum, but to avoid spreading the contagion of degeneracy. Like previous asylum doctors, he also suggested scientific authority was inherently masculine and that middle-class women's natures prepared them to care for the insane (in this case as ideal family care guardians) while still subordinating themselves to a male doctor.

Yet the need for reform also paved the way for some doctors to begin questioning outdated attitudes toward mental illness and family life. In the case of Marandon de Montyel, this meant maintaining his belief in the possibility of cure while rejecting the notion of familial isolation. Like his predecessors and most of his contemporaries, Marandon de Montyel held onto class-based assumptions regarding manual labor and rational self-control. But he also believed his patients' interaction with their families would prove more rehabilitative than isolation from them. The example of Marandon de Montyel's Open Door shows that doctors could question key aspects of the moral treatment regime without giving up on the possibility of welcoming patients back into their communities. This was a first essential step—an admittedly small one—toward breaking down the asylum's walls and the ideological edifice that had helped sustain them since the late eighteenth century.

Conclusion

The "Mad" Woman in a Man's World

THE RELATIONSHIP BETWEEN GENDER and psychiatry that emerged in the late eighteenth century and continued to develop throughout the nineteenth reveals the instability of dominant notions of masculinity, femininity, and mental illness. The psychiatric theories and practices developed by Pinel and his immediate successors, in particular, simultaneously gave scientific credence to notions of gender difference and exposed the contradictions intrinsic to both medical and gender ideologies. Doctors constructed their own personae with an eye toward embodying the ideals of rational masculine self-control and used these same notions in the name of patient cure, with varying degrees of success on both counts. The emphasis alienists placed on the naturalness of bourgeois gender values also provided opportunities for women practitioners to take on uncharacteristically authoritative roles in private asylums because of the widespread celebration of feminine domesticity. Furthermore, even as asylum doctors steadily gained social, cultural, and legal stature after 1838, they faced pushback from multiple directions, particularly from male patients whose internments reflected long-term shifts in the foundation of masculine authority and exposed the vulnerability of psychiatric power to gender-based attacks. By 1900, owing in large part to the sense of malaise engendered by the Franco-Prussian War and the Paris Commune, doctors themselves had abandoned the use of gender scripts as a method of rehabilitation.

On hopeful days I interpret this narrative as proof that asylum doctors were doomed to fail in their attempts to naturalize differences between men and women, that the conceit of bourgeois, masculine rationality was a façade whose influence would eventually disappear because its power had always been based on fiction. On less hopeful days, I realize this book could just as easily have been about the persistence of these myths rather than their weaknesses. Considering the sheer numbers of people hurt by the asylum system and its underlying assumptions about men, women, and madness from the eighteenth century to the present day, does it even make sense to emphasize the limitations of psychiatric or masculine power?

As Judith Surkis points out, gender instability—in and of itself—is not necessarily subversive (especially because gender is *always* unstable). In her analysis of sex and citizenship in late nineteenth-century France, she argues that indications of masculinity in "crisis" actually provided powerful impetus for the policing of gender boundaries, in that "instability fueled the regulatory logic by which an idealized masculinity and a specific configuration of social and political power were articulated and maintained."[1] This appears to have been the case among French doctors, whose abandonment of the moral treatment's understanding of gender-as-cure constituted a reactionary response to widespread challenges posed to bourgeois authority by those who did not embody the rational, masculine ideal in one way or another. It arguably became more difficult to sustain longstanding assumptions regarding masculine self-control and feminine domesticity when evidence of the unnaturalness of bourgeois gender norms abounded in the fin-de-siècle. Yet many medical commentators seemed to hold onto these beliefs more strongly than ever before. Degeneration theorists, for example, continued to insist that behaviors that ran counter to bourgeois expectations—such as masturbation, impotence, same-sex sexual activity, or sadism and masochism—represented evidence of pathology.[2] But because they conceived of the signs of degeneration as congenital rather than circumstantial, they perpetuated the stigma associated with both gender nonconformity and mental illness to an even greater degree than earlier psychiatric practitioners had done.[3]

The work of neurologist Jean-Martin Charcot, whose scientific influence reached its apogee in the 1880s, likewise exhibited these tendencies. He argued that the origins of hysteria were physical rather than psychological, insisting that this quintessentially nineteenth-century pathology was not actually a mental illness at all. For Charcot, hysteria involved the weakening of the nervous system. Such enervation resulted in a variety of physical manifestations, most of which involved the loss of bodily control (including symptoms as seemingly diverse as catatonia and spontaneous blindness to insomnia, upset stomach, and sexual dysfunction). Charcot argued that there were multiple possible causes for an individual's development of hysteria. Some cases were purely hereditary while others involved hereditary predisposition combined with situational trauma of either a physical or emotional variety.[4] Charcot's patients were mostly women, as his clinic was housed in the Parisian women's institution La Salpêtrière, but he rejected the idea that hysteria was connected to organs specific to the female sex, and he argued that the historically feminized disease could also present itself in men (mainly those of the popular classes).[5]

Charcot nevertheless accepted the far more conventional notion that overt expressions of sexual desire among women hysterics represented evidence of their conditions and, like practitioners of the moral treatment, this most famous of French doctors envisioned medicine as a performance. In Charcot's case this was far more literal, with select women patients dramatically revealing and suspending their symptoms under hypnosis for groups of men in Charcot's surgical theater.[6] However, as in the case of the community care system promoted by his student Charles Féré, nothing about these stagings suggested that Charcot's patients might be "cured" by participating in them. Cure was not even their purpose, which was ostensibly to educate those in the audience (although the act of watching women patients in sexually suggestive states of powerlessness likely served to titillate them as well). Once again, the late nineteenth-century obsolescence of the moral treatment indicated the emergence of even less flexible medical attitudes regarding gender performance and the possibility of rehabilitation, ones which nonetheless upheld bourgeois values as insistently as ever.

That said, doctors' decision to transition away from the moral treatment actually reflected the relative vulnerability of bourgeois masculine power at this time. While medical men continued to promote theories of the mind that implied gender conformity and physical health were one and the same, they did so in a society in which ever greater numbers of individuals appeared to reject these notions outright. Women whose claims and lifestyles contradicted the ideal of feminine domesticity in one way or another posed the most obvious challenge. Such women included suffragists who, by and large, embraced the cultural equation of ideal femininity with domestic motherhood while using the symbolic power of the nurturing woman to demand public authority.[7] Even more threatening were New Women who chose to work for a living and sometimes avoided marriage or child-rearing altogether despite their middle-class backgrounds.[8] Bourgeois men also increasingly rejected traditional expectations concerning gender and family at this time. Some engaged in homosexual activities more overtly than earlier in the century or, at the very least, medical discourse and police surveillance surrounding such activities became more pronounced.[9] Others chafed at the restrictions imposed by conventional heterosexual marriages and chose bachelorhood or imperialist adventuring instead.[10] Most significantly, many cultural commentators expressed concern that the conditions of modern life actually caused mental and physical deterioration, particularly among the same bourgeois men whose rationality supposedly signaled their right to rule (and whose "natural" superiority epitomized that of their class and nation, and even that of the West itself).[11] An overemphasis on sedentary intellectual pursuits—i.e., the cultivation of rational self-control, of intellect over physicality—seemed to have broken the most worthy of men, while women boldly demanded rights as intellectual equals. In other words, gender ideology was in the process of revealing itself *as* ideology in no uncertain terms.

And as gender boundaries blurred, so too did other forms of class distinction. With the emergence of the Third Republic, universal male suffrage established itself in France once and for all. Workers not only voted, but they marched, organized, and demanded better working conditions and pay. Inequality remained rampant, but it was also challenged by socialist movements and even spectacular acts of anarchist terrorism.[12] The specter of the Commune lingered and served to remind bourgeois France that its place atop the social ladder could not be taken for granted. No less dramatically, the beginnings of urban mass culture dissolved distinctions between classes, with individuals of all backgrounds comingling in public spaces as never before. From city parks to the Paris morgue, the dividing lines between the bourgeoisie and the rest of French society gradually but persistently eroded.[13]

Alienists unsurprisingly continued to naturalize bourgeois gender norms under these circumstances, but their attempts appear increasingly desperate in hindsight. The kleptomania diagnosis, for example, gained prominence as a medical excuse for elite women's thievery, which had become a source of concern alongside the rise of glittering, crowded department stores.[14] Unlike working women who stole, kleptomaniacs were considered "sad," not "bad." This perspective conveniently allowed the French bourgeoisie to hold onto traditional ideas about women's natures—and the class hierarchies those beliefs helped to sustain—rather than confront the possibility that the "angel in the house" could be a criminal. The diagnosis also conveniently implied wealthy women should be careful to avoid new sites of mass culture where they would dangerously mix with those below their station (women did not tend to heed this warning, yet another sign of changing times). In this context, the notion that bourgeois gender and family values might prove curative lost much of its force, not to mention its rationale. While doctors at the start of the century acted as though the values of their own class had the potential to integrate French society in a genuine, albeit still hierarchical, fashion, many at the end of the century feared this result.

Suffice it to say, the contributions of degeneration theorists to late nineteenth-century psychiatric thinking constituted powerful cultural responses to these various transformations. Yet their efforts often muddled class distinctions even further, although in different ways and to different effect than the actions of their forebears. The pessimism exhibited by someone such as Féré broke down medical faith in cure, but it also diminished the cultural elevation of the bourgeois family: in a world threatened by the ever-lurking and often hidden dangers of degeneration, markers of class status provided the social body very little protection. Even the more optimistic Charcot—who never lost faith that he would find a cure for hysteria even when his ideas fell out of fashion in the 1890s—imagined the family as a source of pathology rather than refuge. The theories of Sigmund Freud, although mostly outside the scope of this project, also served to chip away the symbolic authority of bourgeois family values in the late nineteenth and early twentieth centuries (while simultaneously perpetuating notions of women's natural sexual passivity).[15] For Freud, even "normal" families were the source of neuroses, especially those of a sexual nature. He and the degeneration theorists approached the question of mental illness from very different vantage points—and Freud's patients were not usually candidates for long-term institutionalization—but both of their perspectives undercut traditional asylum psychiatry and the sanctity of the bourgeois family alike. In this way, among others, the fate of the moral treatment and that of the French bourgeoisie were inexorably intertwined, the fall of one preceding but also presaging the inevitable decline of the other.

Thus, while cultural conceptions of masculinity, femininity, and family were never fixed in the century following the French Revolution, the meaning of this uncertainty changed over time. The consequences of such instability also differed depending on an individual's class, gender, and disability status. We have seen how medical practices and gender expectations combined in ways that allowed male patients to resist psychiatric power and allowed women *directrices* to uncharacteristically wield it. We have likewise seen how the behaviors of male doctors were shaped and circumscribed by these same forces, even if the expression of key attributes of ideal masculinity—from personal honor to benevolent paternalism—also helped medical men rebuild their reputations in times of distress.

But what of women patients? They have admittedly received less attention than their male counterparts in this book, in large part because so much has already been written about their encounters with the psychiatric system. Furthermore, despite popular perceptions to the contrary, women did not constitute a significant majority of asylum patients in nineteenth-century France. They were nonetheless uniquely victimized when familial and medical authorities aligned against them to secure their unwilling sequestration. It therefore makes sense to end this book by taking stock of their experiences and what they might suggest about the long-term transformation of familial power.

The mutually reinforcing nature of medical and gender ideologies denied women the opportunity to use their gender against the psychiatric system in the ways men could, and it was more difficult for women to come across sympathetically given the constraints posed by bourgeois domesticity. Authoritarian family dynamics and those associated with the bourgeoisie each revolved around women's subordination to their husbands and fathers. While the nineteenth-century transition to a bourgeois family ideal increased the vulnerability of men considered mad, it also gave them powerful tools with which to challenge asylum commitment. Conversely, women committed against their wills were condemned twice over. If they failed to conform to dominant beliefs regarding women's proper roles, doctors deemed them insane. Yet even if they did embody the feminine ideal, this hardly served as proof of rationality. In fact, it could be seen as the opposite—as in the many cases where the pressures of pregnancy, marriage, and child-rearing supposedly drove women to the madhouse. Bourgeois family values hurt "mad" men, but supported the authority of men as a whole. "Mad" women were doubly marginalized and thus had few weapons with which to combat the psychiatric system.

The case of the unwillingly committed Marie Esquiron makes for a poignant comparison of the options available to male versus female patients. Her experiences also shed light on some of the potential effects of doctors' efforts to institutionalize gender with respect to the attainment of women's rights, the emergence of more egalitarian family dynamics, and the role played by cultural conceptions of rationality and madness in each of these processes. In January 1893, Esquiron (née de Gasté) published a scathing report chronicling the details of her unwilling sequestration at the private asylum of one Dr. Goujon. The forty-six-year-old feminist activist was admitted to the Parisian institution in 1890 and had already lived there for nearly three years when she sent an appeal to the Minister of Justice in an effort to force her release.[16] This was the second time Esquiron had found herself locked away against her will, having been sent to the famous Maison Blanche in 1866 at the age of twenty-one by her father, a wealthy former deputy of the Finistère department named Joseph de Gasté. The events of Esquiron's second internment—in which the enterprising woman sought to overcome the burden of her sex by convincing her interlocutors she was a reasonable person in spite of it—elucidate the ways that gendered conceptions of madness and reason remained bulwarks of psychiatric power at the end of the century.

Esquiron's appeal paints a disturbing picture of life with her father, a man who raised his young daughter on his own following his wife's premature death. Esquiron possessed a vast fortune willed to her by her mother, and she argued that Gasté sought to keep her from spending the money by arranging her commitment in an asylum.[17] One scholar has suggested that a history of sexual abuse might have contributed to Gasté's cruel intentions toward his daughter.[18] An article published by *Le Temps* reported that Esquiron herself implied this at her interdiction hearing, where she recounted a childhood physical confrontation over the keys to her bedroom door and stated that her father "taught her things at seven years old that only a married woman should know."[19]

It would be easy to assume that Gasté harbored traditional beliefs regarding paternal authority and, by extension, the role of women within the family and society. But he was well-known in feminist circles and even introduced a proposition during his time as a legislator to grant women the right to vote. He also noted with frustration that his daughter had supposedly sought to besmirch his reputation with the women's rights advocate Marie-Rose Astié de Valsayre, who was the focus of considerable press attention at this time for advocating women's participation in duels.[20] Gasté's progressive politics did not keep him from using harmful assumptions about women's irrational natures to undercut his daughter's testimony, and he claimed her ability to reason could not be trusted because she spent money foolishly on everything from her toilette to ill-advised land investments. Commentators seemed to have little trouble believing Gasté's interpretation of his daughter's state of mind. Although he was not successful in his attempt to have himself appointed as administrator of Esquiron's 900,000-franc estate, he did persuade the judge to uphold his daughter's institutionalization despite her vigorous protests.[21]

In a twist one could deem ironic if it were not so typical, medical and legal authorities also condemned Esquiron for her apparent desire to conform to gender expectations (when her own life story provides indisputable evidence of the repercussions women faced when they failed to do so). The tale of her 1866 incarceration stands out in the narrative presented by her accusers not only because it was used against her nearly a quarter of a century later but also because it underscores how gendered definitions of irrationality particularly disadvantaged bourgeois women. In her early twenties Esquiron had supposedly focused on marriage to a point of obsession. It seems not to have occurred to doctors that this might be a perfectly rational attitude considering Esquiron's desire to gain independence from her father. Multiple articles referred to her extravagant spending habits during this time, noting she wore elaborate ball gowns while going about her daily routine and that, one day, a *pâtissier* proposed to her. She accepted, according to *Le Matin*, tempted "by the possibility of never again making a brioche."[22] Doctors soon declared Esquiron insane, resulting in her internment at the Maison Blanche for approximately six months.

Esquiron's second institutionalization also pertained to marriage, this time her desire to divorce her inventor husband, a man she had initially married against her father's wishes who later colluded with him to lock Esquiron away. Both men claimed Esquiron's loss of money in a land deal constituted proof of insanity, which they used as a pretext to arrange her institutionalization. Alienists diagnosed her with *délire de persécution*, a common diagnosis for patients interned against their wills, the onset of which had supposedly followed a sudden bout of vomiting. Esquiron believed she had been poisoned, and doctors admitted this was a possibility, yet they still found proof of an unhealthy obsession in her conviction that her sickness had been the work of those conspiring against her.

Perhaps Esquiron's greatest hindrance was the fact that she had recently demanded a divorce. She insisted that the men in her life orchestrated her sequestration because she sought to leave her husband, who she claimed had failed to live up to his marital duties to protect and provide for his household. A divorce would enable Esquiron's financial independence by giving her complete control over her inheritance. Furthermore, it would leave her husband penniless, as he had no real career of his own. If she were interned in an asylum, however, Esquiron would be unable to secure the divorce or spend her money as she pleased. This result satisfied both her father, who might eventually gain control over her estate, and her husband, whom Gasté had agreed to support financially as long as he served as a witness against Esquiron.

Esquiron depicted her decision to seek a divorce as perfectly rational, but it was not difficult for doctors to frame this decision as proof of madness, specifically evidence of a rash temperament and a persistent case of *délire de persécution*.[23] That 9,675 other women and men filed for divorce or separation in the five years following the legalization of at-fault divorce in 1884 did not seem to enter into their equation.[24] There were several legal justifications for the initiation of divorce proceedings, but it was not clear whether Esquiron's situation met any of these standards, and doctors readily determined that her desire to leave her husband indicated a flighty and inconsistent state of mind, especially in conjunction with her purported youthful obsession with marriage.

Gender undoubtedly complicated Esquiron's attempt to persuade powerful men to set her free. As a woman, particularly one who sought to flee her marriage and sever communication with her father, she needed to develop distinct strategies of argumentation in order to combat her institutionalization. She sought to prove her sanity in her attempts to convince judicial authorities to release her, but she needed to do so in a style that would overcome their likely assumptions about women and irrationality. Both Esquiron's womanliness and her perceived mental state worked against her efforts to present herself as rational, particularly when the medical men whose opinions she sought to undermine were paragons of masculine, professional expertise.[25] She therefore presented herself as exceptionally logical—she never admitted to bouts of confusion, as had male victims of unjust institutionalization—and she tended to avoid discussion of emotions in favor of the detailed presentation of evidence in a point-counterpoint fashion. She believed simplicity to be her best defense, writing "I know myself better than the alienists know me, especially after having met me only three times. They got everything wrong—my character, my feelings, my actions past and present, my ideas, my affairs, my whole life. It is not difficult for me to set the record straight, and I have no need to do anything but state the truth simply."[26]

Esquiron sought to prove that her womanliness did not negate her rationality, but her efforts failed to convince those hearing her case in 1893, who upheld the court's earlier decision based on the testimony of medical men. Her ultimate fate is unknown, and perhaps unknowable, but I fear Esquiron never regained her freedom.[27] The symptoms her doctors read as evidence of insanity were the very same traits—in extreme form—that many men at the turn of the century ascribed to all members of the opposite sex who sought equality. This fact, in addition to details particular to Esquiron's family history, proved too great a liability for her to overcome. The strategy she used to counter psychiatric experts nonetheless foretold twentieth-century transformations in gender relations. In time, the decoupling of rationality from manliness would lead to greater equality within the family and beyond, albeit too late to make a difference for the courageous Esquiron.

Not coincidentally, and quite understandably, Esquiron's plan involved doubling down on the alterity of madness by distancing herself from its stigma. Her efforts to secure her personal emancipation thus reveal something essential about the emancipation of women more broadly: namely, that the historical development of relative equality between the sexes owes quite a bit to the continued subordination of those considered insane. This can also be seen, from a different angle, in the histories of male mental patients, especially those bourgeois men whose predicaments were created—or at least exacerbated—by subtle shifts in the basis of masculine authority that took place in the wake of the French

Revolution. We should therefore hesitate in celebrating our own attitudes towards gender equality and condemning those of the nineteenth century. For one, the more egalitarian family structure of today is indebted to that which developed in the century following the French Revolution. More important, what we have absorbed from the nineteenth century—uncritically, for the most part—is the persistent dehumanization of "mad" people in exchange for the piecemeal expansion of human rights for everyone else. If we have finally demolished the cultural linkage between femininity and irrationality (which is itself debatable), the next essential step is the eradication of rationality's equation with personhood.

This will likely prove even more difficult, but if the story of the asylum's relationship to gender teaches us anything, it is that possibilities for resistance and subversion exist in even the most oppressive of circumstances and within the most seemingly intractable ideologies. The cultural authority of asylum psychiatry and that of the French bourgeoisie were both in decline by the end of the 1800s; this is precisely why most doctors chose to abandon the moral treatment while still insisting that women and workers were less rational than middle-class men. Yet, as this book has shown, distinctions of gender, class, and psychiatric disability that supported the interests of the powerful in nineteenth-century France could never be taken for granted. The interdependence of medical and gender ideologies perpetuated by doctors and fostered by the postrevolutionary French state undeniably helped sustain the power of elite men, and the conflation of femininity and irrationality was nothing if not persistent (one need only reflect on the fact that French women did not earn the vote until the end of World War II to understand this truth). But this very interconnectedness also undermined the status quo by exposing supposedly natural class and gender distinctions as cultural constructs. Marie Esquiron knew this, and used it to press for her release in the face of terrible odds. Decades would pass before French society as a whole truly questioned women's "natural" inequality, but the seeds of destruction had been present from the start.

Introduction

1. François Leuret, *Du Traitement moral de la folie* (Paris: J.-B. Baillière, 1840), 423.

2. Leuret, *Du Traitement moral de la folie*, 427.

3. Michel Foucault, *Psychiatric Power: Lectures at the Collège de France, 1973–1974*, trans. Graham Burchell (New York: Picador, 2006), 148.

4. I use "psychiatry" in reference to the field dedicated to the study and treatment of those diagnosed with mental alienation, but will generally use "alienist" or "asylum doctor" for those we would now call psychiatrists.

5. Judith Butler introduced the concept of gender performance and its power to subvert structures of power in *Gender Trouble: Feminism and the Subversion of Identity* (New York and London: Routledge, 1990), 183–193; the concept has been applied by French historians of gender, most notably in Jo Burr Margadant, ed., *The New Biography: Performing Femininity in Nineteenth-Century France* (Berkeley: University of California Press, 2000). I do not consider gender performativity necessarily subversive, although it has subversive potential (a question pursued in this book's conclusion).

6. This statement is not meant to deny the existence of mental illness or minimize the consequences of psychological distress, but rather to highlight the paradoxical behaviors of asylum doctors vis-à-vis their patients in nineteenth-century France. I make no diagnostic claims in this book.

7. The most comprehensive work on the moral treatment in France is Jan Goldstein, *Console and Classify: The French Psychiatric Profession in the Nineteenth Century*, 2nd ed. (Chicago: University of Chicago Press, 2001); see also Robert Castel, *The Regulation of Madness: The Origins of Incarceration in France*, trans. W. D. Halls (Berkeley: University of California Press, 1988) and Ian Dowbiggin, *Inheriting Madness: Professionalization and Psychiatric Knowledge in Nineteenth-Century France* (Berkeley: University of California Press, 1991); for England see Roy Porter, Mind-Forg'd Manacles: A History of Madness in England from the Restoration to the Regency (London: Athlone, 1987); for the United States see Nancy Tomes, *The Art of Asylum-Keeping: Thomas Story Kirkbride and the Origins of American Psychiatry* (Philadelphia: University of Pennsylvania Press, 1994). The emergence of the moral treatment ends Michel Foucault's *Histoire de la folie à l'âge classique* (Paris: Gallimard, 1972).

8. Jean-Étienne-Dominique Esquirol, *Des Établissements des aliénés en France, et des moyens d'améliorer le sort de ces infortunés* (Paris: Imprimerie de Madame Huzard, 1819), 8.

9. *Annuaire statistique de la France,* vol. 20 (Paris: Imprimerie Nationale, 1900), 111.

10. In addition to Dowbiggin, the most thorough account of nineteenth-century anti-psychiatry is a three-volume dissertation: Aude Fauvel, "Témoins Aliénés et Bastilles Modernes: Une histoire politique, social, et culturelle des asiles en France (1800–1914)" (PhD diss., École des Hautes Études en Sciences Sociales, 2005).

11. Robert A. Nye, *Crime, Madness, and Politics in Modern France: The Medical Concept of National Decline* (Princeton, NJ: Princeton University Press, 1984); Daniel Pick, *Faces of Degeneration: A European Disorder, c.1848–c.1918* (Cambridge: Cambridge University Press, 1989); Jean-Christophe Coffin, *La Transmission de la folie, 1850–1914* (Paris: L'Harmattan, 2003).

12. I define disability broadly for the purposes of this book and am admittedly less interested in producing a list of impairments that "counted" as disability in nineteenth-century France than exploring the ways in which changing attitudes toward psychological difference intersected with emergent notions of class and gender. Disability constitutes both a lived experience, the meaning of which has changed over time, and a category of analysis. The cultural valence of all forms of disability shifted in the wake of the Enlightenment and industrialization as the standardized body and mind came to be viewed as prerequisites for productive labor and active citizenship. See Henri-Jacques Striker, *A History of Disability,* trans. William Sayers (Ann Arbor, MI: University of Michigan Press, 1999) and Kim E. Nielsen, *A Disability History of the United States* (Boston: Beacon Press, 2012) as examples of histories that successfully examine commonalities among various types of disability without neglecting the differences between them.

13. Laure Murat, *The Man Who Thought He Was Napoleon: Toward a Political History of Madness,* trans. Deke Dusinberre (Chicago: University of Chicago Press, 2014), 1.

14. I use the term bourgeois not in a Marxian sense, but in reference to a postrevolutionary elite whose social ascendancy was based on wealth and shared values rather than noble birth. As many historians have noted, the middle classes were an incredibly diverse group whose social circumstances discouraged cohesion. For discussion of this historiography see Sarah Maza, *The Myth of the French Bourgeoisie* (Cambridge, MA: Harvard University Press, 2003).

15. Michel Foucault, *History of Madness,* trans. Jonathan Murphy and Jean Khalfa (London: Routledge, 2006), 44–77. For a standard—though I would argue excessive—critique of Foucault, see Edward Shorter, *A History of Psychiatry: From the Era of the Asylum to the Age of Prozac* (New York: John Wiley and Sons, 1997), especially the introduction.

16. Roy Porter, "The Patient's View: Doing Medical History from Below," *Theory and Society* 14, no. 2 (1985): 175–198, http://www.jstor.org/stable/657089. Alexandra Bacopoulos-Viau and Aude Fauvel, "The Patient's Turn: Roy Porter and Psychiatry's

Tales, Thirty Years on," *Medical History* 60, no. 1 (2016): 1, https://doi.org/10.1017/mdh.2015.65. The authors point out that the most forceful critique of recent historiography comes from Flurin Condrau, "The Patient's View Meets the Clinical Gaze," *Social History of Medicine* 20, no. 3 (2007): 526, https://doi.org/10.1093/shm/hkm076.

17. Bacopoulos-Viau and Fauvel, "The Patient's Turn," 12.

18. My approach is indebted to mad studies, which emphasizes the lived experiences of mad people beyond their status as patients (among other imperatives). Although this book remains a work of medical history, I too aim to interpret sources in ways that acknowledge the multiple facets of identity that comprised the nineteenth-century "patient." See Brenda A. LeFrançois, Robert Menzies, Geoffrey Reaume, eds., *Mad Matters: A Critical Reader in Canadian Mad Studies* (Toronto: Canadian Scholars' Press, 2013).

19. P. Bru, *Histoire de Bicêtre* (Paris: Lecrosnié et Babé, 1890), 454–459; Scipion Pinel, *Traité complète du régime sanitaire des aliénés* (Paris: Mauprivez, 1836), 56.

20. Dora Weiner, *The Citizen-Patient in Revolutionary and Imperial Paris* (Baltimore: Johns Hopkins University Press, 1993), 247–248.

21. For the legal status of the interned, see Castel, *The Regulation of Madness*.

22. On gender and the Revolution see Anne Verjus, *Le bon mari. Une histoire politique des hommes et des femmes à l'époque révolutionnaire* (Paris: Fayard, 2010); Joan B. Landes, *Women and the Public Sphere in the Age of the French Revolution* (Ithaca, NY: Cornell University Press, 1988).

23. Christopher Forth, *Masculinity in the Modern West: Gender, Civilization and the Body* (New York: Palgrave Macmillan, 2008), 22–29.

24. On the Enlightenment origins of women's inequality, see Lieselotte Steinbrügge, *The Moral Sex: Woman's Nature in the French Enlightenment*, trans. Pamela E. Selwyn (Oxford: Oxford University Press, 1995), 3–9.

25. On gender, reason, and citizenship see Joan Wallach Scott, *Only Paradoxes to Offer: French Feminists and the Rights of Man* (Cambridge, MA: Harvard University Press, 1997) and Geneviève Fraisse, *Reason's Muse: Sexual Difference and the Birth of Democracy*, trans. Jane Marie Todd (Chicago: University of Chicago Press, 1994).

26. William M. Reddy, *The Invisible Code: Honor and Sentiment in Postrevolutionary France, 1814–1848* (Berkeley: University of California Press, 1997). See the preface and introduction in particular.

27. Michelle Perrot, ed., *Histoire de la vie privée*, vol. 4, *De la révolution à la grande guerre* (Paris: Ed. Du Seuil, 1985); Bonnie Smith, *Ladies of the Leisure Class: The Bourgeoises of Northern France in the Nineteenth Century* (Princeton, NJ: Princeton University Press, 1981).

28. Dr. Legrand du Saulle, *Les Hysteriques: État physique et état mental, actes insolites, délictueux et criminels* (Paris: J.-B. Baillière et fils, 1883).

29. On meritocracy during the Revolution, see Rafe Blaufarb, *The French Army, 1750–1820: Careers, Talent, Merit* (Manchester: Manchester University Press, 2002) and John Carson, *The Measure of Merit: Talents, Intelligence, and Inequality in the French and American Republics, 1750–1940* (Princeton, NJ: Princeton University Press, 2007).

On an earlier period, see Christy Pichichero, "Le Soldat Sensible: Military Psychology and Social Egalitarianism in the Enlightenment French Army," *French Historical Studies* 31, no. 4 (Fall 2008): 553–580, https://doi.org/10.1215/00161071-2008-006.

On the related problem of ambition in postrevolutionary France, see Kathleen Kete, *Making Way for Genius: The Aspiring Self in France from the Old Regime to the New* (New Haven, CT: Yale University Press, 2012). Kete points out that Pinel and Esquirol identified excessive ambition as an inspiration for insanity (77–81).

30. Carson, *The Measure of Merit*, 14–20.

31. From a sociological perspective, the most comprehensive study of the myth of meritocracy in France is Pierre Bourdieu, *La Noblesse d'état: Grandes écoles et l'esprit de corps* (Paris: Les Éditions de Minuit, 1989).

32. For discussion of this wider process see Annette F. Timm and Joshua A. Sanborn, *Gender, Sex, and the Shaping of Modern Europe: A History from the French Revolution to the Present Day,* 2nd ed. (London: Bloomsbury, 2016), especially the introduction.

33. Timm and Sanborn, *Gender, Sex, and the Making of Modern Europe*, 3. Also see Carole Pateman, *The Sexual Contract* (Palo Alto: Stanford University Press, 1988) and Lynn Hunt, *The Family Romance of the French Revolution* (Berkeley: University of California Press, 1992).

34. Rachel Fuchs, *Contested Paternity: Constructing Families in Modern France* (Baltimore: Johns Hopkins University Press, 2008). See especially chapter 2 ("Seduction and Courtroom Encounters in the Nineteenth Century") and chapter 3 ("Find the Fathers, Save the Children, 1870–1912").

35. Elaine Showalter, *The Female Malady: Women, Madness and English Culture, 1830–1980* (New York: Pantheon, 1985); Yannick Ripa, *La Ronde des folles: Femmes, folie, et enfermement au XIXe siècle* (Paris: Aubier, 1987). More recent works addressing the feminization of madness include Lisa Appignanesi, *Mad, Bad and Sad: A History of Women and the Mind Doctors from 1800 to the Present* (London: Virago, 2008) and Susannah Wilson, *Voices from the Asylum: Four French Women Writers, 1850–1920* (Oxford: Oxford University Press, 2010). A notable exception to this trend is Mark Micale, *Hysterical Men: The Hidden History of Male Nervous Illness* (Cambridge, MA: Harvard University Press, 2008). Jann Matlock also examines women and various disciplining structures including the asylum, but draws attention to opportunities for resistance. Jann Matlock, *Scenes of Seduction: Prostitution, Hysteria, and Reading Difference in Nineteenth-Century France* (New York: Columbia University Press, 1994).

36. Catherine Kudlick, "Disability History: Why We Need Another 'Other,'" *American Historical Review* 108 (June 2003): 763–93, https://doi.org/10.1086/ahr/108.3.763; Douglas Baynton, "Disability and the Justification of Inequality in American History," *The New Disability History: American Perspectives*, Paul K. Longmore and Lauri Umansky, eds. (New York: New York University Press, 2001) and *Defectives in the Land: Disability and Immigration in the Age of Eugenics* (Chicago: University of Chicago Press, 2016); Susan Burch and Lindsey Patterson, "Not Just Any Body: Disability, Gender, and History," *Journal of Women's History* 25, no. 4 (Winter 2013): 122–137, doi:10.1353

/jowh.2013.0060. On disability, race, and slavery, see Dea H. Boster, *African American Slavery and Disability: Bodies, Property, and Power in the Antebellum South, 1800–1860* (New York: Routledge, 2013).

37. Baynton, "Disability and the Justification of Inequality in American History," 43–45.

38. The 1913 image can be viewed in the online collections of the Victoria and Albert Museum: http://collections.vam.ac.uk/item/O75893/what-a-woman-may-be-poster-suffrage -atelier/.

39. Margadant, ed., *The New Biography: Performing Femininity in Nineteenth-Century France,* especially the introduction; Mary Louise Roberts, *Disruptive Acts: The New Woman in Fin-de-Siècle France* (Chicago: University of Chicago Press, 2002); Andrea Mansker, *Sex, Honor and Citizenship in Third Republic France* (London: Palgrave Macmillan, 2011); Jennifer Popiel, *Rousseau's Daughters: Domesticity, Education, and Autonomy in Modern France* (Durham, NH: University of New Hampshire Press, 2008).

40. In addition to Forth, see Micale, *Hysterical Men* and Robert A. Nye, *Masculinity and Male Codes of Honor in Modern France* (Berkeley: University of California Press, 1993).

41. Aude Fauvel, "Madness: a 'female malady'? Women and Psychiatric Institutionalisation in France" in Vulnerabilities, social inequalities and health in perspective, eds. Patrice Bourdelais and John Chircop (Évora: Ediçoes Colibri, 2010), 61–75. For the United Kingdom and Ireland, see Jonathan Andrews and Anne Digby, *Sex and Seclusion, Class and Custody: Perspectives on Gender and Class in the History of British and Irish Psychiatry* (Amsterdam: Rodopi, 2004).

42. Mary Louise Roberts, "Beyond 'Crisis' in Understanding Gender Transformation," *Gender & History* 28, no. 2 (2016): 358–366, https://doi.org/10.1111/1468-0424.12212.

Another powerful critique comes from Judith Surkis, *Sexing the Citizen: Morality and Masculinity in France, 1870–1920* (Ithaca, NY: Cornell University Press, 2006).

43. Roberts, "Beyond 'Crisis' in Understanding Gender Transformation," 364.

44. Toby L. Ditz, "The New Men's History and the Peculiar Absence of Gendered Power: Some Remedies from Early American Gender History," *Gender & History* 16, no. 1 (2004): 3, https://doi.org/10.1111/j.0953-5233.2004.324_1.x.

45. On French colonial psychiatry, see Richard C. Keller, *Colonial Madness: Psychiatry in French North Africa* (Chicago: University of Chicago Press, 2007) and Claire Edington, *Beyond the Asylum: Mental Illness in French Colonial Vietnam* (Ithaca, NY: Cornell University Press, 2019); also see Erik Linstrum, *Ruling Minds: Psychology in the British Empire* (Cambridge, MA: Harvard University Press, 2016).

Chapter 1: Gender and the Founding "Fathers" of French Psychiatry

1. Camille Robcis, *The Law of Kinship: Anthropology, Psychoanalysis, and the Family in France* (Ithaca, NY: Cornell University Press, 2013), 17–25.

2. For example, Jean-Étienne Dominique Esquirol, *Des Maladies mentales,* vol. 1 (Paris: J.-B. Baillière, 1838), 122.

3. Jean-Étienne Dominique Esquirol, *Des Passions considérées comme causes, symptômes et moyens curatifs de l'aliénation mentale* (Paris: l'Imprimerie de Didot Jeune, 1805), 6.

4. Philippe Pinel, *L'Aliénation mentale ou la manie: Traité médico-philosophique* (Paris: L'Harmattan: 2006), 14. This is a reprint of Pinel's classic text, originally published in 1800.

5. Philippe Pinel, *Traité médico-philosophique sur l'aliénation mentale,* 2nd edition (Paris: Brosson, 1809), x.

6. Esquirol, *Des Passions,* 14.

7. Felix Voisin, *Des causes morales et physiques des maladies mentales et de quelques autres affections nerveuses telle que l'hystérie, la nymphomanie et le satyriasis* (Paris: J.-B. Baillière, 1826), 16.

8. On contemporary attitudes on hysteria and the biological progression of the female life cycle see Jan Goldstein, *Hysteria Complicated by Ecstasy: The Case of Nanette Leroux* (Princeton NJ: Princeton University Press, 2010).

9. Esquirol, *Des Passions,* 17.

10. Étienne-Jean Georget, *De la folie. Considérations sur cette maladie.* (Paris: Crevot, 1820), 163.

11. Georget, *De la Folie,* 260.

12. Georget, *De la Folie,* 291–292.

13. Esquirol, *Des Passions,* 22.

14. Philippe Pinel, *Recherches et observations sur le traitement moral des aliénés* (Paris: n.d.), 37–38.

15. Esquirol's 1819 promotion of psychiatry was the most serious of these efforts. See Goldstein, *Console and Classify,* 129–147.

16. Goldstein, *Console and Classify,* 279.

17. Jean-Étienne Dominique Esquirol, *Des Établissements des aliénés en France et des moyens d'améliorer le sort de ces infortunés* (Paris: Imprimerie de Madame Huzard, 1819).

18. Pinel, *L'Aliénation mentale ou la manie: Traité médico-philosophique,* 41.

19. Pinel, *L'Aliénation mentale ou la manie: Traité médico-philosophique,* 222–223.

20. Josef Ehmer, "Marriage," *Family Life in the Long Nineteenth Century, 1789–1913,* eds. David I. Kertzer and Mario Barbagli (New Haven, CT: Yale University Press, 2002), 292–300.

21. Michelle Perrot, *A History of Private Life,* vol. 4, *From the Fires of Revolution to the Great War* (Cambridge, MA: Harvard University Press, 1990), 342–344.

22. Loftur Guttormsson, "Parent-Child Relations," *Family Life in the Long Nineteenth Century, 1789–1913,* eds. David I. Kertzer and Mario Barbagli. (New Haven, CT: Yale University Press, 2002), 268.

23. Jean-Étienne-Dominique Esquirol, *Des Maladies mentales,* vol.2 (Paris: J.-B. Baillière, 1838), 745.

24. Esquirol, *Des Maladies mentales,* 2: 745.

25. Esquirol, *Des Maladies mentales*, 2: 745.

26. Esquirol, *Des Maladies mentales*, 2: 755.

27. Foucault refers to this situation as "recognition by mirror," one of several key methods through which practitioners of the moral treatment sought to inculcate self-discipline in patients. Michel Foucault, *Madness and Civilization* (Vintage Books, 1988), 262.

28. Esquirol, *Des Maladies mentales*, 1: 124.

29. Esquirol, *Des Maladies mentales*, 1: 124.

30. Esquirol, *Des Maladies mentales*, 1: 121.

31. Esquirol, *Des Maladies mentales*, 2: 755.

32. Esquirol, *Des Maladies mentales*, 2: 762.

33. Goldstein, *Console and Classify*, 290–291.

34. See chapter 4 for an extended discussion of the legal transformation of familial authority in the eighteenth and nineteenth centuries.

35. As we will see in later chapters, this process was neither straightforward nor uncontested.

36. Esquirol, *Des Maladies mentales*, 1: 121.

37. Esquirol, *Des Maladies mentales*, 1: 121.

38. Esquirol, *Des Maladies mentales*, 1: 122.

39. Esquirol, *Des Maladies mentales*, 1: 122.

40. Esquirol, *Des Passions*, 38.

41. Esquirol, *Des Passions*, 59–60.

42. Pinel, *L'Aliénation mentale ou la manie: Traité médico-philosophique*, 213.

43. Scipion Pinel, *Physiologie de l'homme aliéné: appliquée à l'analyse de l'homme social* (Paris: Librairie des Sciences Médicales, 1833), v.

44. Goldstein, *Console and Classify*, 86.

45. Goldstein, *Console and Classify*, 132.

46. Goldstein, *Console and Classify*, 133.

47. Esquirol, *Des Maladies mentales*, 1: 127.

48. Esquirol, *Des Maladies mentales*, 1: 120.

49. Esquirol, *Des Maladies mentales*, 2: 781.

50. Esquirol, *Des Maladies mentales*, 1: 127.

51. Goldstein, *Console and Classify*, 86.

52. Pinel, *L'Aliénation mentale ou la manie: Traité médico-philosophique*, 103.

53. Pinel, *L'Aliénation mentale ou la manie: Traité médico-philosophique*, 103.

54. Pinel, *L'Aliénation mentale ou la manie: Traité médico-philosophique*, 103.

55. Pinel, *L'Aliénation mentale ou la manie: Traité médico-philosophique*, 103.

56. Pinel, *L'Aliénation mentale ou la manie: Traité médico-philosophique*, 92.

57. Pinel, *L'Aliénation mentale ou la manie: Traité médico-philosophique*, 94–95.

58. Pinel, *L'Aliénation mentale ou la manie: Traité médico-philosophique*, 99–103.

59. On complementarity, see Londa Schiebinger, *The Mind Has No Sex? Women in the Origins of Modern Science* (Cambridge, MA: Harvard University Press, 1991) and

Suzanne Desan, *The Family on Trial in Revolutionary France* (Berkeley: University of California Press).

60. Scipion Pinel, *Traité complet du régime sanitaire des aliénés* (Paris: Mauprivez, 1836), preface iii.

61. Scipion Pinel, *Traité complet*, 42–43.

Chapter 2: Medical Controversy and Honor among (Mad)Men

1. Details of the incident can be found in the *Journal des débats*, January 20, 1839.

2. Esprit Blanche, *Du danger des rigueurs corporelles dans le traitement de la folie* (Paris: A. Gardembas, 1839), 40–41.

3. *Journal des débats,* January 20, 1839.

4. Goldstein, *Console and Classify*, 277–280.

5. Jo Burr Margadant, "Gender, Vice, and the Political Imaginary in Postrevolutionary France: Reinterpreting the Failure of the July Monarchy, 1830–1848," *American Historical Review* 104, no. 5 (1999): 1461–96, https://www.jstor.org/stable/2649346.

6. The methods were called *placement d'office* (internment instigated by the prefecture) and *placement volontaire* (institutionalization of a patient by their family members).

7. Goldstein, *Console and Classify*, 285–292.

8. Goldstein mentions early criticisms in a footnote, 281. For discussions of the elaborate anti-alienism campaigns of the Second Empire see Fauvel, *Témoins aliénés et 'Bastilles modernes'* and Thomas Mueller, "Le placement familiale des aliénés en France. Le Baron Mundy et L'Exposition universelle de 1867," *Romantisme* 3, no. 141 (2008): 37–50, https://doi.org/10.3917/rom.141.0037.

9. The only historian who has analyzed the debate in detail is Ian Dowbiggin, *Inheriting Madness*, 38–53, whose interpretation I address at the end of this chapter. Goldstein mentions the controversy briefly in a footnote (288) as does Laure Murat in her study of the Maison Blanche, *La Maison du Docteur Blanche: histoire d'un asile et de ses pensionnaires, de Nerval à Maupassant* (Paris: JC Lattès, 2001), 55–59.

10. See Robert A. Nye, "Medicine and Science as Masculine 'Fields of Honor,'" *Osiris* 12, no. 2 (1997): 60–79, https://www.jstor.org/stable/301899. He writes, "In terms of our contemporary notions of professional ethics, there is little evidence that ethical considerations played much of a role in the activities of either scientists or liberal professionals. Instead, their clubs and organizations appear to have been content to operate under the aegis of the honor culture and of the honor code that governed masculine relations in the larger public sphere. The rather general statutes many of them adopted, and what we know about their criteria for admission and expulsion, suggest that they were informed in such matters by the tacit knowledge their members possessed in their capacity as men of a certain class. In other words, the 'ethical' standard that guided them was really the ethos of the upper-class male honor culture adapted to the tasks at hand" (67).

11. Robert A. Nye, *Masculinity and Male Codes of Honor in Modern France*, 8.

12. Reddy, *The Invisible Code*, xiii.

13. Anonymous, *Histoire d'une maladie: Fragment relatif à son traitement par le malade* (Béziers: Imprimerie Auguste Malinas, 1870), 13. Chapter 4 of this book contains extended discussion of the patient perspective.

14. Philippe Pinel, *L'Aliénation mentale ou la manie: Traité médico-philosophique*, 275–276.

15. Pinel, *L'Aliénation mentale ou la manie: Traité médico-philosophique*, 276.

16. François Leuret, *Du Traitement des idées ou concecptions délirantes* (Paris: Everat, 1837).

17. Charles Hecquet, *Notice biographique sur la vie et les travaux du docteur Leuret, médecin en chef de l'hospice d'aliénés de Bicêtre, par Charles Hecquet* (Nancy: Grimblot et Veuve Raybois, 1852), 9.

18. Goldstein quotes the physical anthropologist Paul Broca's impressions of Leuret: "I, like everyone else, admired the power of fascination that he exercises over our madmen" (Goldstein, *Console and Classify*, 133). The original remark can be found in Paul Broca, *Correspondance*, vol. 1 (Paris: Typographie Paul Schmidt, 1886), April 4, 1845, 291.

19. François Leuret, "Mémoires sur l'emploi des douches, et des affusions froides dans le traitement de l'aliénation mentale," *Archives generales de médecine* 3, no. 4 (Paris: Béchet jeune, 1839): 283.

20. Laure Murat is the best source of biographical information on the Blanche family. She describes Blanche as an extremely well-respected private asylum director; *La Maison du Docteur Blanche*, 11–13.

21. François Leuret, "Mémoire sur le traitement moral de la folie," *Mémoires de l'academie royale de médecine* 7 (1838): 72.

22. Goldstein notes the continued influence of religious authority on the treatment of insanity long after the passage of the law of 1838; *Console and Classify*, 197–230.

23. On this *encombrement*, see Goldstein, *Console and Classify*, 147–151; George D. Sussman, "The Glut of Doctors in Mid-Nineteenth-Century France," *Comparative Studies in Society and History* 19 (1977): 287–304, https://doi.org/10.1017/S0010417500008720.

24. Reddy, *The Invisible Code*, xiii.

25. Leuret, "Mémoire sur le traitement moral de la folie," 60–75; Blanche, *Du danger des rigueurs corporelles dans le traitement de la folie*, 30–35.

26. Leuret, "Mémoire sur le traitement moral de la folie," 65.

27. Leuret, "Mémoire sur le traitement moral de la folie," 70.

28. Leuret, "Mémoire sur le traitement moral de la folie," 72.

29. Ian Dowbiggin focuses on this aspect of the debate in *Inheriting Madness*, arguing that Leuret was controversial because his contemporaries were beginning to understand madness in physical rather than "moral" (or strictly mental) terms, 38–53.

30. Leuret, "Mémoires sur l'emploi des douches," 75.

31. Blanche, *Du Danger des rigeurs corporelle dans le traitement de la folie*, 12.

32. Pinel, *L'Aliénation mentale ou la manie: Traité médico-philosophique,* 214; Scipion Pinel, *Traité complet du regime sanitaire des aliénés,* 216.

33. Goldstein, *Console and Classify,* 99–100.

34. Desan, *The Family on Trial in Revolutionary France,* 283–310.

35. Jean Delumeau and Daniel Roche, *Histoire des pères et de la paternité* (Paris: Larousse, 1990), 288–305.

36. Blanche, *Du Danger des rigeurs corporelle dans le traitement de la folie,* 34.

37. Blanche, *Du Danger des rigeurs corporelle dans le traitement de la folie,* 45.

38. Blanche, *Du Danger des rigeurs corporelle dans le traitement de la folie,* 51.

39. Blanche, *Du Danger des rigeurs corporelle dans le traitement de la folie,* 6.

40. Blanche, *Du Danger des rigeurs corporelle dans le traitement de la folie,* 10.

41. As Goldstein shows, most alienists who considered themselves members of the influential Esquirol circle had diverse but decidedly bourgeois backgrounds (*Console and Classify,* 139). Carol Harrison's study of emulation among provincial men in various homosocial settings—scientific clubs, philanthropic societies, and the like—makes a similar point regarding the need to bond members of the bourgeoisie when economic and political conditions worked against this end result. Carol E. Harrison, *The Bourgeois Citizen in Nineteenth-Century France: Gender, Sociability, and the Uses of Emulation* (Oxford: Oxford University Press, 1999).

42. Reddy, *The Invisible Code,* especially chapters 4 and 5 (on bureaucrats and journalists, respectively).

43. Andrea Mansker also emphasizes the malleability of the honor code by focusing on its use by French women; Andrea Mansker, *Sex, Honor and Citizenship in Early Third Republic France* (London: Palgrave Macmillan, 2011).

44. Pinel, *L'Aliénation mentale ou la manie: Traité médico-philosophique,* 273.

45. Blanche, *Du Danger des rigeurs corporelle dans le traitement de la folie,* 46.

46. Blanche, *Du Danger des rigeurs corporelle dans le traitement de la folie,* 46.

47. For discussion of the case study as a genre, see Matt Reid, "'La Manie d'Ecrire': Psychology, Auto-Observation, and the Case History," *Journal of the Behavioral Sciences* 40, no. 3 (2004): 265–284, https://doi.org/10.1002/jhbs.20021.

48. Blanche, *Du Danger des rigueurs corporelles dans le traitement de la folie,* 46.

49. Blanche, *Du Danger des rigueurs corporelles dans le traitement de la folie,* 46–47.

50. Blanche, *Du Danger des rigueurs corporelles dans le traitement de la folie,* 46.

51. Blanche used similar tactics with a woman patient who refused to eat after losing her husband to early death. In order to persuade her to start eating again, he said he would require a servant to watch her at all times, even in her bedroom. Blanche rightly assumed that her feminine "modesty" would force the woman to begin eating so as to avoid the unwanted gaze of her guardian (*Du Danger des rigueurs corporelles dans le traitement de la folie,* 49). Chapter 3 of this book takes up the question of bourgeois femininity and psychiatric practice in detail.

52. Blanche, *Du Danger des rigueurs corporelles dans le traitement de la folie,* 48.

53. Blanche, *Du Danger des rigueurs corporelles dans le traitement de la folie,* 48.

54. Blanche, *Du Danger des rigueurs corporelles dans le traitement de la folie,* 48.

55. Blanche, *Du Danger des rigueurs corporelles dans le traitement de la folie,* 48.

56. Leuret, "Mémoire sur le traitement moral de la folie," 555.

57. Leuret, "Mémoire sur le traitement moral de la folie," 555.

58. Leuret, "Mémoire sur le traitement moral de la folie," 555.

59. Leuret, "Mémoire sur le traitement moral de la folie," 556.

60. Leuret, "Mémoire sur le traitement moral de la folie," 556.

61. Leuret, "Mémoire sur le traitement moral de la folie," 558.

62. Leuret, "Mémoire sur le traitement moral de la folie," 558.

63. Leuret also consulted with a private asylum in Paris, although the examples I relate in this chapter mainly come from his experiences at Bicêtre.

64. Leuret, *Du Traitement des idées ou concecptions délirantes,* 5.

65. Leuret, *Du Traitement des idées ou concecptions délirantes,* 5.

66. Leuret, *Du Traitement des idées ou concecptions délirantes,* 5–6.

67. Leuret, *Du Traitement des idées ou concecptions délirantes,* 7.

68. Leuret, *Du Traitement des idées ou concecptions délirantes,* 8.

69. J. E. D. Esquirol, "Rapport," in Blanche, *Du danger des rigueurs corporelles,* 54.

70. Esquirol, "Rapport," in Blanche, *Du danger des rigueurs corporelles,* 55.

71. Esquirol, "Rapport," in Blanche, *Du danger des rigueurs corporelles,* 62.

72. Esquirol, "Rapport," in Blanche, *Du danger des rigueurs corporelles,* 55.

73. Dowbiggin, *Inheriting Madness,* 42; Ulysse Trélat, "Notice sur François Leuret," *Annales d'hygiène publique et de médecine légale* 45 (1851): 258; Alexandre Brierre de Boismont, "Notice biographique sur M. François Leuret," *Annales médico-psycholoquiques* 3 (1851): 525.

74. A. Donné, *Journal des Débats, politiques et littéraires,* September 2, 1842.

75. Londe, "Du délire," *Bulletin de l'Académie nationale de médecine* (1854): 951.

76. Forth, *Masculinity in the Modern West,* 4.

77. Leuret, "Mémoire sur le traitement moral de la folie," 558.

78. Leuret, "Mémoire sur le traitement moral de la folie," 558.

79. Leuret, "Mémoire sur le traitement moral de la folie," 558.

Chapter 3: Domesticating Madness in the Family Asylum

1. Alexandre Brierre de Boismont, *De l'Utilité de la vie de famille dans le traitement de l'aliénation mentale et plus specialement de ses formes tristes* (Paris: Imprimerie de E. Martinet, 1866), 1.

2. I have chosen to refer to Alexandre Brierre de Boismont as Dr. Brierre de Boismont while I refer to his wife by her full name, Athalie Brierre de Boismont (so as not to diminish her role as a historical actor independent of her husband by calling her "Madame").

3. The most comprehensive source of information on Brierre de Boismont's background is Enric J. Novella and Rafael Huertas, "Alexandre Brierre de Boismont and the

origins of the Spanish psychiatric profession," *History of Psychiatry* 22, no. 4 (December 2011): 387–402, https://doi.org/10.1177/0957154X10390440. Mention of his marriage is found on p. 389.

4. Brierre de Boismont, *De l'Utilité de la vie de famille*, 2.

5. Brierre de Boismont, *De l'Utilité de la vie de famille*, 4.

6. Scholars have begun to examine alternatives to institutionalization in large public asylums during the nineteenth century. For France see Murat, *La Maison du docteur Blanche*. Also see Akihito Suzuki, *Madness at Home: The Psychiatrist, the Patient, and the Family in England, 1820–1860* (Berkeley: University of California Press, 2006); Peter Bartlett and David Wright, eds., *Outside the Walls of the Asylum: The History of Care in the Community, 1750–2000* (London: Athlone Press, 1999); Pamela Michael, *Care and Treatment of the Mentally Ill in North Wales, 1800–2000*, (Cardiff: University of Wales Press, 2003).

7. I use the terms "private asylum" (*asile privé*) and *maison de santé* interchangeably, as do my sources. While there were many *maisons de santé* that did not cater to the alienated, those examined here did unless otherwise noted.

8. Alexandre Brierre de Boismont, *Des Hallucinations ou Histoire raisonée des apparitions, des visions, des songes, de l'extase, du magnétisme et du somnabulisme* (Paris: Germer Baillière, 1845); *Du suicide et de la folie suicide* (Paris: Germer Baillière, 1856); "Mémoire pour l'établissement d'un hospice d'aliénés," *Annales d'hygiène publique et de médecine légale* (1836), 39–120.

9. He began writing contributions for the journal's second issue.

10. Brierre de Boismont, *De l'Utilité de la vie de famille*, 9.

11. Alexandre Brierre de Boismont, "Maison de santé du docteur Brierre du Boismont" (undated pamphlet), 1.

12. Brierre de Boismont, "Maison de santé du docteur Brierre du Boismont," 2.

13. C. Sachaile de la Barre, *Les Médecins de Paris jugés par leurs oeuvres* (Paris: Auteur, 1845), 150.

14. Drs. Constans, Lunier, et Dumesnil, *Rapport Général à M. le Ministre de l'Intérieur sur le service des aliénés en 1874* (Paris: Imprimerie National, 1878), 153. According to the same report, there were 40,804 patients living in public institutions at this time.

15. *Almanach-Bottin du commerce de Paris, des départements de la France et des principales villes du monde* (Paris: Bureau de l'Almanach du Commerce, 1842), 214; *Annuaire-Almanach du commerce et de l'industrie, ou almanach des 500,000 addresses de Paris, des départements et des pays étrangers*, (Paris: Chez Fermin Didot Frères, Fils, et Cie., 1862), 915. Unfortunately, the later volume does not distinguish private facilities dedicated to mental healthcare from those dedicated to the treatment of physical ailments. Thus, the figure of eleven private asylums in 1862 is a conservative estimate based only on those *maisons de santé* that earlier editions had already established as private mental institutions.

16. Brierre de Boismont, *De l'Utilité de la vie de famille*, 4.

17. Brierre de Boismont, "Maison de santé du docteur Brierre du Boismont," 1.

18. See Perrot, ed., *Histoire de la vie privée,* vol. 4, *De la révolution à la grande guerre;* Smith, *Ladies of the Leisure Class;* and Martin-Fugier, *La Place des bonnes.*

19. Marie Rivet, *Les Aliénés dans la famille et dans la maison de santé: Etude pour les gens du monde* (Paris: 1875), 111.

20. Rivet, *Les Aliénés dans la famille et dans la maison de santé,* 111.

21. Rivet, *Les Aliénés dans la famille et dans la maison de santé,* 112.

22. Brierre de Boismont, *De l'Utilité de la vie de famille,* 9.

23. Smith, *Ladies of the Leisure Class,* 34–49.

24. For the gender implications of the Civil Code, see Desan, *The Family on Trial,* 283–310.

25. On women and charity, see Christine Adams, *Poverty, Charity, and Motherhood: Maternal Societies in Nineteenth-Century France* (Urbana: University of Illinois Press, 2010); Evelyne Lejeune-Resnick, *Femmes et associations (1830–1880), vraies democrates ou dames patronnesses?* (Paris: Publisud, 1991); Susan Grogan, "Philanthropic Women and the State: The Société de Charité Maternelle in Avignon, 1802–1917," *French History* 14, no. 3 (2000), 295–231, https://doi.org/10.1093/fh/14.3.295.

26. For discussion of the cultural backlash against "bourgeois" values in the postrevolutionary era, see Maza, *The Myth of the French Bourgeoisie.*

27. Castel, *The Regulation of Madness,* 14–45.

28. Brierre de Boismont, *De l'Utilité de la vie de famille,* 24.

29. Brierre de Boismont, *De l'Utilité de la vie de famille,* 24.

30. In this he agreed with his mentor, Esquirol; see especially Esquirol, *Des Maladies mentales,* vol. 1, 116–135.

31. Brierre de Boismont, *De l'Utilité de la vie de famille,* 26.

32. Brierre de Boismont, *De l'Utilité de la vie de famille,* 14.

33. Brierre de Boismont, *De l'Utilité de la vie de famille,* 14.

34. Brierre de Boismont, *De l'Utilité de la vie de famille,* 14.

35. Brierre de Boismont, *De l'Utilité de la vie de famille,* 15.

36. The key secondary source on Rousseau's promotion of domestic motherhood is Popiel, *Rousseau's Daughters.*

37. Brierre de Boismont, *De l'Utilité de la vie de famille,* 11.

38. Brierre de Boismont, *De l'Utilité de la vie de famille,* 11.

39. Brierre de Boismont, *De l'Utilité de la vie de famille,* 11.

40. Brierre de Boismont, *De l'Utilité de la vie de famille,* 12.

41. Rivet, *Les Aliénés dans la famille et dans la maison de santé,* 108.

42. Rivet, *Les Aliénés dans la famille et dans la maison de santé,* 108.

43. Michèle Plott, "The Rules of the Game: Respectability, Sexuality, and the *Femme Mondaine* in Late Nineteenth-Century Paris," *French Historical Studies* 25 no. 3 (2002), 535, https://www.muse.jhu.edu/article/11931.

44. See Ripa's *La Ronde des folles* for examples of women's internment on the basis of "deviant" sexual behavior in the case of France; see Showalter, *The Female Malady* for English examples.

45. Rivet, *Les Aliénés dans la famille et dans la maison de santé,* 174.

46. Rivet notes that many male patients arrived at the family asylum after losing their jobs; *Les Aliénés dans la famille et dans la maison de santé,* 118.

47. Brierre de Boismont, *De l'Utilité de la vie de famille,* 5–6.

48. Brierre de Boismont, *De l'Utilité de la vie de famille,* 6.

49. Popiel, *Rousseau's Daughters,* 6.

50. Her sister, Mathilde, married the vicomte d'Arlincourt in 1854; when he died she married an editor of a political journal and had one child, a girl who eventually married a doctor and professor at the Faculté de Médecine, Simon Duplay. Rivet's brother Albert also opened a *maison de santé* in Saint-Mandé after having been employed for some time by the Banque de France. Dr. Rire, "Brierre de Boismont," *L'Intermédiaire des chercheurs et curieux,* no. 1073 (1905): 579.

51. Rivet, *Les Aliénés dans la famille et dans la maison de santé,* 102. See also Brierre de Boismont, *Annales d'hygiène publique et de médecine légale* 2, no. 44 (1875): 468.

52. See fichier V3E/M879 of the État Civil records of the Archives de Paris. Jean Baptiste Rivet's occupation is unknown. Curiously, Rivet never mentions him in her book.

53. There is some ambiguity in the historical record regarding the ownership of the Saint-Mandé institution, always referred to in promotional materials as the "Maison de Santé de Mme. Rivet, née Brierre de Boismont" [see the advertisement in the *Gazette Medicaux de Paris* 21 (1866) for an example]. The few historians who have referenced the *maison de santé* have repeated the assertion of René Semelaigne, author of a compendium of biographical sketches of noteworthy personalities in the history of nineteenth-century French psychiatry, who claimed Alexandre Brierre de Boismont founded the institution in 1860 but it was directed by his daughter. [René Semelaigne, *Les pionniers de la psychiatrie francaise avant et après Pinel,* vol. 1 (Paris: J.-B. Baillière et fils, 1930), 239.] This is probably inaccurate for several reasons. Court records located at the Bibliothèque Nationale indicate that Rivet was involved in a legal dispute with the city of Paris over her decision to stop leasing a building on the Rue Neuve-Sainte-Geneviève (where she had run an asylum since 1850) and purchase the facility in Sainte-Mandé. Alexandre Brierre de Boismont was not named in the suit, and Rivet's lawyers noted that the new buildings purchased in Saint-Mandé were not for her father. Rivet's husband was named in the suit, but the text of their defense refers only to "Madame Rivet" when discussing the asylum's operations. See Jean-Baptiste Boudin de Vesvres, *Réponse pour M. et Mme. Rivet à la plaidoirie du défenseur de M. le préfet de la Seine* (Paris: L. Martinet, 1859), 2. I have not discovered anything written by Rivet or her father suggesting that the Saint-Mandé facility belonged to, or was even founded by, Alexandre Brierre de Boismont. An advertisement from 1869 does list him as a "médecin consultant" (one Dr. Musset was listed as the "médecin attaché a l'établissement"): *Annuaire thérapeutique, de matière médicale, de pharmacie, et de toxicologie* 29 (1869).

54. Rivet, *Les Aliénés dans la famille et dans la maison de santé,* 75. Rivet never mentioned the role of her husband in her book, suggesting he did not participate in the asylum's affairs.

55. *Réponse pour M. et Mme. Rivet à la plaidoirie du défenseur de M. le Préfet de la Seine*, 5; *Statistique Générale de la France* (Paris: Berger-Levrault et Cie., 1885), 198–199.

56. *Réponse pour M. et Mme. Rivet à la plaidoirie du défenseur de M. le préfet de la Seine*, 5.

57. *Almanach Bottin* (1842), 214. Later editions of the commercial almanac failed to clearly distinguish psychiatric asylums from other medical institutions. For example, the 1862 edition mentions four woman directors aside from Marie Rivet, but there is no reason to believe their facilities focused on the treatment of madness. *Almanach Bottin* (1862), 915.

58. Rivet, *Les Aliénés dans la famille et dans la maison de santé*, i.

59. Rivet, *Les Aliénés dans la famille et dans la maison de santé*, i.

60. Felicia Gordon, *The Integral Feminist: Madeleine Pelletier, 1874–1939, Feminism, Socialism, and Medicine* (Minneapolis: University of Minnesota Press, 1990), 27. For more on the first generation of European women doctors, see Thomas Neville Bonner, *To the Ends of the Earth: Women's Search for Education in Medicine* (Cambridge, MA: Harvard University Press, 1992).

61. Gordon, *The Integral Feminist*, 63; Bonner, *The Ends of the Earth*, 71.

62. Gordon, *The Integral Feminist*, 54–58. Other medical specialties won the battle for women's hospital internships in 1885; Bonner, *The Ends of the Earth*, 73.

63. See Ulysse Robert, *Notes historiques sur Saint-Mandé* (Saint-Mandé: A. Beucher, 1889), 137. Rivet also advertised her services in the *Gazette Médicaux de Paris* 21 (1866) as did her brother, who operated another *maison de santé* on the same street in Saint-Mandé.

64. Sylvain-Christian David, *Philoxène Boyer: un sale ami de Baudelaire* (Paris: Ramsay, 1987), 246–253.

65. Philoxene Boyer, *Deux Saisons* (Paris: A. Lemerre, 1867), 47–48. The poem is titled "La Marquise Aurore."

66. "Marc Fournier," *Le Figaro*, January 8, 1879, 3.

67. The relevant excerpts from Hugo's journals are reproduced in Henri Guillemin, *L'Engloutie, Adele fille de Victor Hugo 1830–1915* (Paris: Editions du Seuil, 1985), 151–152. For a comprehensive discussion of the life and historiography related to Adèle Hugo, see Alana Eldridge, "Adèle Hugo: A Bibliographical Note," *Nineteenth-Century French Studies* 32 (Fall-Winter 2003–2004), 138–143, https://www.jstor.org/stable/23538156.

68. Historians have paid significant attention to how women in the nineteenth century constructed their identities in ways that pushed the boundaries of bourgeois femininity while also attempting to maintain respectability, including Margadant, ed., *The New Biography: Performing Femininity in Nineteenth-Century France,* especially the introduction; Roberts, *Disruptive Acts*; Accampo, *Blessed Motherhood, Bitter Fruit*; Felicia Gordon, "French Psychiatry and the new woman: the case of Dr. Constance Pascale, 1877–1937," *History of Psychiatry* 17, no. 2 (2006), 159–182, 10.1177/0957154X06056601.

69. Rivet, *Les Aliénés dans la famille et dans la maison de santé*, i.

70. Rivet, *Les Aliénés dans la famille et dans la maison de santé*, i.

71. Rivet, *Les Aliénés dans la famille et dans la maison de santé*, i.

72. Rivet, *Les Aliénés dans la famille et dans la maison de santé*, 1.

73. See chapter 5 for more discussion of Rivet and the Commune.

74. Goldstein, *Console and Classify*, 291. See footnote 46.

75. Robert A. Nye, "Honor, Impotence, and Male Sexuality in Nineteenth-Century French Medicine," *French Historical Studies* 2 (1989), 53. 10.2307/286433. See also Thomas Laqueur, *Solitary Sex: A Cultural History of Masturbation* (Cambridge, MA: Zone Books, 2003).

76. There is a vast historiography related to the demographic crisis and its cultural effects following the Prussian defeat of France in 1871. Key works include Elinor Accampo, Rachel Fuchs, and Mary Lynn Stewart, eds., *Gender and the Politics of Social Reform in France, 1870–1914*; Joshua Cole, *The Power of Large Numbers: Population, Politics and Gender in Nineteenth-Century France* (Ithaca, NY: Cornell University Press, 2000).

77. Rivet, *Les Aliénés dans la famille et dans la maison de santé*, 124.

78. Rivet, *Les Aliénés dans la famille et dans la maison de santé*, 124.

79. Rivet, *Les Aliénés dans la famille et dans la maison de santé*, 124.

80. Rivet, *Les Aliénés dans la famille et dans la maison de santé*, 55.

81. Rivet, *Les Aliénés dans la famille et dans la maison de santé*, 55.

82. On household education in nineteenth-century France see Popiel, *Rousseau's Daughters*.

83. Rivet, *Les Aliénés dans la famille et dans la maison de santé*, 59.

84. Rivet, *Les Aliénés dans la famille et dans la maison de santé*, 59.

85. Rivet, *Les Aliénés dans la famille et dans la maison de santé*, 59. Italics in original.

86. Rivet, *Les Aliénés dans la famille et dans la maison de santé*, 60.

87. This was certainly the case for someone like François Leuret, who supported the use of corporal methods to inspire patients' obedience. Yet even those who were critical of physical intimidation as a form of treatment insisted that patients should never be allowed to behave or to speak in an illogical fashion.

88. *Chicago Journal of Nervous and Mental Disease* 2, no. 1 (January 1875).

89. M. L., *L'Union médicale: journal des intérêts scientifiques et practiques, moraux et professionnels du corps medical*, series 3, no. 19 (Paris: 1875), 234.

90. M. L., *L'Union médicale*, 235.

91. Brierre de Boismont, *Annales d'hygiène publique et de médecine légale*, série 2, no. 44 (Paris: J.-B. Baillière et fils, 1875), 469–479.

92. Dowbiggin, *Inheriting Madness*, 106–109.

93. Brierre de Boismont, *Annales d'hygiène publique et de médecine légale*, 472.

94. Aimé-Jean Linas, *Gazette hebdomadaire de la médecine et de chirurgie* 29 (July 1875), 463.

95. Linas, *Gazette hebdomadaire de la médecine et de chirurgie*, 463.

96. Linas, *Gazette hebdomadaire de la médecine et de chirurgie*, 463.

97. Linas, *Gazette hebdomadaire de la médecine et de chirurgie*, 463.

98. Linas, *Gazette hebdomadaire de la médecine et de chirurgie*, 463.

99. Linas specifically mentioned that the Seine asylums Sainte-Anne, Bicêtre, and the Salpêtrière were all under threat of losing funding for their services at this time (464).

100. Linas, *Gazette hebdomadaire de la médecine et de chirurgie*, 463.

101. *La Croix Supplementaire*, no. 3853S (November 21,1895): 3. Rivet had retired several years earlier. Her name disappeared from the *Annuaire Statistique's* list of private asylums after 1888; the record for 1889 lists Henri Dagonet, the former *médecin en chef* of the public Parisian asylum Sainte-Anne, as director of a private asylum for women in Saint-Mandé, suggesting he probably took over for Rivet at that time.

102. Ambroise Tardieu, *Étude médico-légale sur les attentats aux moeurs* (Paris: J.-B. Baillière et fils, 1857).

103. Rivet, *Les Aliénés dans la famille et dans la maison de santé*, 176.

104. Rivet, *Les Aliénés dans la famille et dans la maison de santé*, 176.

Chapter 4: Scandalous Asylum Commitments and Patriarchal Power

1. E., *Le Pourvoyeur d'une maison d'aliénés, discussion-drame en quatre actes en prose. Par un philanthrope. Ouvrage dédié aux magistrates, notamment à ceux chargés de la surveillance des maisons d'insensés et aux partisans de l'emancipation intellectuelle* (Paris: L'Imprimerie de Decourchant, 1840), 37.

2. Fauvel, *Témoins Aliénés et Bastilles Modernes*. Also see Ian Dowbiggin, *Inheriting Madness*, 101–102.

3. Fauvel has identified numerous instances of unwilling sequestration and sixteen cases between the passage of the 1838 law and World War 1 that generated considerable written historical evidence. Of these sixteen, ten were clearly "family affairs" related to issues of spousal incompatibility or inheritance. The rest of the cases involved a wide variety of causes, including political motivations, anti-clericalism, international diplomacy, and confrontations between individuals and specific agents of the police. Family drama thus proved to be the most common inspiration for scandalous asylum commitments. See the appendix of her dissertation for brief summaries of each case.

4. On counternarratives see Aude Fauvel, "A World-Famous Lunatic: Baron Raymond Seillière (1845–1911) and the Patient's View in Transnational Perspective" in *Transnational Psychiatries: Social and Cultural Histories of Psychiatry in Comparative Perspective c. 1800–2000*, ed. Waltraud Ernst and Thomas Mueller (Newcastle: Cambridge Scholars Publishing), 200–208.

5. Jann Matlock, "Doubling Out of the Crazy House: Gender, Autobiography, and the Insane Asylum System in Nineteenth-Century France," *Representations* 34 (Spring 1991): 166–195, https://doi.org/10.2307/2928774. On the famous case of Hersilie Rouy, also see Yannick Ripa, *L'Affaire Rouy: Une femme contre l'asile* (Paris: Tallandier, 2010).

6. Standard legal histories argue that French family law remained relatively unchanged throughout the nineteenth century until the implementation of early social welfare initiatives and the legalization of divorce during the Third Republic. Lloyd

Bonfield, "European Family Law" in The History of the European Family vol. 2, *Family Life in the Long Nineteenth Century, 1789–1913,* ed. David Kertzer and Marzio Barbagli (New Haven, CT: Yale University Press, 2002), 118.

7. Robert Castel also makes this point in *The Regulation of Madness,* 15–25.

8. Gilbert Shapiro and John Markoff, *Revolutionary Demands: A Content Analysis of the Cahiers de Doléances of 1789* (Stanford: Stanford University Press, 1998), 277–278.

9. The term was used in a pamphlet published by the "Younger sons of Provence" during the Revolution. See Desan, *The Family on Trial in Revolutionary France,* 1.

10. Margaret H. Darrow, "Popular Concepts of Marital Choice in Eighteenth-Century France," *Journal of Social History* 19: 2 (1985), 263-264; Bonfield, "European Family Law," 133.

11. For another perspective see Kristen Childers, *Fathers, Families, and the State in France, 1914–1945* (Ithaca, NY: Cornell University Press, 2003). Childers shows that fathers retained some of the rights previously associated with the *lettre de cachet* under the Civil Code of 1804, in that heads of household could incarcerate rebellious children under the age of fifteen for renewable one-month periods through *correction paternelle* (12–13, 15, 18–20). Despite the authority fathers held over their children throughout the nineteenth century, I argue that those deemed insane were significantly more vulnerable to familial control than the typical child (as evidenced by the numbers of those incarcerated in asylums and the long duration of their stays). Furthermore, while *correction paternelle* applied only to children, asylum commitment could affect any member of the family—including the father himself.

12. Desan, *The Family on Trial,* 141–177.

13. Desan, *The Family on Trial,* 305.

14. Bonfield, "European Family Law," 139. He cites article 913 of the Civil Code.

15. Law of 30 June 1838 Concerning the Insane, section 1, article 8.

16. Law of 1838, section 1, article 13.

17. Law of 1838, section 1, article 14.

18. Law of 1838, section 4, article 29.

19. Law of 1838, section 2, article 18.

20. Law of 1838, section 2, article 18.

21. Law of 1838, section 2, article 20.

22. Law of 1838, section 4, article 31.

23. Law of 1838, section 4, article 32.

24. Law of 1838, section 4, article 37.

25. Law of 1838, section 4, article 38.

26. This was two years before Jean was to reach the age of majority.

27. One can reconstruct this chain of events by reading a collection of documents published by Jean Mistral's defenders in 1886, entitled *47 Années de sequestration, Jean Mistral de Saint-Rémy en 1838, L'Homme aux soixante millions n'est pas fou* (Marseille: Imprimerie Génerale Achard et Cie., 1886).

28. Adolphe Dumas, in *47 Années de sequestration,* 11–16.

29. François-Joseph Mistral, in *47 Années de sequestration*, 17–20.

30. François-Joseph Mistral, *47 Années de sequestration*, 18.

31. Christopher H. Johnson, *Becoming Bourgeois: Love, Kinship, and Power in Provincial France, 1670–1880* (Ithaca, NY: Cornell University Press, 2015), 5–18.

32. The issue of inheritance, which had played such a significant role in his initial sequestration, would also play a part in his release. Two sides of the family became embroiled in legal machinations following the death of the elder Mistral. When a cousin discovered Jean's situation he labored to have him set free and help him to regain his rightful inheritance. The case gained widespread publicity and the press dubbed Jean "le fou aux soixante millions," or, "The Madman with Sixty Million"—referring to the vast riches at the root of his tragic fate. Jean was finally set free in 1886, but died shortly thereafter.

33. This can be seen in the history of paternity suits. Rachel Fuchs points out in *Contested Paternity* that paternity suits were technically not allowed during the nineteenth century, an indication of the persistence of fatherly authority vis-à-vis women and children, but that jurisprudence nonetheless indicated more sympathy toward the rights of those born out of wedlock than a strict reading of the legal codes would suggest. The law on paternity suits was overturned in 1912.

34. Ernest Faligan, *Le Gouvernement occulte de la France* (Brussels: A. N. LeBégue et Cie., 1880), 7 and 26–27.

35. Ernest Faligan, *Les Sequestrations arbitraries et le droit de pétition* (Paris: Librairie Generale, 1879), *Le Gouvernment occulte de la France*, and *La Police, juge, et partie* (undated).

36. Faligan's *La Police, juge, et partie* is the best source for background information.

37. Faligan, *La Police, juge, et partie*, 5.

38. Henri Legrand du Saulle, *La délire des persecutions* (Paris: Plon, 1871).

39. Faligan, *La Police, juge, et partie*, 14–15.

40. Faligan, *Les Sequestrations arbitraires*, 6–7.

41. *L'Interdiction* has not been the focus of extensive scholarship. An exception is Michel Lichté, *Balzac, le texte et la loi* (Paris: Presses de l'Université Paris-Sorbonne, 2012), 205–220.

42. Honoré de Balzac, *Le Colonel Chabert,* suivi de *Honorine* et de *L'Interdiction* (Paris: Classiques Garnier, 1964), 219.

43. Balzac, *L'Interdiction*, 219.

44. Balzac, *L'Interdiction*, 302.

45. Balzac, *L'Interdiction*, 299.

46. Balzac, *L'Interdiction*, 303.

47. Castel, *The Regulation of Madness*, 15.

48. Fauvel, "Madness: a 'female malady'? Women and Psychiatric Institutionalisation in France," 61–75.

49. He admits authorship in a later publication, *Les Bastilles modernes: nécessité de leur destruction: recueil d'articles parus dans L'Union Républicaine* (Béziers: Imprimerie du Commerce, 1886), 5.

50. Hippolyte Delas, *Les Bastilles modernes: nécessité de leur destruction.*

51. Hippolyte Delas, *Histoire d'une maladie* (Béziers: Imprimerie Auguste Malinas, 1870), 2.

52. Delas, *Histoire d'une maladie*, 2.

53. Delas, *Histoire d'une maladie*, 7.

54. Delas, *Histoire d'une maladie*, 5.

55. Delas, *Histoire d'une maladie*, 25.

56. John Tosh nicely sums up the role of the home in middle-class conceptions of masculinity in Victorian England: "Domesticity supposedly allowed workhorses and calculating machines to become men again, by exposing them to human rhythms and human affections." John Tosh, *A Man's Place: Masculinity and the Middle-Class Home in Victorian England* (New Haven, CT: Yale University Press, 1999), 6.

57. Delas, *Histoire d'une maladie*, 36.

58. Delas, *Histoire d'une maladie*, 44.

59. *New York Times*, "The Story of an Eccentric Character," April 3, 1875.

60. "Crispino," "Société protectrice des aliénés," *La Revue comique*, December 3, 1871.

61. *Le Galois*, February 28, 1870. Cited in Fault du Puyparlier, *Affaire du Fault du Puyparlier, Pensées au courant de la plume* (Paris: Typographie et Lithographie Renou et Maulde, 1870), 4.

62. Dowbiggin, *Inheriting Madness*, 97.

63. Faulte du Puyparlier, *Regime des aliénés en France, Asile de Charenton* (Paris: Imprimerie Nouvelle, 1870), 15–16.

64. Dowbiggin, *Inheriting Madness*, 98.

65. *New York Times*, "Story of an Eccentric Character."

66. *New York Times*, "Story of an Eccentric Character."

67. Puyparlier, *Régime des aliénés*, 7.

68. Puyparlier, *Régime des aliénés*, 9.

69. Puyparlier, *Régime des aliénés*, 7–8.

70. Puyparlier, *Régime des aliénés*, 5–6.

71. Puyparlier, *Régime des aliénés*, 42.

72. Puyparlier, *Affaire Fault du Puyparlier*, 3.

73. Puyparlier, *Affaire Fault du Puyparlier*, 3.

74. Puyparlier, *Régime des aliénés*, 7–8.

Chapter 5: Rehabilitating a Profession Under Siege

1. Henri Bonnet, *"La Baronne* (à l'Odéon): Lettre à M. l'Inspecteur Général Lunier," *Annales médico-psychologiques* 5, no. 8 (1872): 73.

2. Examples include: Achille Foville, *Les Aliénés, étude pratique sur la législation et l'assistance qui leur sont applicables* (Paris: J.-B. Baillière et fils,1870); Henri Taguet, *Étude de la loi sur les aliénés du 30 juin 1838* (Paris: Imprimerie de E. Donnaud, 1875);

Henri Taguet, *Les Aliénés persécuteurs* (Paris: Imprimerie de E. Donnaud, 1876); Alexandre Brierre de Boismont, *Responsabilité légale des médecins en Espagne. Procès en detention arbitraire de Dona Juana Sagreda* (Paris: Imprimerie de E. Martinet, 1864); Alexandre Brierre de Boismont, "Appréciation médico-légale du regime des aliénés en France," *Annales médico-psychologiques* 4, no. 6 (1865). References to anti-alienism abound in the issues of the *Annales médico-psychologiques* from approximately1860 until the end of the century. Bonnet, *"La Baronne,"* 81.

3. Delas, *Histoire d'une maladie*, 9.

4. Dowbiggin, *Inheriting Madness*, 93.

5. For a vivid account of the conservatism of the early Third Republic, see John M. Merriman, *The Dynamite Club: How a Bombing in Fin-de-Siècle Paris Ignited the Age of Modern Terror*, 2nd ed. (New Haven, CT: Yale University Press, 2016).

6. See Jack D. Ellis, *The Physician-Legislators of France: Medicine and Politics in the Early Third Republic, 1870–1914* (Cambridge: Cambridge University Press, 1990).

7. Paul Cère, *Les populations dangereuses et les misères sociales* (Paris: Librairie de la sociéte des gens de letters, 1872), 124–125.

8. For an excellent description of the operation of Sainte-Anne in the late nineteenth century, see Patricia E. Prestwich, "Family Strategies and Medical Power: 'Voluntary' Committal in a Parisian Asylum, 1876–1914," *Journal of Social History* 27, no. 4 (1994): 799–818, https://doi.org/10.1353/jsh/27.4.799

9. Louis Gustave Bouchereau and Valentin Magnan, *Statistique des malades entrés en 1870 et en 1871 au bureau d'admission des aliénés de la Seine* (Paris: Imprimerie de E. Donnaud, 1872), 3.

10. Bouchereau and Magnan, *Statistiques des malades*, 3.

11. Bouchereau and Magnan, *Statistiques des malades*, 4.

12. Bouchereau and Magnan, *Statistiques des malades*, 5.

13. Bouchereau and Magnan, *Statistiques des malades*, 4.

14. Ludgar Lunier, "Influence des événéments de 1870–1871 sur le mouvement de l'aliénation mentale en France," *Annales Médico-Psychologiques* 5, no. 8 (1872): 174.

15. Lunier, "Influence des événéments de 1870–1871," 179.

16. See Dr. Bergeret, "Cas nombreaux d'aliénation mentale d'une particulière ayant pour cause la perturbation politique et sociale de février 1848," *Annales d'hygiene publique et de medecine legale* 2, no. 20 (July 1863) for examples. Laure Murat's *The Man Who Thought He Was Napoleon* addresses this theme extensively.

17. See Bertrand Taithe's *Defeated Flesh: Welfare, warfare, and the making of modern France* (Manchester University Press, 1999), especially pages 180–229, for an extended discussion of the medical language used to narrate the events.

18. Lunier, "Influence des événéments de 1870–1871," 180.

19. Lunier, "Influence des événéments de 1870–1871," 180.

20. Lunier, "Influence des événéments de 1870–1871," 181.

21. On families' reluctance to commit their relatives, see Prestwich, "Family Strategies and Medical Power."

22. See chapter 3 for an analysis of Brierre de Boismont's attempt to replicate the habits and power relations of the bourgeois home inside his private asylum.

23. Alexandre Brierre de Boismont, "A Lunatic Asylum during the Siege of Paris," *The Lancet,* (March 4, 1872): 301.

24. Brierre de Boismont, "A Lunatic Asylum during the Siege of Paris," 301.

25. Brierre de Boismont, "A Lunatic Asylum during the Siege of Paris," 301.

26. Brierre de Boismont, "A Lunatic Asylum during the Siege of Paris," 301.

27. Brierre de Boismont, "A Lunatic Asylum during the Siege of Paris," 301.

28. Brierre de Boismont, "A Lunatic Asylum during the Siege of Paris," 301.

29. Brierre de Boismont, "A Lunatic Asylum during the Siege of Paris," 302.

30. As seen in chapter 3, Brierre de Boismont was very attuned to the reputation of the psychiatric profession, a point he emphasized in his review of his daughter's soon-to-be published book on private asylum psychiatry.

31. For biographical information on Winslow and his son, see Judith Walkowitz, *City of Dreadful Delight: Narratives of Sexual Danger in Late Victorian London* (Chicago: University of Chicago Press, 1992), 173–174.

32. Brierre de Boismont, "A Lunatic Asylum during the Siege of Paris," 301.

33. Brierre de Boismont, "A Lunatic Asylum during the Siege of Paris," 302.

34. For a description of the evacuation of Ville-Evrard, see Dr. Eugène Billod, *Les aliénés de Vaucluse et de Ville-Evrard pendant le siège de Paris* (Paris: Librairie de l'Academie de Médecine, 1872), 12–14.

35. Billod, *Les aliénés de Vaucluse et de Ville-Evrard pendant le siège de Paris*, 11.

36. Billod, *Les aliénés de Vaucluse et de Ville-Evrard pendant le siège de Paris*, 16.

37. Billod, *Les aliénés de Vaucluse et de Ville-Evrard pendant le siège de Paris*, 18.

38. Billod, *Les aliénés de Vaucluse et de Ville-Evrard pendant le siège de Paris*, 18.

39. Billod, *Les aliénés de Vaucluse et de Ville-Evrard pendant le siège de Paris*, 18.

40. Billod, *Les aliénés de Vaucluse et de Ville-Evrard pendant le siège de Paris*, 60.

41. Billod, *Les aliénés de Vaucluse et de Ville-Evrard pendant le siège de Paris*, 60.

42. Billod, *Les aliénés de Vaucluse et de Ville-Evrard pendant le siège de Paris*, 60.

43. Venita Datta, *Heroes and Legends of Fin-de-Siècle France: Gender, Politics, and National Identity* (Cambridge: Cambridge University Press, 2011), 67.

44. Forth, *Masculinity in the Modern West*, especially introduction.

45. On similar tendencies among intellectuals during the Dreyfus affair, see Venita Datta, *Birth of a National Icon: The Literary Avant-Garde and the Origins of the Intellectual in France* (Albany, NY: State University of New York Press, 1999); Christopher E. Forth, *The Dreyfus Affair and the Crisis of French Manhood* (Baltimore: Johns Hopkins University Press, 2004).

46. See Nye, *Crime, Madness, and Politics in Modern France*, especially chapter 7, "The Boundaries of Responsibility: Asylum Law and Legal Medicine in an Era of Social Defense," 227–264.

47. J. V. Laborde, *Les hommes et les actes de l'insurrection de Paris devant la psychologie morbide* (Paris: Germer Baillière, 1872), iii.

48. Murat, *The Man Who Thought He Was Napoleon*, 168.

49. See Paul Lidsky, *Les écrivains contre la Commune* (Paris: Maspero, 1970).

50. For biographical information see Jacques Poirier, "Jean-Baptiste Vincent Laborde (1830–1903), forgotten neurologist and neurophysiologist," *Gériatrie et psychologie neuropsychiatrie du vieillissement* 13 (2015): 73–82.

51. Laborde, *Les hommes et les actes de l'insurrection de Paris devant la psychologie morbide*, 38. I will focus most of my analysis of the Commune on Laborde, in part because his ideas were widely debated and therefore serve as a useful entry point into a range of psychiatric opinions, but also because Murat has already written an excellent chapter on the Commune that need not be replicated here.

52. Laborde, *Les hommes et les actes de l'insurrection de Paris devant la psychologie morbide*, 81.

53. Laborde, *Les hommes et les actes de l'insurrection de Paris devant la psychologie morbide*, 16.

54. Murat, *The Man Who Thought He Was Napoleon*, 215.

55. Dr. Baume, *Annales Médico-Psychologiques* 5, no. 7 (1872): 306.

56. The reviewer for *L'Union Médicale*, for example, disliked Laborde's suggestion that society itself had "gone mad" during the Commune, but agreed many Communards were in fact insane. *L'Union Médicale: Journal des intérêts scientifiques et pratiques moraux et professionnels du corps médical* 3, no. 98 (21 Novembre 1871): 733–734.

57. Francisque Sarcey, *Le Gaulois*, June 13, 1871. Cited by Gay L. Gullickson, *Unruly Women of Paris: Images of the Commune* (Ithaca, NY: Cornell University Press, 1996), 176.

58. Edmond and Jules Goncourt, *Journal*, May 26, 1871, 814. Cited by Gullickson, *Unruly Women of Paris*, 174.

59. Brierre de Boismont, "A Lunatic Asylum during the Siege of Paris," 302.

60. Marie Rivet, *Les Aliénés dans la famille et dans la maison de santé: Etude pour les gens du monde* (Paris: 1875), 269.

61. Rivet, *Les Aliénés dans la famille et dans la maison de santé*, 241.

62. Rivet, *Les Aliénés dans la famille et dans la maison de santé*, 242.

63. Laborde, *Les hommes et les actes de l'insurrection de Paris devant la psychologie morbide*, 9.

64. Bouchereau and Magnan, *Statistiques des malades*, 5–6.

65. Billod, *Les aliénés de Vaucluse et de Ville-Evrard pendant le siège de Paris*, 41.

66. Laborde, *Les hommes et les actes de l'insurrection de Paris devant la psychologie morbide*, 113.

67. Laborde, *Les hommes et les actes de l'insurrection de Paris devant la psychologie morbide*, 114.

68. Laborde, *Les hommes et les actes de l'insurrection de Paris devant la psychologie morbide*, 115.

Chapter 6: Reforming the Asylum and Reimagining the Family

1. J. Manier, *Les Bastilles modernes, mystères des asiles d'aliénés,* (Paris: Dépot chez M. Block, 1886).

2. Manier, *Les Bastilles modernes, mystères des asiles d'aliénés*, 10.

3. Léopold Turck, *Pétition au Sénat sur le régime des aliénés en France* (Imprimerie de A. Roux, 1865), 88–89. Jacques-Joseph Moreau, *Lettres médicales sur la colonie d'aliénés de Ghéel (Belgique)* (Paris: Imprimerie de Bourgogne et Martinet, 1845).

4. Charles Féré, *Le Traitement des aliénés dans les familles* (Paris: Ancienne Librairie Germer Baillière et cie., 1889), 21.

5. Manier, *Les Bastilles modernes, mystères des asiles d'aliénés*, 10.

6. Alexandre Brierre de Boismont, "Etude bibliographique et pratique sur la colonisation appliquée au traitement des aliénés," *Annales d'hygiène publique et de médecine légale*, 2, no. 12 (1862): 387. He quotes Ferrus at length.

7. Brierre de Boismont, "Etude bibliographique et pratique sur la colonisation appliquée au traitement des aliénés," 387. Again, Brierre de Boismont quotes Ferrus.

8. Brierre de Boismont, "Etude bibliographique et pratique sur la colonisation appliquée au traitement des aliénés," 388–389. Brierre de Boismont summarizes his earlier opinions on family colonization, referring to the years 1845 and 1852. I have not been able to track down the first publication, but his later observations were recorded in the 1852 edition of the *Annales médico-psychologiques*.

9. Jules Falret, "Rapport de M. Jules Falret, au nom de la commission de Gheel," *Annales médico-psychologiques* 8 (1862): 139.

10. Falret, "Rapport de M. Jules Falret, au nom de la commission de Gheel," 140.

11. Falret, "Rapport de M. Jules Falret, au nom de la commission de Gheel," 143.

12. Falret, "Rapport de M. Jules Falret, au nom de la commission de Gheel,"149.

13. Falret, "Rapport de M. Jules Falret, au nom de la commission de Gheel," 157.

14. Falret, "Rapport de M. Jules Falret, au nom de la commission de Gheel," 166.

15. Distrust of the working classes would increase after the Commune. On earlier attitudes see Louis Chevalier, *Laboring Classes and Dangerous Classes in Paris During the First Half of the Nineteenth Century*, trans. Frank Jellinek (New York: Howard Fertig, 2000).

16. Billod, "Discussion sur la colonisation des aliénés. Séance du 26 mai 1862" in *Des Maladies mentales et nerveuses. Pathologie, médecine légale, administration des asiles d'aliénés, etc. Tome 2* (Paris: Masson, 1882), 183–184. Originally published in *Annales médico-psychologiques*, 1862.

17. Billod, "Discussion sur la colonisation des aliénés. Séance du 26 mai 1862," 184.

18. Billod, "Discussion sur la colonisation des aliénés. Séance du 26 mai 1862," 184.

19. Falret, "Rapport de M. Jules Falret, au nom de la commission de Gheel," 165.

20. Falret, "Rapport de M. Jules Falret, au nom de la commission de Gheel," 163.

21. Falret, "Rapport de M. Jules Falret, au nom de la commission de Gheel," 164.

22. Falret, "Rapport de M. Jules Falret, au nom de la commission de Gheel," 164.

23. Daniel Pick notes that Zola's asylum doctor is based on Magnan. Pick, *Faces of Degeneration*, 86–87.

24. Nye, *Crime, Madness, and Politics in Modern France*.

25. Charles Féré, *La famille névropathique, 2nd ed.* (Paris: F. Alcan, 1898).

26. Féré, *Le Traitement des aliénés dans les familles*, 91.

27. Féré, *La Famille névropathique*, 8.

28. Féré, *La Famille névropathique*, 321–330.

29. Féré, *Le Traitement des aliénés dans les familles*, 3.

30. Féré, *Le Traitement des aliénés dans les familles*, 94–95.

31. Féré, *Le Traitement des aliénés dans les familles*, 96.

32. Féré, *Le Traitement des aliénés dans les familles*, 96.

33. Féré, *Le Traitement des aliénés dans les familles*, 62.

34. Joseph Arthaud, *De la Possibilité et de la convenance de faire sortir certaines catégories d'aliénés des asiles spéciaux et de les placer soit dans des exploitations agricoles, soit dans leurs propres familles* (Lyon: Imprimerie d'A. Vingtrinier, 1865), 16–17.

35. Féré, *Le Traitement des aliénés dans les familles*, 98.

36. Féré, *Le Traitement des aliénés dans les familles*, 97.

37. Féré, *Le Traitement des aliénés dans les familles*, 97.

38. Féré, *Le Traitement des aliénés dans les familles*, 97.

39. Féré, *Le Traitement des aliénés dans les familles*, 99.

40. Féré, *Le Traitement des aliénés dans les familles*, 99.

41. Féré, *Le Traitement des aliénés dans les familles*, 99.

42. Féré, *Le Traitement des aliénés dans les familles*, 102.

43. Féré, *Le Traitement des aliénés dans les familles*, 108.

44. Féré, *Le Traitement des aliénés dans les familles*, 109.

45. Féré, *Le Traitement des aliénés dans les familles*, 111.

46. Dr. Viallon, *Augmentation progressive du nombre des aliénés dans le Rhône, assistance a domicile et colonies familiales* (Lyon: Imprimerie Emmanuel Vitte, 1901), 3.

47. Viallon, *Augmentation progressive du nombre des aliénés dans le Rhône*, 2.

48. For more on the family colonies, see Fauvel, "Les fous en liberté. La naissance des 'colonies familiales' de la Seine," *Revue de la Société française d'histoire des hôpitaux* 136 (2009), 16–22; Juliette Rigondet, *Un village pour aliénés tranquilles* (Paris: Fayard, 2019).

49. On reformist psychiatry in the 1890s, see Aude Fauvel, "Aliénistes contre psychiatres: La médecine mentale en crise (1890-1914)," *Psychologie clinique* 17 (2004): 61–76; Elizabeth Nelson, "Running in Circles: A Return to an Old Idea about Asylum Reform in Nineteenth-Century France," *The Journal of the Western Society for French History* 42 (2014). http://hdl.handle.net/2027/spo.0642292.0042.011

50. M. H. Colin, "Des asiles d'aliénés à portes ouvertes (suite)," *Annales médico-psychologiques* 6 (1897): 289–291.

51. Évariste Marandon de Montyel, "L'Open Door et le Congrès de Nancy," *Annales médico-psychologiques* 4 (1896): 390, 405.

52. For Marandon de Montyel's obituary, see *Annales médico-psychologiques* 7 (1908): 465–466.

53. Marandon de Montyel, "Des asiles d'aliénés à portes ouvertes (suite)," *Annales médico-psychologiques* 6 (1897): 275–281. Marandon de Montyel sent out a survey to the public asylum directors of France, seventy-one of whom responded. He discovered that only four used the "liberty method" similar to his own, but that only three rigorously applied isolation. The vast majority of asylums fell somewhere in-between.

54. Marandon de Montyel, "Des asiles d'aliénés à portes ouvertes (suite)," 283.

55. Marandon de Montyel, "Des asiles d'aliénés à portes ouvertes (suite)," 270.

56. Marandon de Montyel, "L'Open Door et le Congrès de Nancy," *Annales médico-psychologiques* 4 (1896): 393.

57. Marandon de Montyel, "La Nouvelle hospitalization des aliénés par la méthode de liberté et son application en Ville-Évrard," *Annales médico-psychologiques* 3 (Paris: Masson, 1896): 65.

58. Waltraud Ernst, ed., *Work, psychiatry, and society, c. 1750–2015* (Manchester: Manchester University Press, 2016).

59. Billod, "Discussion sur la colonisation des aliénés. Séance du 26 mai 1862," 187.

60. Billod, "Discussion sur la colonisation des aliénés. Séance du 26 mai 1862," 188.

61. Brierre de Boismont, "Préface," *L'aliéné devant lui-même: l'appréciation légale, la législation, les systèmes, la société et la famille par H. Bonnet* (Paris: Masson, 1865), xv.

62. Louis Gustave Bouchereau and Valentin Magnan, *Statistiques des malades entrés en 1870 et 1871 au bureau d'admission des aliénés de la Seine* (Paris: Imprimerie de E. Donnaud, 1872), 4.

63. Marandon de Montyel, "La Nouvelle hospitalisation des aliénés par la méthode de liberté et son application en Ville-Évrard," 69.

64. Marandon de Montyel, "La Nouvelle hospitalisation des aliénés par la méthode de liberté et son application en Ville-Évrard," 70.

65. A. Marie, *Note historique sur la colonisation familiale de la Seine* (Anvers: J. E. Buschmann, 1902), 19.

66. M. H. Colin, "Des asiles d'aliénés à portes ouvertes," *Annales médico-psychologiques* 6 (1897): 183–299. Dr. Toulouse, "Des asiles d'aliénés à portes ouvertes," *Annales médico-psychologiques* 6 (1897): 482.

67. M. Febvre, "Des asiles d'aliénés à portes ouvertes," *Annales médico-psychologiques* 6 (1897): 138.

68. Gregory M. Thomas, *Treating the Trauma of the Great War: Soldiers, Civilians, and Psychiatry in France, 1914–1940* (Baton Rouge, LA: Louisiana State University Press, 2009), 146–170.

Conclusion: The "Mad" Woman in a Man's World

1. Judith Surkis, *Sexing the Citizen: Morality and Masculinity in France, 1870–1920* (Ithaca, NY: Cornell University Press, 2006), 12.

2. On sadism and masochism, see Moore, *Sexual Myths of Modernity: Sadism, Masochism, and Historical Teleology.*

3. Susan Ashley has drawn attention to the ways in which degeneration theorists, including those interested in so-called sexual deviants, distinguished between "born" degenerates and individuals considered "accidental misfits." Those in the latter category deserved social support, while those in the former required incarceration. Such thinking marginalized both these groups, albeit to different degrees. Susan Ashley, *"Misfits" in Fin-de-Siècle France and Italy: Anatomies of Difference* (London: Bloomsbury, 2017).

4. Ashley, *"Misfits" in Fin-de-Siècle France and Italy*, 92–93.

5. Micale, *Hysterical Men*; Daniela S. Barberis, "Hysteria in the Male: Images of Masculinity in Late Nineteenth-Century France," in *Phallacies: Historical Intersections of Disability and Masculinity*, ed. Kathleen M. Brian and James W. Trent Jr. (New York: Oxford University Press, 2017), 173–193. Charcot opened a ward for male hysterics at the Salpêtrière in 1882.

6. Asti Hustvedt, *Medical Muses: Hysteria in Nineteenth-Century Paris* (New York: W. W. Norton, 2011).

7. On French feminism see Karen Offen, *Debating the Woman Question in the French Third Republic, 1870–1920* (Cambridge: Cambridge University Press, 2017); on the ways conceptions of ideal motherhood constrained women's activism, see Accampo, *Blessed Motherhood, Bitter Fruit.*

8. Roberts, *Disruptive Acts.*

9. Michel Foucault, *The History of Sexuality, Vol. 1: An Introduction,* trans. Robert Hurley (New York: Vintage Books, 1990). Foucault points to 1870 as the point when the notion of homosexual identity emerged in French medical discourse: "The sodomite had been a temporary aberration; the homosexual was now a species" (43). See Andrew Israel Ross, *Public City/Public Sex: Homosexuality, Prostitution, and Urban Culture in Nineteenth-Century Paris* (Philadelphia: Temple University Press, 2019) on the visibility of homosexual activity in the nineteenth-century capital.

10. John Tosh examines aspects of this phenomenon in late nineteenth-century England in *A Man's Place: Masculinity and the Middle-Class Home in Victorian England,* 2nd ed. (New Haven, CT: Yale University Press, 2007). See especially Part 3, "Domesticity Under Strain, c. 1870–1900." On French imperialism see Christelle Taraud, "Virility in the Colonial Context," in *A History of Virility*, ed. Alain Corbin, Jean-Jacques Courtine, and Georges Vigarello, trans. Keith Cohen (New York: Columbia University Press, 2016).

11. Forth, *Masculinity and the Modern West*, especially Chapter 6 ("Modern Primitives: Manhood and Metamorphosis around 1900").

12. John Merriman, *The Dynamite Club: How a Bombing in Fin-de-Siècle Paris Ignited the Age of Modern Terror* (New Haven, CT: Yale University Press, 2016).

13. See Vanessa Schwartz, *Spectacular Realities: Early Mass Culture in Fin-de-Siècle Paris* (Berkeley: University of California Press, 1999); Susanna Barrows, *Distorting Mirrors: Visions of the Crowd in Late Nineteenth-Century France* (New Haven, CT: Yale University Press, 1981); David Harvey, *Paris: Capital of Modernity* (New York: Routledge, 2005); Michael B. Miller, *The Bon Marché: Bourgeois Culture and the Department Store, 1869–1920* (Princeton, NJ: Princeton University Press, 1981).

14. Patricia O'Brien, "The Kleptomania Diagnosis: Bourgeois Women and Theft in Late Nineteenth-Century France," *Journal of Social History* 17, no. 1 (1983): 65–77. http//: www.jstor.org/stable/3787239.

15. Feminist criticism of Freud constitutes a field unto itself. Simone de Beauvoir, *The Second Sex,* trans. Constance Borde and Sheila Malovany-Chevallier (New York: Vintage, 2011) is a good place to start.

16. She spoke at the 1889 *Congrès français et international du droit des femmes* about unfair inheritance policies.

17. Marie Esquiron, née Gasté, *Memoire adressé à monsieur le minstre de la justice* (Paris: Imprimerie Henon, 1893), 5–6.

18. This is literary scholar Susannah Wilson's contention. Wilson, *Voices from the Asylum*, 96. Esquiron's doctors dwelled on her narration of childhood experiences, particularly the assertion that her father supposedly taught her about the "breeding habits of animals."

19. *Le Temps,* August 1, 1890, 6. Unlike some other cases of unjust sequestration, Esquiron's plight received considerable press attention. *Le Temps* was the only newspaper that detailed Esquiron's accusations against her father, particularly those of a sexual nature; most focused instead on his testimony against her.

20. *Le Temps*, August 1, 1890. On Valsayre, see Andrea Mansker, "The Female Point of Honor in *Fin-de-Siècle* France," in *Honor in the Modern World: Interdisciplinary Perspectives,* ed. Laurie M. Johnson and Dan Demetriou (Lanham, MD: Lexington Books, 2016), 208–218.

21. The court chose a presumably less biased individual, a bailiff named Lebrysois, instead.

22. *Le Matin*, March 19, 1891, 3.

23. Esquiron, *Mémoire*, 10–11.

24. Sully Ledermann, "Les divorces et les séparations de corps en France," *Population* (French edition) 3, no. 2 (April-June 1948), 313–344. Cited in Mansker, *Sex, Honor, and Citizenship*, 91.

25. Murat makes a similar point in her interpretation of Esquiron's case in *La Maison du Docteur Blanche: Histoire d'un asile et de ses pensionnaires de Nerval à Maupassant* (Paris: J. C. Lattès, 2001), Kindle, location 3528–3673.

26. Esquiron, *Mémoire,* 6.

27. While Fauvel mentions in the appendix of *Bastilles Modernes* that Esquiron

eventually gained her freedom, I believe she mixed up the outcomes of Esquiron's first and second institutionalizations. (Murat indeed notes in *La Maison du Docteur Blanche* that Esquiron's 1866 incarceration ended after approximately six months when she was sent to live with a cousin). My research suggests that Esquiron never left the asylum—a Pauline-Marie Esquiron is recorded as having died on March 7, 1912, in the twelfth arrondissement (the location of Goujon's asylum, where he served as mayor and even has a street named after him).

BIBLIOGRAPHY

Archives

Archives de l'Assistance Publique – Hôpitaux de Paris
Archives Municipales de Saint-Mandé
Archives de Paris

Periodicals

Annales d'hygiène publique et de médecine légale
Annales médico-psychologiques
Gazette médicaux de Paris
Journal des débats
La Croix supplementaire
Le Figaro
Le Gaulois
Le Matin
La Revue comique
Le Temps
L'Union médicale
New York Times

Printed Primary Sources

47 années de sequéstration, Jean Mistral de Saint-Remy en 1838, L'Homme aux soixante millions n'est pas fou. Marseille: Imprimerie Générale Achard et Cie., 1886.
Almanach-Bottin du commerce de Paris, des départements de la France et des principales villes du monde. Paris: Bureau de l'Almanach du Commerce, 1842.
Annuaire-Almanach du commerce et de l'industrie, ou almanach des 500,000 addresses de Paris, des départements et des pays étrangers. Paris: Chez Fermin Didot Frères, Fils, et Cie., 1862.

Anonymous, *Histoire d'une maladie: Fragment relatif à son traitement par le malade.* Béziers: Imprimerie Auguste Malinas, 1870.

Arthaud, Joseph. *De la Possibilité et de la convenance de faire sortir certaines catégories d'aliénés des asiles spéciaux et de les placer soit dans des exploitations agricoles, soit dans leurs propres familles.* Lyon: Imprimerie d'A. Vingtrinier, 1865.

Balzac, Honoré de. *Le Colonel Chabert,* suivi de *Honorine,* et de *L'Interdiction.* Paris: Classiques Garnier, 1964.

Bergeret, Dr. "Cas nombreaux d'aliénation mentale d'une particulière ayant pour cause la perturbation politique et sociale de février 1848." *Annales d'hygiene publique et de médecine legale* 2, no. 20 (July 1863).

Billod, Eugène. *Les aliénés de Vaucluse et de Ville-Évrard pendant le siège de Paris.* Paris: Librairie de l'Academie de Médecine, 1872.

——. "Discussion sur la colonisation des aliénés. Séance du 26 mai 1862." In *Des Maladies mentales et nerveuses, pathologie, médecine légale, administration des asiles d'aliénés, etc. Tome 2.* Paris: Masson, 1882.

Blanche, Esprit. *Du danger du rigueurs corporelles dans le traitement de la folie.* Paris: A. Gardembas, 1839.

Bonnet, Henri. *"La Baronne* (à l'Odéon): Lettre à M. l'Inspecteur Général Lunier." *Annales médico-psychologiques* 5, no. 8 (1872).

Bouchereau, Louis Gustave and Valentin Magnan. *Statistiques des malades entrés en 1870 et 1871 au bureau d'admission des aliénés de la Seine.* Paris: Imprimerie de E. Donnaud, 1872.

Boudin de Vesvres, Jean-Baptiste. *Réponse pour M. et Mme. Rivet à la plaidoirie du défenseur de M. le préfet de la Seine.* Paris: L. Martinet, 1859.

Boyer, Philoxene. *Deux saisons.* Paris: A. Lemerre, 1867.

Brierre de Boismont, Alexandre. *De l'Utilité de la vie de famille dans le traitement de l'aliénation mentale et plus spécialement de ses formes tristes.* Paris: Imprimerie de E. Martinet, 1866.

——. "Préface," *L'aliéné devant lui-même: l'appréciation légale, la législation, les systèmes, la société et la famille par H. Bonnet.* Paris: Masson, 1865.

——. "Notice biographique sur M. François Leuret." *Annales médico-psychologiquiques* 3 (1851).

——. *Maison de santé du docteur Brierre du Boismont* (undated pamphlet).

——. *Des hallucinations ou Histoire raisonnée des apparitions, des visions, des songes, de l'extase, du magnétisme et du somnabulisme.* Paris: G. Baillière, 1845.

——. *Du suicide et de la folie suicide.* Paris: G. Baillière, 1856.

——. "Mémoire pour l'établissement d'un hospice d'aliénés." *Annales d'hygiène publique et de médecine légale* (1836).

——. *Responsabilité légale des médecins en Espagne. Procès en detention arbitraire de Dona Juana Sagreda.* Paris: Imprimerie de E. Martinet, 1864.

——. "A Lunatic Asylum during the Siege of Paris." *The Lancet* (March 4, 1872).

——. "Appreciation médico-légale du régime des aliénés en France." *Annales médico-psychologiques* 4, no. 6 (1865).

——. "Étude bibliographique et pratique sur la colonisation appliquée au traitement des aliénés." *Annales d'hygiène publique et de médecine légale,* 2, no. 12 (1862).

Bru, P. *Histoire de Bicêtre.* Paris: Lecrosnier et Babé, 1890.

Cère, Paul. *Les populations dangereuse et les misères sociales.* Paris: Librairie de la société des gens de letters, 1872.

Colin, M. H. "Des asiles d'aliénés à portes ouvertes." *Annales médico-psychologiques* 6 (1897).

Constans, Lunier, and Dumesnil, Drs. *Rapport Général à M. le Ministre de l'Intérieur sur le service des aliénés en 1874.* Paris: Imprimerie National, 1878.

Delas, Hippolyte. *Les Bastilles modernes: Nécessité de leur Destruction, recueil d'articles parus dans L'Union Républicaine.* Béziers: Imprimerie de Commerce, 1886.

——. *Histoire d'une maladie.* Béziers: Imprimerie Auguste Malinas, 1870.

E., *Le Pourvoyeur d'une maison d'aliénés, discussion-drame en quatre actes en prose. Par un Philanthrope. Ouvrage dédié aux magistrats, notamment à ceux chargés de la surveillance des maisons d'insensés et aux partisans de l'émancipation intellectuelle.* Paris: L'Imprimerie de Decourchant, 1840.

Esquirol, Jean-Étienne-Dominique. *Des Établissements des aliénés en France et des moyens d'améliorer le sort de ces infortunés.* Paris: Imprimerie de Madame Huzard, 1819.

——. *Des Maladies mentales.* Vol. 1. Paris: J.-B. Baillière et fils, 1838.

——. *Des Maladies mentales,* Vol. 2. Paris: J.-B. Baillière et fils, 1838.

——. *Des Passions considérées comme causes, symptômes et moyens curatifs de l'aliénation mentale.* Paris: l'Imprimerie de Didot Jeune, 1805.

Esquiron, Marie. *Mémoire adressé à monsieur le ministre de la justice.* Paris: Imprimerie Henon, 1893.

Faligan, Ernest. *Le Gouvernement occulte de la France.* Brussels: A. N. LeBégue et Cie., 1880.

——. *Les Police, juge, et partie.*

——. *Les Séquestrations arbitraries et le droit de pétition.* Paris: Librairie Générale, 1879.

Falret, Jules. "Rapport de M. Jules Falret, au nom de la commission de Gheel." *Annales médico-psychologiques*, no. 8 (1862).

Febvre, M. "Des asiles d'aliénés à portes ouvertes." *Annales médicos-psychologiques* 6 (1897).

Féré, Charles. *La famille névropathique.* Paris: F. Alcan, 1898.

——. *Le Traitement des aliénés dans les familles.* Paris: Ancienne Librairie Germer Baillière et Cie., 1889.

Foville, Achille. *Les Aliénés, étude pratique sur la législation et l'assistance qui leur sont applicables.* Paris: J. B. Baillière et fils, 1870.

Georget, Étienne-Jean. *De la folie. Considérations sur cette maladie.* Paris: Crevot, 1820.

Hecquet, Charles. *Notice biographique sur la vie et les travaux du docteur Leuret, médecin en chef de l'hospice d'aliénés de Bicêtre, par Charles Hecquet.* Nancy: Grimblot et Veuve Raybois, 1852.

Laborde, J. V. *Les hommes et les actes de l'insurrection de Paris devant la psychologie morbide*. Paris: Germer Baillière, 1872.

Legrand du Saulle, Henri. *La délire des persécutions*. Paris: Plon, 1871.

———. *Les Hystériques: État physique et état mental, actes insolites, délictueux et criminels*. Paris: J.-B. Baillière et fils, 1883.

Leuret, François. "Mémoire sur l'emploi des douches, et des affusions froides dans le traitement de l'aliénation mentale." *Archives générales de médecine* 3, no. 4 (1839).

———. "Mémoire sur le traitement moral de la folie." *Mémoires de l'académie royale de médecine* 7 (1838).

———. *Du Traitement des idées ou conceptions délirantes*. Paris: Everat, 1837.

———. *Du Traitement moral de la folie*. Paris: J.-B. Baillière, 1840.

Linas, Aimé-Jean. *Gazette hebdomadaire de la médecine et de chirurgie* 29 (July 1875).

Londe, "Du délire." *Bulletin de l'Académie nationale de médecine* (1854).

Lunier, Ludgar. "Influence des événements de 1870–1871 sur le mouvement de l'aliénation mentale en France." *Annales médico-psychologiques* 5, no. 8 (1872).

Manier, J. *Les Bastilles modernes, mystères des asiles d'aliénés*. Paris: Dépot chez M. Block, 1886.

Marandon de Montyel, Évariste. "Des asiles d'aliénés à portes ouvertes." *Annales médicos-psychologiques* 6 (1897).

———. "La Nouvelle hospitalisation des aliénés par la méthode de liberté et son application en Ville-Évrard." *Annales médicos-psychologiques* 3 (1896).

———. "L'Open Door et le Congrès de Nancy." *Annales médico-psychologiques* 4 (1896).

Marie, A. *Note historique sur la colonisation familiale de la Seine*. Anvers: J. E. Buschmann, 1902.

Pinel, Philippe *L'Aliénation mentale ou la manie: Traité médico-philosophique*. 1st edition. Paris: L'Harmattan, 2006. Originally published 1801 by Chez Richard, Caille, et Ravier.

———. *Traité médico-philosophique sur l'aliénation mentale*. 2nd edition. Paris: Brosson, 1809.

———. *Recherches et observations sur le traitement moral des aliénés*. Paris: n.d.

Pinel, Scipion. *Physiologie de l'homme aliéné: appliquée à l'analyse de l'homme social*. Paris: Librairie des Sciences Médicales, 1833.

———. *Traité complet du régime sanitaire des aliénés*. Paris: Mauprivez, 1836.

Puyparlier, Fault du. *Affaire du Fault du Puyparlier, pensées au courant de la plume*. Paris: Typographie et Lithographie Renou et Maulde, 1870.

———. *Régime des aliénés en France, Asile de Charenton*. Paris: Imprimerie Nouvelle, 1870.

Rire, Dr. "Brierre de Boismont." *L'Intermédiaire des chercheurs et curieux*, no. 1073 (1905).

Rivet, Marie. *Les Aliénés dans la famille et dans la maison de santé: Étude pour les gens du monde*. Paris: Masson, 1875.

Robert, Ulysse. *Notes historiques sur Saint-Mandé*. Saint-Mandé: A. Beucher, 1889.

Sachaile de la Barre, C. *Les Médecins de Paris jugés par leurs oeuvres*. Paris: Auteur, 1845.

Semelaigne, René. *Les pionniers de la psychiatrie française avant et après Pinel. Vol. 1.* Paris: J.-B. Baillière et fils, 1930.

Statistique générale de la France. Paris: Berger-Levrault et Cie., 1885.

Taguet, Henri. *Étude de la loi sur les aliénés du 30 juin 1838.* Paris: Imprimerie de E. Donnaud, 1875.

——. *Les Aliénés persécuteurs.* Paris: Imprimerie de E. Donnaud, 1876.

Tardieu, Ambroise. *Étude médico-légale sur les attentats aux moeurs.* Paris: J.-B. Baillière, 1857.

Toulouse, Dr. "Des asiles d'aliénés à portes ouvertes." *Annales médico-psychologiques* 6 (1897).

Tours, Jacques-Joseph Moreau de. *Lettres médicales sur la colonie d'aliénés de Ghéel (Belgique).* Paris: Imprimerie de Bourgogne et Martinet, 1845.

Trélat, Ulysse. "Notice sur François Leuret." *Annales d'hygiène publique et de médecine légale* 45 (1851).

Turck, Léopold. *Pétition au Sénat sur le régime des aliénés en France.* Imprimerie de A. Roux, 1865.

Viallon, Dr. *Augmentation progressive du nombre des aliénés dans le Rhône, assistance a domicile et colonies familiales.* Lyon: Imprimerie Emmanuel Vitte, 1901.

Voisin, Felix. *Des causes morales et physiques des maladies mentales et de quelques autres affections nerveuses telle que l'hystérie, la nymphomanie et le satyriasis.* Paris: J.-B. Baillière, 1826.

Zola, Emile. *L'Assomoir.* Paris: Hachette, 1996. Originally published 1877 by Charpentier.

Secondary Sources

Accampo, Elinor Ann. *Blessed Motherhood, Bitter Fruit: Nelly Roussel and the Politics of Female Pain in Third Republic France.* Baltimore: Johns Hopkins University Press, 2006.

Accampo, Elinor Ann, Rachel Ginnis Fuchs, and Mary Lynn Stewart. *Gender and the Politics of Social Reform in France, 1870–1914.* Baltimore: Johns Hopkins University Press, 1995.

Adams, Christine. *Poverty, Charity, and Motherhood: Maternal Societies in Nineteenth-Century France.* Champaign: University of Illinois Press, 2010.

Andrews, Jonathan, and Anne Digby. *Sex and Seclusion, Class, and Custody: Perspectives on Gender and Class in the History of British and Irish Psychiatry.* Amsterdam, New York: Rodopi, 2004.

Andrews, Naomi Judith. *Socialism's Muse: Gender in the Intellectual Landscape of French Romantic Socialism.* Lanham, MD: Lexington Books, 2006.

Appignanesi, Lisa. *Mad, Bad and Sad: A History of Women and the Mind Doctors from 1800 to the Present.* London: Virago, 2010.

Ashley, Susan A. *"Misfits" in Fin-de-Siècle France and Italy: Anatomies of Difference*. London: Bloomsbury, 2017.

Bacopoulos-Viau, Alexandra, and Aude Fauvel. "The Patient's Turn Roy Porter and Psychiatry's Tales, Thirty Years On." *Medical History* 60, no. 1 (2016): 1–18, https://doi.org/10.1017/mdh.2015.65.

Barrows, Susanna. *Distorting Mirrors: Visions of the Crowd in Late Nineteenth-Century France*. New Haven, CT: Yale University Press, 1981.

Bartlett, Peter, and David Wright. *Outside the Walls of the Asylum: The History of Care in the Community 1750–2000*. London: Athlone Press, 1999.

Baynton, Douglas C. *Defectives in the Land: Disability and Immigration in the Age of Eugenics*. Chicago: University of Chicago Press, 2017.

Beauvoir, Simone de. *The Second Sex*. Translated by Constance Borde and Sheila Malovany-Chevallier. New York: Vintage, 2011. First published 1949 by Gallimard.

Blaufarb, Rafe. *The French Army 1750–1820: Careers, Talent, Merit*. Manchester: Manchester University Press, 2002.

Boddice, Rob. "The Manly Mind? Revisiting the Victorian 'Sex in Brain' Debate." *Gender & History* 23, no. 2 (2011): 321–340, https://doi.org/10.1111/j.1468-0424.2011.01641.x.

Bonner, Thomas Neville. *To the Ends of the Earth: Women's Search for Education in Medicine*. Cambridge, MA: Harvard University Press, 1992.

Boster, Dea H. *African American Slavery and Disability: Bodies, Property and Power in the Antebellum South, 1800–1860*. New York: Routledge, 2013.

Bourdieu, Pierre. *The State Nobility: Elite Schools in the Field of Power*. Translated by Lauretta C. Clough. Palo Alto: Stanford University Press, 2010. Originally published 1989 by Les Éditions de Minuit.

Bras, Anatole le. *Un enfant à l'asile. Vie de Paul Taesch*. Paris: CNRS Editions, 2018.

Brian, Kathleen M., and James W. Trent Jr., ed. *Phallacies: Historical Intersections of Disability and Masculinity*. Oxford: Oxford University Press, 2017.

Brown, Edward M. "François Leuret: The Last Moral Therapist." *History of Psychiatry* 29, no. 1 (2018): 38–48, https://doi.org/10.1177/0957154X17735782.

Burch, Susan, and Lindsey Patterson. "Not Just Any Body: Disability, Gender, and History." *Journal of Women's History* 25, no. 4 (2013): 122–137, https://doi.org/10.1353/jowh.2013.0060.

Burch, Susan, and Michael Rembis. *Disability Histories*. Champaign: University of Illinois Press, 2014.

Butler, Judith. *Gender Trouble: Feminism and the Subversion of Identity*. New York: Routledge, 1990.

Cabanès, Jean-Louis. *Le corps et la maladie dans les récits réalistes (1856–1893)*. Paris: Diffusion Klincksieck, 1991.

Cabanès, Jean-Louis, Jacqueline Carroy, and Nicole Edelman. *Psychologies fin de siècle*. Nanterre: Centre des sciences de la littérature française de l'université de Paris ouest, 2008.

Carroy, Jacqueline. *Hypnose, suggestion et psychologie. L'invention de sujets.* Paris: Presses Universitaires de France, 1991.

Carroy, Jacqueline, Annick Ohayon, and Régine Plas. *Histoire de la psychologie en France.* Paris: La Découverte, 2006.

Carson, John. *The Measure of Merit: Talents, Intelligence, and Inequality in the French and American Republics, 1750–1940.* Princeton, NJ: Princeton University Press, 2007.

Castel, Robert. *The Regulation of Madness: The Origins of Incarceration in France.* Berkeley: University of California Press, 1988.

Chevalier, Louis. *Laboring Classes and Dangerous Classes in Paris during the First Half of the Nineteenth Century.* Translated by Frank Jellinek. New York: H. Fertig, 1973. Originally published 1958 by Plon.

Childers, Kristen Stromberg. *Fathers, Families, and the State in France, 1914–1945.* Ithaca, NY: Cornell University Press, 2003.

Clark, Linda L. *Women and Achievement in Nineteenth-Century Europe.* Cambridge: Cambridge University Press, 2008.

Coffin, Jean-Christophe. *La transmission de la folie: 1850–1914.* Paris: Editions L'Harmattan, 2003.

Cole, Joshua. *The Power of Large Numbers: Population, Politics, and Gender in Nineteenth-Century France.* Ithaca, NY: Cornell University Press, 2000.

Coleborne, Catharine. "White Men and Weak Masculinity: Men in the Public Asylums in Victoria, Australia, and New Zealand, 1860s–1900s." *History of Psychiatry* 25, no. 4 (2014): 468–476, https://doi.org/10.1177/0957154X14543758.

Condrau, Flurin. "The Patient's View Meets the Clinical Gaze." *Social History of Medicine* 20, no. 3 (2007): 525–540, https://doi.org/10.1093/shm/hkm076.

Copley, Antony. *Sexual Moralities in France, 1780–1980: New Ideas on the Family, Divorce, and Homosexuality: An Essay on Moral Change.* London: Routledge, 1992.

Corbin, Alain, Jean-Jacques Courtine, and Georges Vigarello. *A History of Virility.* New York: Columbia University Press, 2016.

Counter, Andrew J. *The Amorous Restoration: Love, Sex, and Politics in Early Nineteenth-Century France.* Oxford: Oxford University Press, 2016.

——. "Bad Examples: Children, Servants, and Masturbation in Nineteenth-Century France." *Journal of the History of Sexuality* 22, no. 3 (2013): 403–425.

Courtin, Roger. *Charles Féré (1852–1907), Médecin de Bicêtre, et le néo-psychologie.* Paris: Connaisances et Savoirs, 2007.

Datta, Venita. *Birth of a National Icon: The Literary Avant-Garde and the Origins of the Intellectual in France.* Albany, NY: State University of New York Press, 1999.

——. *Heroes and Legends of Fin-de-Siècle France: Gender, Politics, and National Identity.* Cambridge: Cambridge University Press, 2011.

David, Sylvain-Christian. *Philoxène Boyer: Un sale ami de Baudelaire.* Paris: Ramsay, 1987.

Davidson, Denise Z. *France after Revolution: Urban Life, Gender, and the New Social Order.* Cambridge, MA: Harvard University Press, 2007.

Desan, Suzanne. *The Family on Trial in Revolutionary France*. Berkeley: University of California Press, 2006.

Ditz, Toby L. "The New Men's History and the Peculiar Absence of Gendered Power: Some Remedies from Early American Gender History." *Gender & History* 16, no. 1 (2004): 1–35, https://doi.org/10.1111/j.0953-5233.2004.324_1.x.

Dodman, Thomas. *What Nostalgia Was: War, Empire, and the Time of a Deadly Emotion*. Chicago: University of Chicago Press, 2018.

Doerner, Klaus. *Madmen and the Bourgeoisie: A Social History of Insanity and Psychiatry*. London: Blackwell, 1984.

Donzelot, Jacques. *The Policing of Families*. Baltimore: Johns Hopkins University Press, 1997.

Doron, Claude-Olivier. "Félix Voisin and the Genesis of Abnormals." *History of Psychiatry* 26, no. 4 (2015): 387–403, https://doi.org/10.1177/0957154X15604789.

Dowbiggin, Ian Robert. *Inheriting Madness: Professionalization and Psychiatric Knowledge in Nineteenth-Century France*. Berkeley: University of California Press, 1991.

Edelman, Nicole. *Histoire de la voyance et du paranormal. Du XVIIIe siècle à nos jours*. Paris: Le Seuil, 2014.

——. "Hommes/femmes dans l'histoire, l'enjeu des catégories construites. L'invention de l'hystérie par l'école de la Salpêtrière et les transformations de la catégorie femme (années 1850–années 1890)." *Revue d'histoire du XIXe siècle. Société d'histoire de la révolution de 1848 et des révolutions du XIXe siècle*, no. 13 (1996), https://doi.org/10.4000/rh19.99.

——. *Les métamorphoses de l'hystérique: Du début du XIXe siècle à la Grande Guerre*. Paris: La Découverte, 2013.

——. "L'espace hospitalier des aliénistes et des neurologues: un laboratoire pour penser les foules citadines (années 1850–années 1880)?" *Revue d'histoire du XIXe siècle. Société d'histoire de la révolution de 1848 et des révolutions du XIXe siècle*, no. 17 (December, 1998). https://doi.org/10.4000/rh19.140.

Edington, Claire. *Beyond the Asylum: Mental Illness in French Colonial Vietnam*. Ithaca, NY: Cornell University Press, 2019.

Eldridge, Alana. "Adèle Hugo: A Bibliographical Note." *Nineteenth-Century French Studies* 32, no. 1/2 (2003): 138–143. https://www.jstor.org/stable/23538156.

Ellis, Jack D. *The Physician-Legislators of France: Medicine and Politics in the Early Third Republic, 1870–1914*. Cambridge: Cambridge University Press, 1990.

Ernst, Waltraud. *Work, Psychiatry and Society, c. 1750–2015*. Manchester: Manchester University Press, 2016.

Ernst, Waltraud, and Thomas Mueller, eds. *Transnational Psychiatries: Social and Cultural Histories of Psychiatry in Comparative Perspective c. 1800–2000*. Cambridge: Cambridge Scholars Publishing, 2010.

Estienne, Jeanne Mesmin d'. "La folie selon Esquirol. Observations médicales et conceptions de l'aliénisme à Charenton entre 1825 et 1840." *Revue d'histoire du XIXe siècle. Société d'histoire de la révolution de 1848 et des révolutions du XIXe siècle*, no. 40 (2010): 95–112, https://doi.org/10.4000/rh19.3994.

Fauvel, Aude. *Témoins aliénés et "Bastilles modernes." Une histoire politique, sociale, et culturelle des asiles en France (1800–1914)*. PhD diss, Paris EHESS, 2005.

——. "'En dehors des murs.' Pour une histoire renouvelée des institutions de la folie à l'époque contemporaine." *Scienza e Filosofia* 13 (2015): 58–74.

——. "A World-Famous Lunatic: The 'Seillière Affair' (1887–1889) and the Circulation of Anti-Alienists' Views in the Nineteenth Century." In *Transnational Psychiatries: Social and Cultural Histories of Psychiatry in Comparative Perspective c. 1800–2000*, edited by Waltraud Ernst and Thomas Mueller, 200–228.

——. "Le crime de Clermont et la remise en cause des asiles en 1880." *Revue d'histoire moderne et contemporaine* 49, no. 1 (2002): 195–216.

——. "Les fous en liberté. La naissance des 'colonies familiales' de la Seine." *Revue de la Société française d'histoire des hôpitaux* 136 (2010): 16–22.

——. "Madness: A 'Female Malady'?: Women and Psychiatric Institutionalisation in France." In *Vulnerability, Social Inequality, and Health*, ed. Patrice Bourdelais and John Chircop. Lisbon: Edições Colibri, 2010.

——. "Psychiatrie et désobéissance: écrire à l'asile: la France, la Grande-Bretagne et l'exception écossaise (XIXe siècle)." In *Enfermements II. Règles et dérèglements en milieux clos (IVe-XIXe siècle)*. Edited by Isabelle Heullant-Donat, Julie Claustre, Élisabeth Lusset, Falk Bretschneider. Editions de la Sorbonne, 2015.

——. "Gheel, la 'ville des fous': un mythe séculaire, une pratique méconnue (1860–2010)." In *La fin de l'asile? Histoire de la déshospitalisation psychiatrique dans l'espace francophone au XXe siècle*. Edited by Alexandre Klein, Hervé Guillemain and Marie-Claude Thifault. Presses Universitaires de Rennes, 2018.

——. "Aliénistes contre psychiatres: La médecine mentale en crise (1890–1914)." *Psychologie clinique* 17 (2004): 61–76.

Foley, Susan K. *Women in France since 1789: The Meanings of Difference*. New York: Palgrave Macmillan, 2004.

Forth, Christopher E. *Masculinity in the Modern West: Gender, Civilization and the Body*. New York: Palgrave Macmillan, 2008.

——. *The Dreyfus Affair and the Crisis of French Manhood*. Baltimore: Johns Hopkins University Press, 2004.

Foucault, Michel. *Folie et dérasion: histoire de la folie à l'âge classique*. Paris: Plon, 1961.

——. *History of Madness*. Edited by Jean Khalfa and translated by Jonathan Murphy and Jean Khalfa. London: Routledge, 2006. Originally published 1972 by Gallimard.

——. *Psychiatric Power: Lectures at the Collège de France, 1973–1974*. Edited by Jacques Lagrange and translated by Graham Burchell. New York: Macmillan, 2008.

——. *The Birth of the Clinic*. Translated by A. M. Sheridan. London: Routledge, 2002. Originally published 1963 by Presses Universitaires de France.

——. *The History of Sexuality, Vol. 1: An Introduction*. Translated by Robert Hurley. New York: Vintage, 1990. Originally published 1976 by Éditions Gallimard.

——. *Madness and Civilization*. Translated by Richard Howard. New York: Vintage Books, 1988. Originally published 1961 by Librarie Plon.

Fraisse, Geneviève. *Reason's Muse: Sexual Difference and the Birth of Democracy*. Translated by Jane Marie Todd. Chicago: University of Chicago Press, 1994.

Fuchs, Rachel G. *Contested Paternity: Constructing Families in Modern France*. Baltimore: Johns Hopkins University Press, 2010.

Gauchet, Marcel, and Gladys Swain. *Madness and Democracy: The Modern Psychiatric Universe*. Translated by Catherine Porter. Princeton, NJ: Princeton University Press, 1999.

Gilman, Sander L. "Madness as Disability." *History of Psychiatry* 25, no. 4 (December 2014): 441–49, doi:10.1177/0957154X14545846.

Goldstein, Jan. *Console and Classify: The French Psychiatric Profession in the Nineteenth Century*, 2nd edition. Chicago: University of Chicago Press, 2002.

——. "Foucault among the Sociologists: The 'Disciplines' and the History of the Professions." *History and Theory* 23, no. 2 (1984): 170–192, https://doi.org/10.2307/2505005.

——. *Hysteria Complicated by Ecstasy: The Case of Nanette Leroux*. Princeton, NJ: Princeton University Press, 2011.

——. "The Uses of Male Hysteria: Medical and Literary Discourse in Nineteenth-Century France." *Representations* 34 (1991): 134–165. https://doi.org/10.2307/2928773.

Gordon, Felicia. *Constance Pascal*. London: IGRS, University of London, 2013.

——. "French Psychiatry and the New Woman: The Case of Dr Constance Pascal, 1877–1937." *History of Psychiatry* 17, no. 66 part 2 (2006): 159–182, https://doi.org/10.1177/0957154X06056601.

——. *The Integral Feminist: Madeleine Pelletier, 1874–1939: Feminism, Socialism and Medicine*. Minneapolis: University of Minnesota Press, 1991.

Gould, Roger V. *Insurgent Identities: Class, Community, and Protest in Paris from 1848 to the Commune*. Chicago: University of Chicago Press, 1995.

Grogan, Susan. "Philanthropic Women and the State: The Société de Charité Maternelle in Avignon, 1802–1917." *French History* 14, no. 3 (2000): 295–321, https://doi.org/10.1093/fh/14.3.295.

Guillemain, Hervé. "Des institutions privées d'histoire. Enquête sur les archives d'entreprises capitalistes dédiées à la gestion de la folie (France, 1930–1950)." *Santé mentale au Québec* 41, no. 2 (2016): 101–118, https://doi.org/10.7202/1037958ar.

Guillemin, Henri. *L'Engloutie – Adèle, fille de Victor Hugo 1830–1915*. Paris: Editions du Seuil, 1985.

Gullickson, Gay L. *Unruly Women of Paris: Images of the Commune*. Ithaca, NY: Cornell University Press, 1996.

Hahn, H. Hazel. *Scenes of Parisian Modernity: Culture and Consumption in the Nineteenth Century*. London: Palgrave Macmillan, 2009.

Harris, Ruth. *Murders and Madness: Medicine, Law, and Society in the Fin de Siècle*. Oxford: Oxford University Press, 1989.

Harrison, Carol E. *The Bourgeois Citizen in Nineteenth-Century France: Gender, Sociability, and the Uses of Emulation*. Oxford: Oxford University Press, 1999.

Harvey, David. *Paris, Capital of Modernity*. New York: Taylor & Francis, 2003.

Hause, Steven C., and Anne R. Kenney. *Women's Suffrage and Social Politics in the French Third Republic*. Princeton, NJ: Princeton University Press, 1984.

Heuer, Jennifer Ngaire. *The Family and the Nation: Gender and Citizenship in Revolutionary France, 1789–1830*. Ithaca, NY: Cornell University Press, 2005.

——. "'No More Fears, No More Tears'? Gender, Emotion and the Aftermath of the Napoleonic Wars in France." *Gender & History* 28, no. 2 (2016): 438–460, https://doi.org/10.1111/1468-0424.12217.

Hewitt, Jessie. "Married to the 'Living Dead': Madness as a Cause for Divorce in Late Nineteenth-Century France." *Contemporary French Civilization* 40, no. 3 (2015): 311–330, https://doi.org/10.3828/cfc.2015.18.

——. "Women Working 'Amidst the Mad': Domesticity as Psychiatric Treatment in Nineteenth-Century Paris." *French Historical Studies* 38, no. 1 (2015): 105–137, https://doi.org/10.1215/00161071-2822721.

Huertas, Rafael. "Subjectivity in Clinical Practice: On the Origins of Psychiatric Semiology in Early French Alienism." *History of Psychiatry* 25, no. 4 (2014): 459–467, https://doi.org/10.1177/0957154X14543992.

Hunt, Lynn. *The Family Romance of the French Revolution*. Berkeley: University of California Press, 1992.

Hustvedt, Asti. *Medical Muses: Hysteria in Nineteenth-Century Paris*. New York: W. W. Norton, 2011.

Johnson, Christopher H. *Becoming Bourgeois: Love, Kinship, and Power in Provincial France, 1670–1880*. Ithaca, NY: Cornell University Press, 2015.

Johnson, Laurie M., and Dan Demetriou, eds. *Honor in the Modern World: Interdisciplinary Perspectives*. Lanham, MD: Lexington Books, 2016.

Keller, Richard C. *Colonial Madness: Psychiatry in French North Africa*. Chicago: University of Chicago Press, 2007.

Kertzer, David I. and Marzio Barbagli, eds. *The History of the European Family: Family Life in the Long Nineteenth Century (1789–1913)*. New Haven, CT: Yale University Press, 2002.

Kete, Kathleen. *Making Way for Genius: The Aspiring Self in France from the Old Regime to the New*. New Haven, CT: Yale University Press, 2012.

Klein, Alexandre, Hervé Guillemain, and Marie-Claude Thifault. *La fin de l'asile? Histoire de la déshospitalisation psychiatrique dans l'espace francophone au XXe siècle*. Rennes: Presses Universitaires de Rennes, 2018.

Kudlick, Catherine J. "Disability History: Why We Need Another 'Other.'" *American Historical Review* 108, no. 3 (2003): 763–793, https://doi.org/10.1086/ahr/108.3.763.

Landes, Joan B. *Women and the Public Sphere in the Age of the French Revolution*. Ithaca, NY: Cornell University Press, 1996.

Laqueur, Thomas Walter. *Making Sex: Body and Gender from the Greeks to Freud*. Cambridge, MA: Harvard University Press, 1992.

——. *Solitary Sex: A Cultural History of Masturbation*. Boston: Zone Books, 2003.

LeFrançois, Brenda, Robert Menzies, and Geoffrey Reaume, eds. *Mad Matters: A Critical Reader in Canadian Mad Studies*. Toronto: Canadian Scholars Press, 2013.

Lichtlé, Michel, Sophie Vanden Abeele, and Françoise Mélonio. *Balzac, le texte et la loi*. Paris: Presses Universitaires Paris-Sorbonne, 2012.

Lidsky, Paul. *Les écrivains contre la Commune*. Paris: La Découverte, 1999.

Linstrum, Erik. *Ruling Minds: Psychology in the British Empire*. Cambridge, MA: Harvard University Press, 2016.

Longmore, Paul K., and Lauri Umansky. *The New Disability History: American Perspectives*. New York: New York University Press, 2001.

Mackaman, Douglas P. *Leisure Settings: Bourgeois Culture, Medicine, and the Spa in Modern France*. Chicago: University of Chicago Press, 1998.

Mansker, Andrea. *Sex, Honor and Citizenship in Early Third Republic France*. Basingstoke: Palgrave Macmillan, 2011.

Marcus, Sharon. *Apartment Stories: City and Home in Nineteenth-Century Paris and London*. Berkeley: University of California Press, 1999.

Margadant, Jo Burr. "Gender, Vice, and the Political Imaginary in Postrevolutionary France: Reinterpreting the Failure of the July Monarchy, 1830–1848." *American Historical Review* 104, no. 5 (1999): 1461–1496, https://doi.org/10.2307/2649346.

——, ed. *The New Biography: Performing Femininity in Nineteenth-Century France*. Berkeley: University of California Press, 2000.

Martin-Fugier, Anne. *La bourgeoise*. Paris: Grasset, 2014.

——. *La place des bonnes*. Paris: Grasset, 2014.

Matlock, Jann. "Doubling out of the Crazy House: Gender, Autobiography, and the Insane Asylum System in Nineteenth-Century France." *Representations* 34 (1991): 166–195, https://doi.org/10.2307/2928774.

——. *Scenes of Seduction: Prostitution, Hysteria, and Reading Difference in Nineteenth-Century France*. New York: Columbia University Press, 1994.

Maza, Sarah. *Private Lives and Public Affairs: The Causes Célèbres of Prerevolutionary France*. Berkeley: University of California Press, 1995.

——. *Myth of the French Bourgeoisie: An Essay on the Social Imaginary, 1750–1850*. Cambridge: Harvard University Press, 2009.

Merriman, John M. *The Dynamite Club: How a Bombing in Fin-de-Siècle Paris Ignited the Age of Modern Terror*. Reprint edition. New Haven, CT: Yale University Press, 2016.

Micale, Mark S. *Hysterical Men the Hidden History of Male Nervous Illness*. Cambridge, MA: Harvard University Press, 2008.

Micale, Mark S., and Roy Porter, eds. *Discovering the History of Psychiatry*. New York: Oxford University Press, 1994.

Michael, Pamela. *Care and Treatment of the Mentally Ill in North Wales, 1800–2000*. Cardiff: University of Wales Press, 2003.

Miller, Michael Barry. *The Bon Marché: Bourgeois Culture and the Department Store, 1869–1920*. Princeton, NJ: Princeton University Press, 1981.

Mosse, George L. *The Image of Man: The Creation of Modern Masculinity*. Oxford: Oxford University Press, 1998.

Mueller, Thomas. "Le placement familial des aliénés en France. Le baron Mundy et l'Exposition universelle de 1867." *Romantisme* 141, no. 3 (2008): 37–50, https://doi.org/10.3917/rom.141.0037.

Murat, Laure. *La maison du docteur Blanche: Histoire d'un asile et de ses pensionnaires, de Nerval à Maupassant*. Paris: J C Lattès, 2001.

——. *The Man Who Thought He Was Napoleon: Toward a Political History of Madness*. Translated by Deke Dusinberre. Chicago: University of Chicago Press, 2014.

Nelson, Claudia, and Daniel Nelson. *Family Ties in Victorian England*. London: Greenwood Publishing Group, 2007.

Nelson, Elizabeth. "Running in Circles: A Return to an Old Idea about Asylum Reform in Nineteenth-Century France." *The Journal of the Western Society for French History* 42 (2014), http://hdl.handle.net/2027/spo.0642292.0042.011

Nord, Philip G. *The Republican Moment: Struggles for Democracy in Nineteenth-Century France*. Cambridge, MA: Harvard University Press, 1995.

Novella, Enric J., and Rafael Huertas. "Alexandre Brierre de Boismont and the Origins of the Spanish Psychiatric Profession." *History of Psychiatry* 22, no. 4 (December 1, 2011): 387–402, https://doi.org/10.1177/0957154X10390440.

Nye, Robert A. *Crime, Madness, and Politics: The Medical Concept of National Decline*. Princeton, NJ: Princeton University Press, 1984.

——. "Honor, Impotence, and Male Sexuality in Nineteenth-Century French Medicine." *French Historical Studies* 16, no. 1 (1989): 48–71, https://doi.org/10.2307/286433.

——. *Masculinity and Male Codes of Honor in Modern France*. New York: Oxford University Press, 1993.

——. "Medicine and Science as Masculine 'Fields of Honor.'" *Osiris* 12 (1997): 60–79, https://www.jstor.org/stable/301899.

O'Brien, Patricia. "The Kleptomania Diagnosis: Bourgeois Women and Theft in Late Nineteenth-Century France." *Journal of Social History* 17, no. 1 (1983): 65–77, https://doi.org/10.1353/jsh/17.1.65.

Offen, Karen. *Debating the Woman Question in the French Third Republic, 1870–1920*. Cambridge: Cambridge University Press, 2018.

Park, Sun Young. *Ideals of the Body: Architecture, Urbanism, and Hygiene in Postrevolutionary Paris*. Pittsburgh: Pittsburgh University Press, 2018.

Pateman, Carole. *The Sexual Contract*. Palo Alto: Stanford University Press, 1988.

Pedersen, Jean Elisabeth. *Legislating the French Family: Feminism, Theater, and Republican Politics, 1870–1920*. New Brunswick, NJ: Rutgers University Press, 2003.

Perrot, Michelle. *A History of Private Life, Volume 4: From the Fires of Revolution to the Great War*. Cambridge, MA: Harvard University Press, 1990.

Pichichero, Christy. "Le Soldat Sensible: Military Psychology and Social Egalitarianism in the Enlightenment French Army." *French Historical Studies* 31, no. 4 (2008): 553–580, https://doi.org/10.1215/00161071-2008-006.

Pick, Daniel. *Faces of Degeneration: A European Disorder, c. 1848–1918*. Cambridge: Cambridge University Press, 1989.

Plott, Michele. "The Rules of the Game: Respectability, Sexuality, and the Femme Mondaine in Late-Nineteenth-Century Paris." *French Historical Studies* 25, no. 3 (2002): 531–556, https://www.muse.jhu.edu/article/11931.

Poirier, Jacques. "Jean-Baptiste Vincent Laborde (1830–1903), forgotten neurologist and neurophysiologist." *Geriatrie et psychologie neuropsychiatrie du vieillissement* 13 (2015): 73–82, https://doi.org/10.1684/pnv.2015.0518.

Popiel, Jennifer J. *Rousseau's Daughters: Domesticity, Education, and Autonomy in Modern France*. Durham, NH: University of New Hampshire Press, 2008.

Porter, Roy. *A Social History of Madness: Stories of the Insane*. New York: E. P. Dutton, 1989.

——. *Mind-Forg'd Manacles: A History of Madness in England from the Restoration to the Regency*. London: Athlone Press, 1987.

——. "The Patient's View: Doing Medical History from Below." *Theory and Society* 14, no. 2 (1985): 175–198.

Prestwich, Patricia E. "Family Strategies and Medical Power: 'Voluntary' Committal in a Parisian Asylum, 1876-1914." *Journal of Social History* 27, no. 4 (1994): 799–818, https://doi.org/10.1353/jsh/27.4.799.

Quin, Grégory, and Anaïs Bohuon. "Muscles, Nerves, and Sex: The Contradictions of the Medical Approach to Female Bodies in Movement in France, 1847–1914." *Gender & History* 24, no. 1 (2012): 172–186, https://doi.org/10.1111/j.1468-0424.2011.01674.x.

Reddy, William M. *The Invisible Code: Honor and Sentiment in Postrevolutionary France, 1814–1848*. Berkeley: University of California Press, 1997.

——. *The Navigation of Feeling: A Framework for the History of Emotions*. Cambridge: Cambridge University Press, 2001.

Reed, Matt T. "'La manie d'Écrire': psychology, auto-observation, and case history." *Journal of the History of the Behavioral Sciences* 40, no. 3 (2004): 265–284, https://doi.org/10.1002/jhbs.20021.

Reeder, Linda. "Unattached and Unhinged: The Spinster and the Psychiatrist in Liberal Italy, 1860–1922." *Gender & History* 24, no. 1 (2012): 187–204, https://doi.org/10.1111/j.1468-0424.2011.01675.x.

Reiss, Benjamin. *Theaters of Madness: Insane Asylums and Nineteenth-Century American Culture*. Chicago: University of Chicago Press, 2008.

Rembis, Michael A., Catherine Jean Kudlick, and Kim E. Nielsen, eds. *The Oxford Handbook of Disability History*. Oxford: Oxford University Press, 2018.

Resnick, Evelyne. *Femmes et associations, 1830–1880: vraies democrates ou dames patronesses?* Paris: Publisud, 1991.

Rigondet, Juliette, *Un village pour aliénés tranquilles*. Paris: Fayard, 2019.

Ripa, Yannick. *La ronde des folles. Femme, folie et enfermement au XIXe siècle: 1838–1870*.

———. *Women and Madness: The Incarceration of Women in Nineteenth Century France*. Translated by Catherine du Peloux Menagé. Minneapolis: University of Minnesota Press, 1990.

Robcis, Camille. *The Law of Kinship: Anthropology, Psychoanalysis, and the Family in France*. Ithaca, NY: Cornell University Press, 2013.

Roberts, Mary Louise. "Beyond 'Crisis' in Understanding Gender Transformation." *Gender & History* 28, no. 2 (2016): 358–366, https://doi.org/10.1111/1468-0424.12212.

———. *Disruptive Acts: The New Woman in Fin-de-Siècle France*. Chicago: University of Chicago Press, 2005.

Roche, Daniel and Jean Delumeau, eds. *Histoire des pères et de la paternité*. Paris: Larousse, 1990.

Ross, Andrew Israel. *Public City/Public Sex: Homosexuality, Prostitution, and Urban Culture in Nineteenth-Century Paris*. Philadelphia: Temple University Press, 2019.

Schafer, Sylvia. *Children in Moral Danger and the Problem of Government in Third Republic France*. Princeton, NJ: Princeton University Press, 1997.

Schiebinger, Londa. *The Mind Has No Sex? Women in the Origins of Modern Science*. Cambridge, MA: Harvard University Press, 1991.

Schneider, William. "Toward the Improvement of the Human Race: The History of Eugenics in France." *Journal of Modern History* 54, no. 2 (1982): 268–291, https://www.jstor.org/stable/1906158

Schuster, Jean-Pierre, Nicolas Hoertel, and Frédéric Limosin. "The Man behind Philippe Pinel: Jean-Baptiste Pussin (1746–1811)." *British Journal of Psychiatry* 198, no. 3 (March 2011): 241–241, https://doi.org/10.1192/bjp.198.3.241a.

Schwartz, Vanessa R. *Spectacular Realities: Early Mass Culture in Fin-de-Siècle Paris*. Berkeley: University of California Press, 1999.

Scott, Joan W. *Gender and the Politics of History*. New York: Columbia University Press, 1999.

———. *Only Paradoxes to Offer: French Feminists and the Rights of Man*. Cambridge, MA: Harvard University Press, 1997.

Shapiro, Gilbert, Timothy Tackett, Philip Dawson, and John Markoff. *Revolutionary Demands: A Content Analysis of the Cahiers de Doléances of 1789*. Palo Alto: Stanford University Press, 1998.

Shorter, Edward. *A History of Psychiatry: From the Era of the Asylum to the Age of Prozac*. New York: Wiley, 1998.

Showalter, Elaine. *The Female Malady: Women, Madness, and Culture in England, 1830–1980*. New York: Pantheon Books, 1986.

Smith, Bonnie G. *Ladies of the Leisure Class: The Bourgeoises of Northern France in the Nineteenth Century*. Princeton, NJ: Princeton University Press, 1981.

———. *The Gender of History: Men, Women, and Historical Practice*. Cambridge, MA: Harvard University Press, 2000.

Smith, Bonnie G., and Beth Hutchison, eds. *Gendering Disability*. New Brunswick, NJ: Rutgers University Press, 2004.

Steinbrügge, Lieselotte. *The Moral Sex: Woman's Nature in the French Enlightenment*. New York: Oxford University Press, 1995.

Stiker, Henri-Jacques. *A History of Disability*. Translated by William Sayers. Ann Arbor: University of Michigan Press, 1999.

Surkis, Judith. *Sexing the Citizen: Morality and Masculinity in France, 1870–1920*. Ithaca, NY: Cornell University Press, 2006.

Sussman, George D. "The Glut of Doctors in Mid-Nineteenth-Century France." *Comparative Studies in Society and History* 19, no. 3 (July 1977): 287–304, https://doi.org/10.1017/S0010417500008720.

Suzuki, Akihito. *Madness at Home: The Psychiatrist, the Patient, and the Family in England, 1820–1860*. Berkeley: University of California Press, 2006.

Taithe, Bertrand. *Defeated Flesh: Medicine, Welfare, and Warfare in the Making of Modern France*. Lanham, MD: Rowman & Littlefield, 1999.

Thomas, Gregory M. *Treating the Trauma of the Great War: Soldiers, Civilians, and Psychiatry in France, 1914–1940*. Baton Rouge: Louisiana State University Press, 2009.

Timm, Annette F., and Joshua A. Sanborn. *Gender, Sex and the Shaping of Modern Europe: A History from the French Revolution to the Present Day*. 2nd edition. London: Bloomsbury Academic, 2016.

Tomes, Nancy. *The Art of Asylum-Keeping: Thomas Story Kirkbride and the Origins of American Psychiatry*. Philadelphia: University of Pennsylvania Press, 1994.

Topp, Leslie. *Freedom and the Cage: Modern Architecture and Psychiatry in Central Europe, 1890–1914*. University Park: Penn State University Press, 2017.

Tosh, John. *A Man's Place: Masculinity and the Middle-Class Home in Victorian England*. New Haven, CT: Yale University Press, 1999.

——. "Home and Away: The Flight from Domesticity in Late-Nineteenth-Century England Re-Visited." *Gender & History* 27, no. 3 (2015): 561–575, https://doi.org/10.1111/1468-0424.12150.

Traugott, Mark. *The Insurgent Barricade*. Berkeley: University of California Press, 2010.

Verhoeven, Timothy. "Pathologizing Male Desire: Satyriasis, Masculinity, and Modern Civilization at the Fin de Siècle." *Journal of the History of Sexuality* 24, no. 1 (2015): 25–45, https://www.muse.jhu.edu/article/563626.

Verjus, Anne. *Le bon mari: Une histoire politique des hommes et des femmes à l'époque révolutionnaire*. Paris: Fayard, 2010.

Verjus, Anne, and Denise Z. Davidson. *Le roman conjugal: Chroniques de la vie familiale à l'époque de la Révolution et de l'Empire*. Seyssel (Ain): Champ Vallon, 2011.

Wagner, Peter. *A Sociology of Modernity: Liberty and Discipline*. London: Routledge, 2002.

Walkowitz, Judith R. *City of Dreadful Delight: Narratives of Sexual Danger in Late-Victorian London*. Chicago: University of Chicago Press, 1992.

Weiner, Dora B. *The Citizen Patient in Revolutionary and Imperial Paris*. Baltimore: Johns Hopkins University Press, 1993.

Williams, Rosalind H. *Dream Worlds: Mass Consumption in Late Nineteenth Century France*. Berkeley: University of California Press, 1982.

Wilson, Colette. *Paris and the Commune 1871–78: The Politics of Forgetting*. Manchester: Manchester University Press, 2016.

Wilson, Susannah. *Voices from the Asylum: Four French Women, 1850–1920*. Oxford: Oxford University Press, 2010.

Wise, Sarah. *Inconvenient People: Lunacy, Liberty, and the Mad-Doctors in England*. London: Counterpoint, 2013.

Woloch, Isser. *The New Regime: Transformations of the French Civic Order, 1789–1820s*. New York: W. W. Norton, 1995.

absolutism: and imprisonment of mad people, 20–21; and patriarchal power, link between, 96; replacement of, and gendering of reason, 9–10; and unjust asylum commitment, 33, 96, 107

affective family ties: disturbance of, as symptom of insanity, 11, 27; idealization of, bourgeois families and, 11, 19, 29. *See also* sentimental family

age, and onset of insanity, 23

agricultural labor: as form of treatment, 121, 127, 145; in Open Door treatment method, 160

alcoholism, hereditary, studies of, 151

alienists (asylum doctors): alliance with state, 92, 95, 132, 139, 141; bourgeois backgrounds of, 7, 186n41; challenges to reputation of, concerns about, 41, 48, 92, 117; on Communards as mad people, 119, 133, 134–139; crises of 1870–1871 and, 118–127; fatherly authority of, 47, 48, 50–51, 105; financial interest in admitting new patients, 144; and gender ideology, 2, 6, 10, 14–15, 17, 41, 42, 90–91, 166, 169; and honor, seeking to project, 48, 52–54, 64–66, 129–131; and masculine rationality, perpetuation of ideal of, 2, 3, 14, 17, 40, 45, 95, 108; neurologists replacing, 5; opposition to (anti-alienist movement), 53, 92, 150, 164; paternal role of, vision of, 36–37;

performance of authority by, 2, 37–39, 52; performance of strength during times of crisis, 120–127; role in family care model, 154–155, 156; safeguarding of professional prerogatives by, 41, 118–119, 123; self-promotion in aftermath of Franco-Prussian War, 127–132; use of term, 2, 177n4; on women and irrationality, association of, 2, 14, 17, 24, 68. *See also* doctor-patient relationship; psychiatric authority; psychiatric profession

ambition, insanity linked to, 135, 136

anti-alienist movement: emergence of, 53, 92, 150, 164; writings in, 109, 141, 160

Arthaud, Joseph, 154

L'Assomoir (Zola), 149–150

Astié de Valsayre, Marie-Rose, 172

asylum(s): admission process for, 97, 120–121, 184n6; calls for reform of, 53, 93, 141, 143, 144–145; vs. community care, 141, 143; compared to prison (Bastille), 53, 93, 105, 143, 159, 160; depiction in Zola's *L'Assomoir,* 150; as family, early alienists' vision of, 36–37; and family colony, cross-pollination of, 149; during Franco-Prussian War, 120, 121–131; growth in 19th century, 5; as hospitals, vision of, 154; national system of, establishment of, 42, 43, 52, 96; pacification associated with, 139; as place of (curative) seclusion,

28, 29, 31, 34; political liberalism and, 9; reform proposals for, 17, 141–142, 157–163, 164–165; self-reflection in, moral treatment and, 31, 183n27; as temporary homes, Pinel's view of, 36, 151; without walls (Open Door method), 158–160, 165. *See also* private asylums; public asylums; unjust asylum commitment

asylum doctors. *See* alienists

authoritarian family: pathologizing of, 29, 33; transition away from, 16, 44, 93, 95

authority: of nurses/guardians, in family care model, 155, 156; in transition, historical moment of, 51; of women, in psychiatric community, 69, 75–77, 84. *See also* masculine authority; paternal authority; psychiatric authority

Bacopoulos-Viau, Alexandra, 7

Balzac, Honoré de: critique of postrevolutionary family, 106, 107, 114; *L'Interdiction,* 106–109, 114; *Père Goriot,* 10–11

La Baronne (play), 111, 114, 117

Baynton, Douglas, 12

Beard, Charles, 152

Bernhardt, Sarah, 111

Bicêtre asylum, 121; elimination of physical restraints at, 8, 38, 40; Esquirol as director of, 28; Féré as chief physician of, 152, 154, 158; funding constraints on, 193n99; Leuret as director of, 1, 2–4, 46, 47, 49; Pinel as director of, 8, 46, 133; Pussin as overseer of, 8, 38–39

Billod, Eugène: on asylum sequestration as social good, 139; as director of Vaucluse, during Franco-Prussian War, 127–132, 148; on Gheel community care model, 147–149, 161

biological explanations for insanity: rise of, 5, 16, 63–64, 150–151, 164; in women, early alienists on, 23, 24, 27. *See also* hereditary theories of insanity

Bismarck, Otto von, 117

Blanche, Esprit, 43, 47; case histories discussed by, 56, 57–58; on cold shower treatment, 44–45, 47, 48–49, 50, 51–53, 58, 64; treatment regimens devised by, 55, 56, 62, 63, 186n51; and *vie de famille* treatment, 47, 66, 71

Bleynie, M., 43, 44

Bonnet, Henri, 117

Bouchereau, Louis Gustave, 121–122, 138

Bourdieu, Pierre, 180n31

Bourgeois, Alexis, 43

bourgeoisie, French, 2; and affective family ties, idealization of, 11, 19, 29, 100; decline of, fall of moral treatment and, 170; gender values associated with, and psychiatric treatment, 2, 47; and masculine behavior, everyday policing of, 11; use of term, 9, 178n14. *See also* gender ideals, bourgeois

Bourneville, Dr., 162

Boyer, Philoxène, 80

Brierre de Boismont, Alexandre: career of, 69–70; on daughter's memoir, 85–86, 198n30; daughter's praise for, 79; English colleague's support for, 124, 126; fatherly role of, 120, 125; during Franco-Prussian War, 124–126; on Gheel colony, 145–146; infantilization of patients by, 74, 83; on Paris Commune, 133, 137; on placement of mentally ill patients, 161; and *vie de famille* method, 70, 71, 74; wife of, 67

Brierre de Boismont, Athalie (née Maillard), 67, 79; as asylum *directrice,* 67, 71–76; as idealized example of bourgeois womanhood, 76–77, 90

Brierre de Boismont family, 190n50;
family mythology of, 86, 89;
psychiatric treatment method used by,
15, 70, 71–77
Butler, Judith, 177n5

chaining, of mental patients: at Gheel
colony, 145; personal account of, 110;
Pinel and end to, 8, 20, 21, 40, 144
Charcot, Jean-Martin, 5, 152,
167–168, 170
Charenton asylum, 43, 121; cold shower
treatment at, 43; unjust commitments
to, 101, 102, 103, 112
Charles X (King of France), 28
childbirth, and onset of mental
illness, 24
children: absence of mental illness
among, 23; asylum patients compared
to, 37, 48, 49–50, 51, 61, 74, 82–83, 133;
new approaches to rearing of, 29–30;
paternal authority over, persistence in
19th century, 100, 101, 102–103, 195n33;
role in asylum care, *vie de famille*
method and, 70, 75, 76, 78, 79, 83; and
unjust asylum commitment of parents,
109–110, 137; use of asylum system to
discipline, 93
citizenship rights, institutionalization
and loss of, 9, 49, 74
Civil Code of 1804: and loss of citizenship
rights, 49; and paternal authority, 97,
108, 115, 194n11; and restrictions on
women's property rights, 72
class distinctions: alienists and
naturalization of, 6, 61, 164, 169;
blurring of, 169–170; in diagnoses of
Communards, 134, 135–138; French
Revolution and new expectations
regarding, 8, 9; in Gheel colony,
164; myth of meritocracy and, 11; in
onset of insanity, early alienists on,

23, 26, 27; and psychiatric treatment
scenarios, 35, 59–60, 61
cold shower treatment, 46; Blanche
on, 44–45, 47, 48–49, 50, 51–53, 58,
64; debate on, 15, 43, 44–53, 59–63,
92; "energetic moral treatment"
as euphemism for, 48; Esquirol
on, 61–62, 63; Leuret on, 44–45,
46, 47, 48, 58, 59–60, 62, 64–65;
patient response to, 43, 110; Pinel on,
46, 54–55; as threat to psychiatric
profession, 63–64
community care model, 17, 141–142;
vs. asylum system, 141, 143; criticism
of, 145–146, 147–149, 152, 161; and
curability of insanity, loss of faith
in, 142, 157, 168; implementation in
France, 163; moral treatment compared
to, 149. *See also* family colonization
"cottage system," Scottish, 154
curability of insanity: community care
and loss of faith in, 142, 157, 168;
degeneration theory and loss of faith
in, 136, 151, 170; Enlightenment and
faith in, 8; moral treatment and faith
in, 21, 27, 135

Dagonet, Henri, 193n101
Dagron, Jules, 86
Datta, Venita, 131–132
degeneration theory, 136, 143, 151, 167;
on "born degenerates" vs. "accidental
misfits," 203n3; class distinctions
erased by, 170; crises of 1870–1871 and,
152, 164; and curability of insanity,
loss of faith in, 136, 151, 170; and
family isolation, 152, 153, 154, 157; Féré
and, 152–153, 157; moral treatment
compared to, 140, 152
Delas, Hippolyte, 109–110, 114–115, 118
délire de persecution. See persecution
mania

delusions: cold shower method used
to treat, 45, 46, 47, 49, 59–60;
revolutionary upheavals and, 1,
6, 133, 135
dementia: and family colony
placement, 158; unjust asylum
commitment for, 109
depression: family influences worsening,
31–32, 33; surprise used in treatment of,
36; *vie de famille* treatment for, 76–77
Desan, Suzanne, 97
disability: as baseline inequality, 12;
definition of, 178n12; and gender,
mutually constitutive nature of, 6,
13; psychological, used to legitimate
hierarchies, 138
disability history, 12
disobedience, insanity equated with, 100
Ditz, Toby, 13
divorce: abolition in 1816, 113; calls
for legalization of, 113, 114, 115;
legalization of, 173; Napoleonic Civil
Code on, 51; during revolutionary
era, 113; unjust institutionalization of
women seeking, 173
doctor(s), asylum. *See* alienists
doctor-father persona, 51; Pinel (Scipion)
on, 36–37, 50–51; in *vie de famille*
treatment method, 74
doctor-patient relationship: imbalance of
power in, Foucault on, 2; as inherently
authoritarian and abusive, Manier
on, 144; moral treatment and, 4,
34, 36–37; Open Door method and,
162, 163; performance of honor in,
48, 52–54, 64–65; performance of
psychiatric authority in, 2, 37–39, 52
Doctrinaires, 43
domesticity. *See* feminine domesticity
domestic violence, as source of
insanity, 26
Dowbiggin, Ian, 63, 184n9, 185n29

Dumas, Adolphe, 99
Dun-sur-Auron, family colony at, 157–158

Edmond, Charles, 111
education: formal, absence among
women *directrices*, 68, 79; medical,
entry of women in, 79–80; of patients,
moral treatment and, 37, 49, 73, 74;
and professionalization of psychiatry,
40, 88; of young women, and onset of
madness, 25
emotions: family life and aggravation of,
29; healing properties of, early alienists
on, 27, 41; redirecting in normative
fashion, moral treatment and, 21, 27,
35–36; unchecked, as source of insanity,
21–22, 23, 25, 26–27, 57, 135, 136
Enlightenment: disciplining nature of, 6,
9; and faith in curability of insanity, 8
Esquirol, Jean-Étienne-Dominique:
and Brierre de Boismont, 69; case
histories published by, 54; on causes
of madness, 21–22, 25, 26–27; on
cold shower treatment, 61–62, 63;
as director of Bicêtre asylum, 28;
on doctor's authority, 37; gendered
treatment scenarios of, 35–36; on
heads of households afflicted with
mental alienation, 33–34; and humane
treatment of mental patients, 159, 160;
on isolation, 30–34, 37; and law of
1838, 96; and Leuret, 47, 61–62; and
moral treatment, 5; on role of age in
onset of insanity, 23; students of, 47,
145; survey of asylums, 5, 28
Esquiron, Marie, 171–174, 175, 204n18,
204n19, 204n27
eugenics, 153
evolutionary decline, madness as
sign of, 151

Faligan, Ernest, 100–105

Falret, Jules, 146–147, 148, 149, 161
family: affective ties in, 11, 19, 29, 100;
    alienists' suspicion of, 31–32, 161, 162;
    asylum compared to, 36–37; conflicts
    in, and unjust asylum commitments,
    16, 141, 193n3; doctor's, replacing
    patient's family with, 47; egalitarian,
    path to, 174, 175; of madmen, efforts
    to preserve honor of, 65; neuropathic,
    152–153; as partner in treatment,
    Marandon de Montyel on, 162, 163;
    postrevolutionary, Balzac's critique
    of, 106, 107, 114; reincorporation
    of patients into, as goal of moral
    treatment, 26, 32; sentimental, ideal
    of, 11, 12, 19, 93; and social stability,
    during times of political turmoil, 19,
    29, 72; as source of mental illness,
    alienists on, 20, 32–33, 36, 41–42,
    47, 73, 81, 170; transitional moment
    in history of, 4; treatment methods
    modeled on (*vie de famille*), 47, 66,
    70–73. *See also* authoritarian family;
    isolation, family; sentimental family
family colonization, 141–142; asylum
    and, cross-pollination of, 149; class
    and gender dimensions of, 152, 155–156;
    criticism of, 145–146, 147–149, 152;
    doctor's role in, 154–155, 156; Féré on,
    153–157, 164, 168; in France, 157–158;
    Gheel (Belgium) model of, 143–149;
    moral treatment compared to, 149;
    nurses/guardians in, importance of,
    147, 155–157; Scottish model of, 154
family law, in revolutionary era, 95–97,
    193n6; abuse of, 96; and marriage
    choice, 100
family visitations: moral treatment and
    discouragement of, 37; Open Door
    method and, 162, 163
fatherly role, alienist's, 47, 48, 50; Brierre
    de Boismont (Alexandre) and, 120, 125;

disagreement over proper enactment
    of, 50; Franco-Prussian War and, 124,
    133; Pinel (Philippe) on, 36, 50; Pinel
    (Scipion) on, 36–37, 50–51. *See also*
    paternal authority
Fauvel, Aude, 7, 108, 193n3, 204n27
fear, as impetus for cure, 50, 65
feminine domesticity, ideal of: asylum
    doctors and reinforcement of, 2, 6;
    bourgeois home and, 72; challenges
    to, 167, 168; comparative stability of,
    68–69; economic context bolstering,
    9; private asylum *directrices* and, 68,
    166; use in psychiatric treatment
    process, 15, 39–40, 69, 71–72
feminist activists: and challenges to
    feminine domesticity ideal, 168; unjust
    asylum commitment of, 171–174
Féré, Charles, 152; at Bicêtre asylum,
    152, 154, 158; on family colonization,
    153–157, 164, 168; on hereditary
    degeneration, 152–153, 157, 164
Ferrus, Guillaume, 145, 146, 148
finances, loss of control over, during
    asylum stays, 9, 49, 74, 98
financial interests: affective family ties
    and, 100; alienists', in admitting new
    patients, 144; and unjust asylum
    commitment, 93, 98, 99, 101, 109–
    110, 195n32
Forth, Christopher, 9, 64
Foucault, Michel, 2, 6–7, 183n27, 203n9
Fournier, Marc, 80
Foussier, Edouard, 111
Franco-Prussian War, 117; aftermath of,
    133–134; asylums during, 120, 121–131;
    impact on psychiatric profession, 16,
    118, 120–132, 140, 141, 164; loss of,
    and degeneration theory, 151; patients'
    return to families during, 122, 161
French Revolution: meritocratic
    thrust of, and psychological distress,

10–11, 22, 24, 135; and new class
and gender expectations, 8, 9; and
paternal authority, 108, 116; and rise
of psychiatric profession, 8–9, 15,
94–95, 144
Freud, Sigmund, 170
Fuchs, Rachel, 12, 195n33

Galton, Francis, 153
Gambetta, Leon, 134
Gasté, Joseph de, 171–172, 173
gender: centrality to asylum interactions,
2–3; changing notions of, asylum
documents as windows into, 14;
constructed nature of, treatment
approaches highlighting, 3, 69; and
disability, mutually constitutive nature
of, 6, 13; French Revolution and new
expectations regarding, 8–9; and
psychiatric treatment scenarios, 2, 3–4,
14, 35, 39–40, 41; sex and, uncoupling
as evidence of insanity, 1, 3
gender difference: alienists and
naturalization of, 18, 115–116, 164,
166, 169; blurring of boundaries in,
168–169; in onset of insanity, early
alienists on, 23–24
gender ideals, bourgeois, 2, 9–10;
alienists' contradictory relationship
to, 10, 14–15, 42, 90–91, 166, 169;
asylums modeled on, 36–37, 47,
66; constructed nature of, asylum
directrices exposing, 90; flexibility
within, 13; as justification for women's
expert status, 76–77, 78; patient's
acceptance of, as proof of cure, 2, 3;
psychiatric approaches reflecting/
reinforcing, 2, 4, 6, 15, 17–18, 19, 41,
166; psychiatric theories undermining,
170; scandalous asylum commitments
undermining, 94. *See also* feminine
domesticity; masculine rationality

gender instability, premise of, 13, 167, 170
gender nonconformity, as sign of mental
illness, 2, 27, 164, 167
gender performance, concept of, 177n5
Georget, Étienne-Jean, 25–26, 63
Gheel (Belgium) community care model,
143–149; criticism of, 145–146, 147–
149, 152, 161; replicability in France,
146, 147, 148, 154
Goldstein, Jan, 38, 44, 81, 184n9, 186n41
Goncourt, Edmond and Jules de, 137
guardians, in family colonies, 147, 155–157
Guizot, François, 43
Gullickson, Gay, 137
Guttormsson, Loftur, 29

Haussmann, Baron, 120, 145
hereditary theories of insanity: turn
toward, 5, 16, 136, 138, 140, 143, 150–
151, 164. *See also* degeneration theory
home, bourgeois: isolation and threat
posed to image of, 41–42; as refuge
from political turmoil, 19, 29, 72
homosexuality: and challenges to gender
expectations, 168; in French medical
discourse, Foucault on, 203n9;
pathologizing of, 76, 81, 157, 167
honor (honor code): alienists seeking to
project, 48, 52–54, 64–66, 129–131;
appeal to, in efforts to disprove
diagnosis of madness, 104–105;
curative potential of, 54, 57–61, 65;
as double-edged sword for medical
men, 53; vs. ethical standards, 184n10;
families of madmen and efforts to
preserve, 65, 71; Leuret's conception
of, 64–65; malleability of, 54, 186n43;
masculine culture of, and proliferation
of insanity, 15, 54, 56, 57; masculine
rationality and, 45, 65; middle-class
values and, 66; and professionalization
of psychiatry, 63–64; and social

mobility in postrevolutionary France, 45, 53; use in psychiatric treatment, 15, 53, 54, 55, 56, 57–61; women's role in asylum care and, 75–76

hospitals: asylums functioning as, vision of, 154; mental patients housed in, 8, 18, 123

Hugo, Adèle, 80

Hugo, Victor, 80, 112

The Human Comedy (Balzac), 106–108

hysteria: Charcot on causes and treatment of, 167–168; lesbianism conflated with, 81; women's biological predisposition to, claims regarding, 10, 167

impotence, pathologizing of, 157, 167

inheritance: law on, revolutionary-era changes in, 97; unjust institutionalization used to manipulate, 99–100, 109

insanity: biological/somatic explanations for, rise of, 5, 16, 63–64, 150–151, 164; causes of, early alienists on, 21–26, 27, 29; class-and gender-based understandings of, 6, 23–27, 135, 167, 171, 172; contagion of, 153, 164; disobedience equated with, 100; family as source of, theories of, 20, 32–33, 36, 41–42, 47, 73; hereditary basis of, theories of, 5, 16, 136, 138, 140, 143, 150–151, 164; honor code and proliferation among men, 15, 54, 56, 57; medicalization of, 8, 41; meritocratic society and increase in, 10–11, 22, 24, 135; modern life and increased threat of, 152, 168; as "moral" (mental) condition, theories of, 4, 62, 63, 136; objective vs. communal determination of, 104; Paris Commune equated with, 119, 123, 133, 134–139, 140; passions/ unchecked emotions as source of, 21–22, 23, 25, 26–27, 57, 135, 136; patron

saint of, 143; political upheaval/ revolution and, 119, 122, 134–135, 136, 138–139, 140; as sign of evolutionary decline, 151; stigma associated with, perpetuation of, 167; susceptibility to, early alienists on, 21, 136; warfare and proliferation of, 163; in women, early alienists on, 23, 24–26. *See also* curability of insanity

L'Interdiction (Balzac), 106–109, 114

irrationality, women and, doctors perpetuating association of, 2, 14, 17, 24, 68, 175

isolation, family: as central principle of psychiatric treatment, 28–29, 73, 160–161; vs "change of milieu," 162; cold shower treatment compared to, 46; degeneration theory's insistence on, 152, 153, 154, 157; family colonization and, 157; law of 1838 and, 73; moral treatment and, 28–34; and bourgeois home, threat posed to image of, 41–42; and psychiatric profession, legitimation of, 28, 37, 73; rejection of, Marandon de Montyel and, 161–162, 164–165; shock of, 34; *vie de famille* treatment and, 47, 73

Jubline, Marguerite, 39–40

July Monarchy: and bourgeois family values, 41, 73; end of, 93; oversupplied job market of, 41; psychiatric profession during, 30, 43–44, 53

kleptomania diagnosis, 169

labor: class-based assumptions regarding, 160, 165; as form of treatment, 60, 121, 127, 145; in Open Door treatment method, 160

Laborde, Jean-Baptiste Vincent, 133, 134–136, 138, 140, 199n51

law: family, in revolutionary era,
95–97, 193n6; on inheritance, 97; on
marriage/divorce, 51, 100, 113, 173
law on asylum commitment (law of 1838):
calls for reform of, 44, 86, 93, 138;
concept of isolation embedded in, 73;
and disinheritance of children, 97;
doctor's certificate required by, 97,
99; impact on psychiatric profession,
44, 48, 52; *lettre de cachet* compared
to, 99; and loss of citizenship rights/
property control, 49, 74, 98; methods
of sequestration outlined in, 97–98,
184n6; passage of, 5, 43; psychiatric
community's push for, 96; and unjust
institutionalization, 95, 98–99, 193n3
Legrand du Saulle, Henri, 10,
102, 103, 105
lesbianism, pathologizing of, 76, 81
lettre de cachet: abolition of, 96–97;
interdiction compared to, 107; law
of 1838 compared to, 99; and unjust
institutionalization, 96, 107
Leuret, François: Blanche's methods
contrasted with, 62, 66; case histories
discussed by, 58–61; on cold shower
treatment, 44–45, 46, 47, 48, 58,
59–60, 62, 64–65; Esquirol and, 47,
61–62; on fear as impetus for cure,
50; and honor, in doctor-patient
relationship, 64–65; infantilization
of patients by, 61, 83; methods of,
as threat to psychiatric profession,
63–64; powerful sway over patients,
47, 185n18; on psychological vs.
physical bases of insanity, 62, 63;
as self-made *bourgeois,* 1, 46–47;
treatment of Dupré, 1, 2–4; treatment
of Theodor, 49, 51–52; treatment of
Vincent, 58–59
liberty, concept of (*liberté*): and
community care model, 146, 148,

149; and humane treatment of mental
patients, 8, 28, 159; and "Open Door"
model, 160; and psychiatric profession,
28, 95, 133
lifestyle, as cause of insanity, early
alienists on, 23–24
Linas, Aimé-Jean, 86–89
Louis-Napoleon Bonaparte, 93, 117, 119
Louis Philippe I (King of France), 43, 44,
92. *See also* July Monarchy
Lunier, Ludgar, 122–124

madness. *See* insanity
mad people: Communards of Paris
depicted as, 119, 133, 134–139;
compared to children, 37, 48, 49–50,
51, 61, 74, 82–83, 133; as dangerous,
doctors' stake in spreading belief
about, 133, 145; devaluation of, and
opportunities for empowerment of
elite women, 90; hereditary theories
and increased marginalization of, 140;
humane treatment of, early alienists
and, 8, 20, 159, 160; incarceration of,
absolutist state and, 20–21; loss of
citizenship rights/property control
during asylum stays, 9, 49, 74, 98;
persistent dehumanization of, 175;
self-presentation strategies in attempts
to gain release, 109; writings/voices of,
94, 101–102, 103, 109–110
mad studies, 179n18
Magnan, Valentin, 121–122, 138, 150, 151
maisons de santé: use of term, 188n7. *See
also* private asylums
Manier, J., 141, 143, 144
manipulation, in psychiatric treatment,
3–4, 55, 57–60, 64–65, 168;
femininity and, 39–40, 75, 76. *See also*
performance
Marandon de Montyel, Évariste, 158;
backlash against, 163; as director of

Ville-Évrard, 158, 159; on families as
partners in treatment, 162, 163; and
Open Door method, 158–160, 165;
rejection of family isolation by, 161–
162, 164–165

Margadant, Jo Burr, 44

marriage: choice in, forced
institutionalization to deny, 92,
99–100, 101–102; conflicts in, and
unjust asylum commitment, 113, 172–
173; gender complementarity in, belief
in, 40; ideal, 29; middle-class cult of,
114; revolutionary era laws on, 96

masculine authority: alienists'
performance of, 2, 37–39, 47, 52;
asylum doctors bolstering, 14;
characteristics needed for projection
of, 38–39; gendering of reason and
changes in, 11–12; Napoleonic Civil
Code and, 51; rationality vs. physicality
in conception of, 4, 11, 45

masculine rationality/self-control,
ideal of: bourgeoisie and everyday
policing of, 11; economic context
bolstering, 9; and patriarchal power,
11, 115; alienists' reinforcement of,
2, 3, 11, 14, 17, 40, 45, 95, 108, 166;
challenges to, 66, 167; and honor,
45, 65; and vulnerability to unjust
institutionalization, 16, 108, 171

masturbation, insanity linked to,
23, 82, 167

men: insanity in, as psychological
reaction to cultural expectations,
23–24; irrational, women as most
suitable overseers of, 39–40, 69,
74–77. *See also* masculine authority;
masculine rationality

mental illness. *See* insanity

mental patients. *See* mad people

meritocracy: French Revolution and, 10;
myth of, class distinctions maintained

by, 11; and psychological distress,
increase in sources of, 10–11, 22, 24, 135

middle classes: gender expectations as
means of distinction for, 9–10. *See also*
bourgeoisie, French

Mistral, François-Joseph, 99–100, 105

Mistral, Jean, 99, 100, 105, 195n32

Mitchell, Silas Weir, 153

modernity: disciplining nature of, 6; and
insanity, increased threat of, 152, 168

monarchical power: and patriarchal
power, link between, 96. *See also*
absolutism

Monasterio, Antonia, 141

moral treatment, 4–5, 20, 21;
abandonment of, 17, 163–164, 167,
168, 170, 175; community care in
relation to, 142; contradictions in, 50;
criticism of, 5, 93; curative potential
of, belief in, 21, 27, 135; decline of,
16–17, 150, 151; degeneration theory
compared to, 140, 152; doctor-patient
relationship in, 34, 36–37; "energetic,"
48, 63; and familial isolation, 28–34;
gender dimensions of, 42; goal
of, 26, 32, 48, 149; individualized
regimen required by, 5, 56, 186n51;
Leuret's performance of, 60, 65; vs.
medicalization of psychiatry, 64;
mental bases of insanity addressed by,
4, 62; patient's daily life in, 37; role of
strangers in, 31; shock/surprise used in,
34, 36; unjust asylum commitment as
contradiction to, 164

Moreau de Tours,
Jacques-Joseph, 143, 146

Morel, Benedict, 136, 151, 152

Murat, Laure, 6, 133, 134, 184n9,
185n20, 199n51

Napoleonic Civil Code, and masculine
authority, 51

national asylum system: calls for reform
of, 141, 143; establishment of, 42,
43, 52, 96
neurologists, alienists replaced by, 5
neuropathic family, 152–153
New Women, 168
normative instability, stable narrative
built on, 13, 17
Nye, Robert, 45, 151, 184n10

Old Regime: continuities with
19th century, 105, 106; unjust
institutionalization during, 33, 96, 107.
See also absolutism
Open Door method, 158–160, 165;
attacks on, 163; interaction with
families in, 162; support for,
162, 202n53

Paris Commune, 133–134; class prejudice
in assessment of, 134, 135–138; demise
of, 118; female supporters of, sexist
assumptions about, 81, 137–138;
long-term impact of, 169; as madness,
alienists on, 119, 123, 133, 134–139, 140;
and national decline, perception of, 152
Pariset, Étienne, 61, 62
passions. *See* emotions
paternal authority: alienist's role modeled
on, 47, 48, 50–51, 105, 157; Civil Code
of 1804 and, 97, 108, 115, 194n11;
persistence in postrevolutory era,
100, 101, 102–103, 105, 115, 195n33;
revolutionary era and attacks on, 108,
116; and unjust asylum sequestration,
92, 96, 99–105
patients: histories from point of view of,
call for, 7; writings/voices of, 94, 101–
102, 103, 109–110. *See also* mad people
patriarchal power: Civil Code of 1804
and, 97, 194n11; masculine rationality
as justification for, 11, 115; and

monarchical power, link between, 96.
See also paternal authority
patriarchy: definition of, 11, 115;
transition to fraternity from, 11
Pelletier, Madeleine, 80
Père Goriot (Balzac), 10–11
performance: of authority, alienists',
2, 37–39, 47, 52, 66; bourgeois
womanhood as, 90; gender, concept of,
177n5; of honor, alienists', 48, 52–54,
64–66; psychiatric treatment as, 3–4,
55, 57–60, 64–65, 168; of strength
during times of crisis, alienists and,
120–127. *See also* fatherly role, alienists'
persecution mania (*délire de persecution*),
diagnosis of: among revolutionaries,
135; unjust institutionalization based
on, 102, 103, 173
Pinel, Philippe: case histories published
by, 54, 55; on causes of madness,
21–22, 26–27, 29, 151; on cold shower
treatment, 46, 54–55; on curability
of insanity, 21, 27, 151; as director of
Bicêtre asylum, 8, 46, 133; on doctors'
performance of authority, 37, 38; on
fatherly role of asylum doctors, 36, 50;
on fear, 50; and humane treatment
of mental patients, 8, 20, 159; on
ideal asylum overseer, 38–39, 40, 42;
loss of faith in methods of, 164; and
moral treatment, 4, 5, 20, 21, 48, 149;
openness to lay expertise, 40, 41;
and removal of physical restraints, 8,
20, 21, 40, 144, 149; on *surveillante*,
gender-specific skills of, 39–40; on
susceptibility to mental illness, 21, 136
Pinel, Scipion: on doctor-father persona,
36–37, 50–51; on professionalization of
psychiatry, 40
placement d'office, 98, 102, 184n6
placement volontaire, 97, 184n6
Plott, Michèle, 75

politics: exclusion of women from, gendering of reason and, 10, 13; passions unleashed in, and madness, 135; women engaged in, sexist assumptions about, 137

Popiel, Jennifer, 77

Porter, Roy, 7

poverty, as source of insanity, 26

pregnancy, and onset of insanity, 24

primogeniture: affective family ties as substitute for, 100; elimination of, 97

prisons: asylums compared to, 53, 93, 105, 143, 159, 160; placement of mad people in, absolutist state and, 20–21

private asylums (*maisons de santé*), 5; amenities of, 70; families' efforts to preserve honor and placement in, 65, 71; public asylums compared to, 83–84; "salon" in, 71–72, 74–75; statistics on, 71; use of term, 188n7; *vie de famille* method used in, 70, 71; women *directrices* in, 67–68, 71–75, 76–78, 87, 89–90, 156, 166. *See also specific asylums*

property: loss of control over, law of 1838 and, 49, 74, 98. *See also* inheritance

psychiatric authority/power: absolute, alienists' insistence on, 105; abuses of, revelations regarding, 141; assumptions about mad people and, 133; cold shower debate and disagreement over, 48, 50; Foucauldian vision of, 7; fragility of, 2; language of fatherhood and, 47, 48, 50–51; law of 1838 and, 44; performance of, 2, 37–39, 47, 52, 66; projecting during times of crisis, 128, 129; protests against misuse of, 92; women practitioners and, 75–77

psychiatric profession: alliance with state, 92, 95, 132, 139, 141; arbitrary asylum sequestration as threat to, 86, 92, 141, 164; cold shower method as threat

to, 63–64; concept of liberty (*liberté*) and, 28, 95, 133; crises of 1870-1871 and, 16, 118–119, 139, 140, 141, 164, 166; criticism in second half of 19th century, 15–16, 44, 53, 88; "diagnosis" of Communards as public relations strategy for, 138; Franco-Prussian War and, 16, 118, 120–132, 140, 141; French Revolution and rise of, 8–9, 15, 94–95, 144; isolation method and bolstering of, 28, 37, 73; July Monarchy and, 30, 43–44, 53; law of 1838 and, 44, 48, 52, 73, 96; professionalization of, 4, 40, 63; Rivet's defense of, 85–86; safeguarding of reputation of, 41, 53, 121–132; Third Republic and, 16, 119, 138, 141; women in, entry of, 79–80

psychiatric treatment: child-rearing approaches compared to, 29–30; class distinctions and, 35, 59–60, 61; family isolation as central principle of, 28–29, 73, 160–161; feminine ideal used in, 15, 39–40, 69; gendered scenarios for, 2, 3–4, 14, 35, 39–40, 41; labor as form of, 60, 121, 127; Open Door method of, 158–160, 165; performative aspects of, 3–4, 55, 57–60, 64–65, 168; and punishment, blurring of boundaries between, 52–53; revolutionary ideals and, 8–9; threat of violence in, 1, 2, 57, 60, 66; use of honor in, 15, 53, 54, 55, 56, 57–61; *vie de famille* method of, 47, 66, 70–77. *See also* moral treatment

puberty, and onset of insanity, 23

public asylums: admission process for, 102, 120–121; growth of, 5; Linas's defense of, 87–88; overcrowding of, search for solutions to, 144, 153–154, 157, 158; private asylums compared to, 83–84; psychiatric training in, 88, 89; underfunding of, 150, 163–164, 193n99. *See also specific asylums* punishment, psychiatric treatment and, 50; blurring of boundaries between, 52–53; Rivet's decision not to use, 83. *See also* cold shower treatment

Pussin (overseer of Bicêtre asylum), 8, 38–39, 40; authority projected by, 38–39; wife of, 39–40

Puyparlier, Auguste Fault du, 111–114, 115

rationality: alienists' professed faith in, 21; conformity to gender expectations and, 3; vs. sex/physicality, in conception of masculine authority, 4, 11; uncoupling from manliness/personhood, need for, 174, 175. *See also* masculine rationality

reason, gendering of, 3, 171; and exclusion of women from politics, 10, 13; power to upset prevailing dynamics, 17; replacement of absolutism and, 9–10. *See also* masculine rationality; rationality

Reddy, William, 45

revolution: equation with madness, 119, 134–135, 136, 138–139, 140; and susceptibility to delusions, 1, 6, 133, 135. *See also* French Revolution; Paris Commune

Rivet, Arthur Jean Baptiste, 78

Rivet, Marie (née Brierre de Boismont), 67, 77; on asylum patients as children, 82–83; on Communardes, 81, 137–138; critical response to memoir of, 83–89; death of, 89; defense of psychiatric profession, 85–86; as *directrice,* 77–78, 84, 190n53; expertise of, anxiety provoked by, 88–89; memoir of, 78–84; on mother's "salon," 71–72; role in father's private asylum, 75, 76, 79; self-presentation of, contradictions in, 76, 79, 80–81, 89, 90; siblings of, 190n50; during Siege of Paris, 125;

social circle of, 80; subtle critique of bourgeois family values, 85; on theatricality of sanity, 90

Roberts, Mary Louise, 13

Roche-Gandon asylum, 117

Rousseau, Jean-Jacques, 51, 74

Rouy, Hersilie, 141

Sainte-Anne asylum, 121; during Franco-Prussian War, 121–122; during Paris Commune, 138; role in asylum admission process, 102, 120; scenes in Zola's *L'Assommoir,* 150; threat of losing funding, 193n99

Saint-Mandé asylum, 78, 89, 190n53, 193n101

Salpêtrière women's hospital, 121; Charcot's clinic in, 167; freeing of patients in, 8; threat of losing funding, 193n99

Sanborn, Joshua, 11

sanity: as conformity to masculine norms, 61; honor and, cultural associations of, 65; increasingly narrow definitions of, 41; theatricality of, Rivet on, 90

Sarcey, Francisque, 137

scientific positivism, rise of, 150

Scotland: "cottage system" in, 154; "Open Door" method in, 158

Second Republic, 93

self-discipline/control: in child-rearing and psychiatric treatment, 30; Enlightenment and expectation of, 6, 9; lack of, as evidence of insanity, 65; and upward social mobility, 11. *See also* masculine rationality/self-control, ideal of

self-reflection, in asylum setting, 31; Foucault on, 183n27

sentimental family, ideal of, 11, 12, 19, 29; dictatorial family dynamics within,

100, 101, 102–103, 105; emergence
of, 95; therapeutic isolation and, 32;
transition from authoritarian family
to, 44, 93; unjust asylum commitment
undermining, 109–110
sex: and gender, uncoupling of,
as evidence of insanity, 1, 3; vs.
reason, in conception of masculine
authority, 4, 11
sexuality: nonconforming, pathologizing
of, 157; nonreproductive,
stigmatization of, 23, 82; women's
overt expressions of, pathologizing of,
76, 81, 168, 189n44
shame: curative power of, 65; as source of
insanity, 54, 56, 57
shock/surprise: in cold shower treatment,
46; in moral treatment, 34, 36, 37
social mobility: economic barriers
to, framing as personal defects, 11;
honor and, in postrevolutionary
France, 45, 53
state, psychiatric profession's alliance
with, 92, 95, 132, 139, 141
sterilization, forced, 153
strait jackets, use in asylums, 47, 52, 110
suffragists, and challenges to feminine
domesticity ideal, 168
Surkis, Judith, 167
syphilis, 154

Tardieu, Ambroise, 89
Thiers, Adolphe, 134
Third Republic, 117–118; accusations
of medical maltreatment during, 93;
psychiatric profession's allegiance to,
16, 119, 138, 141; relative conservatism
of, 119; universal male suffrage in, 169;
unjust institutionalization during, 105
Timm, Annette, 11
treatment. *See* psychiatric treatment;
specific treatment methods

Turck, Léopold, 143

unjust asylum commitment: absolutism
and, 33, 96, 107; and anti-alienist
movement, 53, 92, 150, 164; and
bourgeois gender ideals, undermining
of, 94; criticism of, 92, 93, 94, 117;
family conflict and, 16, 141, 193n3; of
feminist activists, 171–174; financial
motives for, 93, 98, 99, 101, 109–110,
195n32; of heads of households,
106–115; law of 1838 and, 95, 98–99,
193n3; *lettre de cachet* and, 96, 107;
marital conflicts and, 113; paternal
authority and, 92, 96, 99–105; plays
condemning, 92, 111; during Third
Republic, 105; as threat to psychiatric
profession, 86, 92, 141, 164; of
women, 12, 14, 85, 141, 171–174;
writings of victims of, 94, 101–102,
103, 109–110

Vaucluse asylum, 121; as agricultural
colony, 159; during Franco-Prussian
War, 127–131, 139, 148
vie de famille treatment, 47, 70–77;
Blanche family and, 47, 66, 71; Brierre
de Boismont family and, 15, 70, 71–77;
children's role in, 70, 75, 76, 78, 79,
83; doctor-father persona in, 74;
isolation from biological family and,
47, 73; women's role in, 70, 71–77,
79, 87, 89–90
Ville-Évrard asylum, 121, 127; as
agricultural colony, 159, 160; during
Franco-Prussian War, 127; Marandon
de Montyel as director of, 158, 159
Villejuif asylum, 162
violence: system of care based on,
warning against, 62; threat of, use in
psychiatric treatment, 1, 2, 57, 60, 66
Voisin, Felix, 23, 24, 63

Winslow, Forbes, 126
women: asylum patients, 80, 170–171;
  biological predisposition to hysteria,
  claims regarding, 10, 167; bourgeois
  ideal regarding, 2, 9, 90; causes/onset
  of insanity in, early alienists on, 23,
  24–26, 27; Communardes, diagnosed
  as insane, 137–138; elite, kleptomania
  diagnosis for, 169; elite, opportunities
  for public engagement of, 72, 90;
  entry into medical profession, 79–80;
  exclusion from political sphere,
  gendering of reason and, 10, 13; family
  colony for, 157–158; feminist activists,
  asylum commitment of, 171–174;
  gendered treatment scenarios for,
  35–36; heartless and logical, portrayal
  in scandalous commitment stories,
  106–107, 111–112, 114; involvement
  in public sphere, anxieties associated
  with, 114, 137; and irrationality,
  doctors perpetuating association of, 2,
  14, 17, 24, 68, 175; as nurses/guardians,
  in family care model, 155–156, 164; as
  overseers of irrational men, 39–40, 69,
  74–77; overt expressions of sexuality
  by, pathologizing of, 76, 81, 168,
  189n44; property rights of, Civil Code
  of 1804 and restrictions on, 72; role
  in asylum care, as *directrices,* 67–68,
  71–75, 76–78, 87, 89–90, 156, 166;
  role in asylum care, as *surveillantes,*
  39–40; role in asylum care, *vie de
  famille* method and, 70, 71–77, 79,
  87, 89–90; role in bourgeois home,
  72; unjust asylum commitment of, 12,
  14, 85, 141, 171–174. *See also* feminine
  domesticity, ideal of
World War I, community care after, 163

Zola, Emile, *L'Assomoir,* 149–150

CPSIA information can be obtained
at www.ICGtesting.com
Printed in the USA
LVHW052015031120
670609LV00006B/576